National Key Book Publishing Planning Project of the 13th Five-Year Plan

"十三五"国家重点图书出版规划项目

International Clinical Medicine Series Based on the Belt and Road Initiative

"一带一路"背景下国际化临床医学丛书

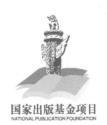

国家出版基金项目
NATIONAL PUBLICATION FOUNDATION

Stomatology

口腔科学

Chief Editor　He Wei　Wang Peng

主编　何　巍　王　鹏

U0340634

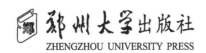

郑州大学出版社
ZHENGZHOU UNIVERSITY PRESS

图书在版编目(CIP)数据

口腔科学 = Stomatology：英文／何巍，王鹏主编. — 郑州：郑州大学出版社，2020. 12(2025.1 重印)

("一带一路"背景下国际化临床医学丛书)

ISBN 978-7-5645-6497-1

Ⅰ. ①口… Ⅱ. ①何…②王… Ⅲ. ①口腔科学 - 英文 Ⅳ. ①R78

中国版本图书馆 CIP 数据核字(2019)第 142155 号

口腔科学 = Stomatology：英文

项目负责人	孙保营　杨秦予	策 划 编 辑	李龙传
责 任 编 辑	陈文静	装 帧 设 计	苏永生
责 任 校 对	张彦勤	责 任 监 制	朱亚君

出版发行	郑州大学出版社	地　　址	河南省郑州市高新技术开发区
出 版 人	卢纪富		长椿路 11 号(450001)
经　　销	全国新华书店	网　　址	http://www.zzup.cn
印　　刷	广东虎彩云印刷有限公司	发行电话	0371-66966070
开　　本	850 mm×1 168 mm　1 / 16		
印　　张	21.5	字　　数	830 千字
版　　次	2020 年 12 月第 1 版	印　　次	2025 年 1 月第 2 次印刷
书　　号	ISBN 978-7-5645-6497-1	定　　价	129.00 元

Staff of Expert Steering Committee

Chairmen

Zhong Shizhen   Li Sijin   Lü Chuanzhu

Vice Chairmen

Bai Yuting   Chen Xu   Cui Wen   Huang Gang   Huang Yuanhua
Jiang Zhisheng   Li Yumin   Liu Zhangsuo   Luo Baojun   Lü Yi
Tang Shiying

Committee Member

An Dongping   Bai Xiaochun   Cao Shanying   Chen Jun   Chen Yijiu
Chen Zhesheng   Chen Zhihong   Chen Zhiqiao   Ding Yueming   Du Hua
Duan Zhongping   Guan Chengnong   Huang Xufeng   Jian Jie   Jiang Yaochuan
Jiao Xiaomin   Li Cairui   Li Guoxin   Li Guoming   Li Jiabin
Li Ling   Li Zhijie   Liu Hongmin   Liu Huifan   Liu Kangdong
Song Weiqun   Tang Chunzhi   Wang Huamin   Wang Huixin   Wang Jiahong
Wang Jiangang   Wang Wenjun   Wang Yuan   Wei Jia   Wen Xiaojun
Wu Jun   Wu Weidong   Wu Xuedong   Xie Xieju   Xue Qing
Yan Wenhai   Yan Xinming   Yang Donghua   Yu Feng   Yu Xiyong
Zhang Lirong   Zhang Mao   Zhang Ming   Zhang Yu'an   Zhang Junjian
Zhao Song   Zhao Yumin   Zheng Weiyang   Zhu Lin

专家指导委员会

Staff of Editor Steering Committee

Chairmen

Cao Xuetao   Wu Jiliang

Vice Chairmen

Chen Pingyan	Chen Yuguo	Huang Wenhua	Li Yaming	Wang Heng
Xu Zuojun	Yao Ke	Yao Libo	Yu Xuezhong	Zhao Xiaodong

Committee Member

Cao Hong	Chen Guangjie	Chen Kuisheng	Chen Xiaolan	Dong Hongmei
Du Jian	Du Ying	Fei Xiaowen	Gao Jianbo	Gao Yu
Guan Ying	Guo Xiuhua	Han Liping	Han Xingmin	He Fanggang
He Wei	Huang Yan	Huang Yong	Jiang Haishan	Jin Chengyun
Jin Qing	Jin Runming	Li Lin	Li Ling	Li Mincai
Li Naichang	Li Qiuming	Li Wei	Li Xiaodan	Li Youhui
Liang Li	Lin Jun	Liu Fen	Liu Hong	Liu Hui
Lu Jing	Lü Bin	Lü Quanjun	Ma Qingyong	Ma Wang
Mei Wuxuan	Nie Dongfeng	Peng Biwen	Peng Hongjuan	Qiu Xinguang
Song Chuanjun	Tan Dongfeng	Tu Jiancheng	Wang Lin	Wang Huijun
Wang Peng	Wang Rongfu	Wang Shusen	Wang Chongjian	Xia Chaoming
Xiao Zheman	Xie Xiaodong	Xu Falin	Xu Xia	Xu Jitian
Xue Fuzhong	Yang Aimin	Yang Xuesong	Yi Lan	Yin Kai
Yu Zujiang	Yu Hong	Yue Baohong	Zeng Qingbing	Zhang Hui
Zhang Lin	Zhang Lu	Zhang Yanru	Zhao Dong	Zhao Hongshan
Zhao Wen	Zheng Yanfang	Zhou Huaiyu	Zhu Changju	Zhu Lifang

编审委员会

Editorial Staff

作者名单

主　编
　　何　巍　　郑州大学第一附属医院
　　王　鹏　　承德医学院附属医院

副主编
　　楚金普　　郑州大学第一附属医院
　　刘　斌　　兰州大学口腔医学院
　　何　伟　　北京大学口腔医院
　　韩　波　　四川大学华西口腔医院

编　委（以姓氏汉语拼音为序）
　　楚金普　　郑州大学第一附属医院
　　付　坤　　郑州大学第一附属医院
　　高　振　　赣南医学院第一附属医院
　　郭竹玲　　海南医学院口腔医学院
　　韩　波　　四川大学华西口腔医院
　　何丽明　　大理大学第一附属医院
　　何　伟　　北京大学口腔医院
　　和晓庸　　大理大学第一附属医院
　　黄　敏　　大理大学第一附属医院
　　康　宏　　兰州大学口腔医学院
　　刘　斌　　兰州大学口腔医学院
　　罗　文　　海南医学院第一附属医院
　　田凯月　　首都医科大学口腔医学院
　　王国芳　　郑州大学第一附属医院
　　许莹莹　　承德医学院附属医院
　　薛　鹏　　郑州大学第一附属医院
　　殷丽华　　兰州大学口腔医学院
　　赵红宇　　郑州大学第一附属医院

Preface

At the Second Belt and Road Summit Forum on International Cooperation in 2019 and the Seventy-third World Health Assembly in 2020, General Secretary Xi Jinping stated the importance for promoting the construction of the "Belt and Road" and jointly build a community for human health. Countries and regions along the "Belt and Road" have a large number of overseas Chinese communities, and shared close geographic proximity, similarities in culture, disease profiles and medical habits. They also shared a profound mass base with ample space for cooperation and exchange in Clinical Medicine. The publication of the International Clinical Medicine series for clinical researchers, medical teachers and students in countries along the "Belt and Road" is a concrete measure to promote the exchange of Chinese and foreign medical science and technology with mutual appreciation and reciprocity.

Zhengzhou University Press coordinated more than 600 medical experts from over 160 renowned medical research institutes, medical schools and clinical hospitals across China. It produced this set of medical tools in English to serve the needs for the construction of the "Belt and Road". It comprehensively coversaspects in the theoretical framework and clinical practices in Clinical Medicine, including basic science, multiple clinical specialities and social medicine. It reflects the latest academic and technological developments, and the international frontiers of academic advancements in Clinical Medicine. It shared with the world China's latest diagnosis and therapeutic approaches, clinical techniques, and experiences in prescription and medication. It has an important role in disseminating contemporary Chinese medical science and technology innovations, demonstrating the achievements of modern China's economic and social development, and promoting the unique charm of Chinese culture to the world.

The series is the first set of medical tools written in English by Chinese medical experts to serve the needs of the "Belt and Road" construction. It systematically and comprehensively reflects the Chinese characteristics in Clinical Medicine. Also, it presents a landmark achievement in the implementation of the "Belt and Road" initiative in promoting exchanges in medical science and technology. This series is theoretical in nature, with each volume built on the mainlines in traditional disciplines but at the same time introducing contemporary theories that guide clinical practices, diagnosis and treatment methods, echoing the latest research findings in Clinical Medicine.

As the disciplines in Clinical Medicine rapidly advances, different views on knowledge, inclusiveness, and medical ethics may arise. We hope this work will facilitate the exchange of ideas, build common ground while allowing differences, and contribute to the building of a community for human health in a broad spectrum of disciplines and research focuses.

Nick Lemoine

Foreign Academician of the Chinese Academy of Engineering

Dean, Academy of Medical Sciences of Zhengzhou University

Director, Barts Cancer Institute, London, UK

6th August, 2020

Foreword

Under the background of more frequent international exchange and the increasing number of international students who want to have medical education in China, the textbooks on oral sciences in English version are badly needed for the internationalization of higher medical education and the bilingual teaching.

This textbook, as an introduction to oral science, is written to provide the general idea and knowledge of anatomy and common diseases of oral and maxillofacial region. It has nearly 300,000 words, which includes 18 chapters: anatomy and physiology of oral and maxillofacial structure, oral and maxillofacial examination, oral healthcare, endodontic diseases, periodontal diseases, common diseases of oral mucosa, local dental anesthesia, tooth extraction, oral implantology, oral and maxillofacial infection, maxillofacial injuries, diseases of temporomandibular joint, tumors of oral and maxillofacial region, maxillofacial nervous disease, dentition defect and edentulism, malocclusions, dentomaxillofacial deformities and orthognathic surgery, and relationship between oral diseases and systemic diseases. The textbook is mainly intended for international students, but it can also be used as a reference for dental students in the process of bilingual teaching. One of the features of the book is that dentomaxillofacial deformities and orthognathic surgery is included to closely keep pace with the trend of oral science and the need of patients.

This textbook is a cooperation work by professors from different schools of stomatology all over China. We express the sincere gratitudes to every author for their meticulous work and contributions. Due to the limited level, there are inevitably shortcomings and errors in the book, and valuable opinions and suggestions are welcome while using.

Authors

Contents

Chapter 1

Anatomy and Physiology of Oral and Maxillofacial Regions

1.1 Introduction

1.1.1 Ranges of oral and maxillofacial regions

Oral and maxillofacial region is the general name of the oralcavity and maxillofacial structure, which is located in the lower 2/3 of the facial region. The face is the area from the hairline to the lower border of mandible or below the chin, bilaterally to the posterior edge of the mandibular ramus or the mastoid process of temporal bone. Clinically, the facial region is often divided into three parts: the upper face, the middle face and the lower, according to the first line crossing into the middle of the two eyebrow bow line, and the second horizontal line of the oral fissure, and the third horizontal line of the hyoid bone.

The upper 1/3 facial region is called craniofacial part, which is to support the surface area where the cranial bone is the main. The maxillofacial region is the region where the maxilla and the mandible are the main bone support. The scope of modern stomatology, especially oral and maxillofacial surgery, has extended to the cranial base and the neck, and has been interdisciplinary with ophthalmology, otorhinolaryngology, neurosurgery, plastic surgery and so on.

The anatomical areas of the maxillofacial region can be divided into frontal area, orbital area, infraorbital region, zygomatic region, nasal region, oral and lip region, chin area, buccal region, parotid masseter area, ear area, temporal area, submental region, submandibular region and upper cervical region.

Oral cavity is located in the maxillofacial region. It is a functional organ composed of teeth, jaws and lips, cheek, palate, tongue, mouth floor and salivary glands. The mouth is a cavity, and it is filled with the tongue when it is closed. The anterior border oral cavity is the upper and lower lip, posterior to the oropharyngeal cavity is the epiglottis. The upper border is the palate, with a dome shaped, apart for the lower nasal meatus, the lower is the slightly depressed muscular floor of the mouth. The floor is occupied by the tongue. Two sides of oral cavity are the cheeks. The anatomical region of the oral cavity can be divided into oral vestibule, tooth and alveolar bone, tongue, palate, and mouth floor.

1.1.2   The main physiological functions of the oral and maxillofacial regions

The tissues and organs of the oral and maxillofacial region have the functions of feeding, chewing, tasting, swallowing, facial expression and auxiliary language and breathing.

As the starting point of the upper digestive tract, the main function of teeth is for chewing, lip for sucking, tongue for swallowing and auxiliary deglutition. Through secreting saliva, the salivary glands complete the preliminary amylase digestion of food by lubricating oral mucosa and mixing food for swallowing easily. When eating, the tongue, cheek and lip coordinate and mix the food with saliva, send them into the upper and lower teeth for chewing, and then swallow the food.

There are many receptors on the tongue. Among them, the taste receptor is used to distinguish the taste of food, such as acid, sweet, bitter, spicy and salty, and can regulate the secretion of saliva through the feedback mechanism of gustatory sense. Other receptors on the body of the tongue can also distinguish cold, heat, mechanical stimulation, and so on.

Oral cavity is an important part of human digestive system. The tooth is an important masticatory organ, and undertaking the task of rough processing of food. The tooth has different shape and function, the incisors for cutting, the canine for tearing, the premolar and molar for chewing and grinding further. At the same time, the tongue coordinates with labial and buccal muscles to mix and transport food to occlusal surface where is needed. After grinding, food is transported to the oropharynx and enters into the esophagus and stomach by swallowing reflex. The initial mechanical process and chemical reaction lays a good foundation for the food digestion. In addition, during the chewing process, the three main salivary glands secrete a variety of digestive enzymes through central nerve reflex. Tooth loss or loose will result in dropping down of chewing efficiency, additionally, coarse food is not only hard to swallow, but also it will increase the burden of gastrointestinal tract digestion, and lead to indigestion and gastrointestinal diseases.

Oral cavity is also one of the important voice organs. The vocal sounds resonate in the oral cavity and under the regulation of the central nerve system, the tongue changes in dimensions and positions will produce resonant cavity changes at the same time. The lips and cheek, soft palate muscles, teeth are also involved in regulating respiratory airflow in the size, velocity, and then develop vocal sounds. Although the oral cavity does not belong to the respiratory system, it has the respiratory function, especially in nasal obstruction, or in physical exercise in order to increase ventilation of the lung. Oral breathing may be needed for the body to provide more air in this conditions. The position of the tongue root will have a direct impact on the dimensions of laryngeal cavity. The mouth floor swelling will make the tongue root move posteriorly and narrow size of the pharyngeal cavity and close the pharyngeal cavity when in serious condition. This may cause obstruction of the upper respiratory tract and threat the patient's life. Therefore, the dentist should always pay attention to the respiratory tract and keep the respiratory tract clear and ensure the patient's life the safe.

In addition to general sensory functions such as pain, temperature, touch and pressure, oral mucosa has a unique function of sense of taste. Taste bud in the mucosa of the posterion of the tongue is oral peculiar taste receptors. It will taste acid, sweet, bitter, spicy, salty and transmit this acute sense to the brain which will decide on the choice of food, and regulate secretion of three salivary glands and the mucous glands through a complex neural refletion. The secretion of saliva will directly participate in the process of food digestion.

The maxilla and mandible are the main framework of the oral cavity and the most important bone structure of the facial contour. The morphology of jaws and the related structures combined with lips and cheek soft tissues determine the different facial features. The middle third of the face is in the center of human vision and the visual focus of people's social communication. The deformity of the lips nose and jaws will seriously affect the human appearance. The defects of maxillofacial soft and hard tissues, such as congenital cleft lip and cleft palate, jaw deformity caused by trauma or tumor or other deformities, may cause the patient's psychological pressure far more than the functional loss of. People are more concerned for facial appearance when existed in hard process and soft maxillofacial deformity than concentrated on chewing and language attention. Therefore, when the surgery treatment planning is determined and implemented, medical workers must follow the maxillofacial surgery principle which both form and function are same importance and follow the basic principles of aesthetics.

1.1.3   Anatomic and physiological characteristics and clinical significance of oral and maxillofacial regions

The special and anatomical characteristics of the oral and maxillofacial region give special clinical significance to them.

1.1.3.1   The location is exposed

The oral and maxillofacial region is exposed and easy to be injured, but after suffering from disease, it is easy to detect early and treatment timely.

1.1.3.2   The blood supply is abundant

The oral and maxillofacial regions are rich in vessels that make tissues and organs have strong ability of anti-infection and the wound healing fast after trauma or operation. But on the other hand, it is because of its abundant blood supply and loose tissue, the bleeding phenomenon and local swelling after injury are more obvious.

1.1.3.3   Anatomical structure is complex

The anatomy of oral and maxillofacial region is complex, involved in facial nerve, trigeminal nerve, salivary gland and its duct. Damages of these organs will lead to complications such as facial paralysis, numbness and salivary gland fistula.

1.1.3.4   Natural skin wrinkles

Facial skin forms natural skin wrinkles in different directions, referred to as skin lines. The direction of the skin lines varies with age. The surgical incision in the maxillofacial region should be designed along the direction of the skin line, and the incision should be chosen in more concealed area. Thus, the scar is not obvious after the wound is healed.

1.1.3.5   The deform and dysfunction of maxillofacial region

The disease of oral and maxillofacial region is often caused by congenital or postnatal diseases, such as cleft lip, palate or burn scar, which cause abnormal facial contours, dysfunction or even facial deformities.

1.1.3.6   The oral maxillofacial disease is easy to spread to adjacent parts

The oral and maxillofacial region is next to brain and pharyngolaryngeal part, it is easily to be involved in brain and pharynlaryngeal part when inflammation, trauma, tumor and other diseases take place.

1.2 The Oral Cavity

The entire oral cavity is lined with mucous membrane tissue. This tissue is highly specialized and adapted to meet the needs of the area it covers. The oral cavity consists of the vestibule and the oral cavity proper. ①The vestibule is the space between the teeth and the inner mucosal lining of the lips and cheeks. ②The oral cavity proper is the space contained the upper and lower dental arches.

1.2.1 Vestibules

The vestibules are lined with mucosal tissue. The texture of the vestibular mucosa is thin, red, loosely bound to the underlying alveolar bone. The inside surface of the cheeks forms the side walls of the oral cavity. The buccal vestibule is the area between the cheeks and the teeth or alveolar ridge. On the inner surface of the cheek, just opposite the second maxillary molar, is a small elevation of tissue called the parotid papillar. The parotid papillar protects the opening of the parotid duct of the parotid salivary gland.

1.2.1.1 Labial and other frenula

A frenum is a narrow band of tissue that connects two structures. The maxillary labial frenum passes from the oral mucosa at the midline of the maxillary arch to the midline of the inner surface of the upper lip. The mandibular labial frenum passes from the oral mucosa at the midline of the mandibular arch to the midline of the inner surface of the lower lip.

In the areas of the first maxillary permanent molar, the buccal frenum passes from the oral mucosa of the outer surface of the maxillary arch to the inner surface of the cheek. The lingual frenum passes from the ventral border of the tongue.

1.2.1.2 Gingiva

The gingiva, commonly referred to as the "gums", is masticatory mucosa that covers the alveolar processes of the jaws and surrounded the necks of the teeth. Normal gingival tissue has the following characteristics.

(1)Gingiva surrounds the tooth like a collar and is self-cleaning.

(2)Gingiva is firm and resistant and tightly adapted to the tooth and bone.

(3)The surfaces of the attached gingiva and interdental papillae are stippled and resemble the rind of an orange.

(4)The color of the gingival surface varies according to the individual's pigmentation.

Unattached gingiva, also known as marginal gingiva, or free gingiva, is the border of the gingiva surrounding the teeth in collar-like fashion.

(1)The unattached gingiva, which is usually light pink or coral colored, is not bound to the underlying tissue of the tooth. It consists of the tissues from the top of the gingival margin to the base of the gingival sulcus. The unattached gingiva is usually about 1 mm wide, and it forms the soft wall of the gingival sulcus.

(2)Interdental gingiva: also known as gingival papillar, is the extension of the free gingiva that fills the interproximal embrasure between two adjacent teeth.

(3)Gingival groove: also known as the free gingival groove, is a shallow groove that runs parallel to the margin of the unattached gingiva and marks the beginning of the attached gingiva.

(4)Attached gingiva: the attached gingiva extends from the base of the sulcus to the mucogingival junction. It is a stippled, dense tissue that is self-protecting, firmly bound, and resilient. The mucogingival junction is the point where the attached gingiva joins the lining mucosa.

1.2.2 The oral cavity proper

Hold your teeth together, with your tongue, feel the areas of the oral cavity proper. The oral cavity proper is the areas inside of the dental arches. In back of your last molar, there is a space that links the vestibule and the oral cavity proper.

1.2.2.1 Hard palate

With your tongue, feel your hard palate, or roof of your mouth. The hard palate separates the nasal cavity above from the oral cavity below. The nasal surfaces are covered with respiratory mucosa, and the oral surfaces are covered with oral mucosa. The mucosa of the hard palate is tightly bound to the underlying bone, which is why submucosal injections into the palate area can be extremely painful.

Behind the maxillary central incisors is the incisive papillar, a pear—shaped pad of tissue that covers the incisive foramen. This is the site of injection for anesthesia of the nasopalatine nerve. Extending laterally from the incisive papillar are irregular ridges or folds of masticatory mucosa called palatal rugae. Running posteriorly from the incisal papillar is the midline platal raphe. Numerous minor palatal glands open onto the palatal mucosa as small pits.

1.2.2.2 Soft palate

Move your tongue to the back of your hard palate, and feel where the soft palate begins. The soft palate is the movable posterior one third of the palate. It has no bony skeleton and hangs like a limp curtain into the pharynx behind it. The soft palate ends posteriorly as a free edge with a hanging projection called the uvula.

The soft palate is supported posteriorly by two arches. The anterior arch runs from the soft palate down to the lateral aspects of the tongue as the palatoglossal arch. The posterior arch is called the free posterior border of the soft palate and is called the palatopharyngeal arch. The opening between the two arches is called the isthmus of fauces and contains the palatine tonsil.

1.2.2.3 Tongue

The tongue is an important organ that is responsible for a lot of functions.

(1) Speaking.

(2) Manipulation and positioning of food.

(3) Sensation of tasting.

(4) Swallowing.

(5) Cleaning of the oral cavity.

After eating, notice how your tongue moves from crevice to crevice. Seeking out and removing bits of retained food in your mouth.

The body of the tongue is the anterior two thirds of the tongue found in the oral cavity. The root of the tongue is the posterior part that turns vertically downward to reside in the pharynx. The dorsum is the superior and posterior roughened aspects of the tongue. It is covered with small papillae of various shapes and colors. The sublingual surface of the tongue is covered with thin, smooth, transparent mucosa through which many underlying vessels can be seen. There are two small papillans on either side of the lingual frenulum just behind the central incisors. Through these papilla into the mouth are the openings of the submandibular ducts. It is through these ducts that saliva enters the oral cavity.

Two smaller, fimbriated folds parallel the midline lingual frenum on either side. Again, lingual frenum is the thin fold of mucous membrane that extends from the floor of the mouth to the underside of the tongue.

1.2.2.4 Taste buds

The taste buds, which are the receptor cells for the sense of taste, are located on the dorsum of the tongue. A substance must be mixed with liquid before it can stimulate the taste buds on the tongue.

The taste buds are located on the fungiform papillar and in the trough of the large vallate papillar, which form a V letter the posterior portion of the tongue. The numerous filiform papillae, which cover the entire surface of the tongue, provide the sense of touch but do not contain taste receptors. Specific areas of the tongue receive each taste sensation, as follows.

(1) Sweet at the tip.

(2) Salty at the anterior sides and tip.

(3) Sour at the sides toward the posterior.

(4) Bitter in the center of the dorsum toward the posterior.

1.2.3 Teeth

Teeth are either single rooted or multirooted and sit in bony sockets, or alveoli, within the alveolar process of the maxilla and mandible. In the mouth a cuff of gingival tissue surrounds the tooth. The portion of the tooth that is visible in the oral cavity is called the crown.

Each tooth consists of crown and one or more roots. The size and shape of the crown and the size and number of roots vary according to the type of tooth.

1.2.3.1 Crown

The crown has dentin covered by enamel, and each root has dentin covered by cementum. The inner portion of the dentin of both the crown and the toot also covers the pulp cavity of the tooth close to the cementenamel junction(CEJ). The CEJ is the external line at the neck or cervix of the tooth where the enamel of the crown and cementum of the root usually meet.

Positions of the crown can be defined as more specific ways. The anatomic crown is the portion of the tooth covered with enamel. The size of the anatomic crown remains constant through the life of the tooth, regardless of the position of the gingiva. The clinical crown is the portion of the tooth that is visible in the mouth. The clinical crown varies in length during the life cycle of the tooth depending on the level of the gingiva. The clinical crown is shorter as the tooth erupts into position and is longer as the surrounding tissues recede.

1.2.3.2 Root

The root of the tooth is the portion normally embedded in the alveolar process and is covered with cementum. Depending on the type of tooth, the root may have one, two, or three branches.

Bifurcation means division into two roots. Trifurcation means division into three roots.

The tapered end of each root tip is known as the apex. Any structure or object that is situated at the apex is called apical. Anything surrounding the apex is called periapical.

1.2.3.3 Enamel

Enamel, which makes up the anatomic crown of the tooth, is the hardest material of the body. This hardness is important because enamel forms the protective covering for the softer underlying dentin. It also provides a strong surface for crushing, grinding, and chewing food.

Enamel can withstand crushing stresses to about 100,000 pounds per square inch. Although enamel is strong, it is also very brittle. And this brittleness may cause the enamel to fracture or chip. Along with enamel's strength, however, the crushing effect of the dentin and the springlike action of the periodontium enable enamel to withstand most of the pressures brought against it.

Enamel is translucent and ranges from yellow to grayish white in color. These variations in shade are caused by differences in the thickness and translucency of the enamel and in the color of the dentin beneath it.

Enamel, which is formed by ameloblasts, consists of 99% inorganic matter and only 1% – 4% organic matrix. Hydroxyapatite, which consists primarily of calcium, is the most abundant mineral component. Hydroxyapatite is the material that is lost in the process of dentin decay.

1.2.3.4　Dentin

Dentin makes up the main portion of the tooth structure and extends almost the entire length of the tooth. It is covered by enamel on the crown and by cementum on the toot.

In the deciduous teeth, dentin is very light yellow. In permanent teeth, it is light yellow and somewhat transparent. The color may darken with age.

Dentin is a mineralized tissue that is harder than bone and cementrum but not as hard as enamel. Dentin is composed of 70% inorganic material and 30% organic matter and water.

Dentin is capable of continued growth and repair, dentin consists of primary dentin, secondary dentin and tertiary dentin(reparative dentin).

1.2.3.5　Cemntum

Cementum covers the root of the tooth. It overlies the dentin and joins the enamel at the CEJ. A primary function of cementum is to anchor the tooth to the bony socket with attachment fibers in the periodontium.

Cementum is light yellow and easily distinguishable from enamel by its lack of luster and darker hue. It is somewhat lighter in color than dentin.

Unlike bone, cementum does not resorb and form again. The difference is important because it makes orthodontic treatment possible. However, cementum is still capable of some repair by the deposition of new layers.

1.2.3.6　Pulp

The inner aspect of the dentin forms the boundaries of the pulp chamber. As with the dentin surrounding it, the contour of the pulp chamber follows the contours of the exterior surface of the tooth.

The part of the pulp lies within the crown portion is called the coronal pulp. The other portion of the pulp is more apically located and is referred to as the radicular pulp, or the root pulp. During the development of the root, the continued deposition of dentin causes this area to become longer and narrower. The radicular portion of the pulp in each root is continuous with the tissues of the periapical area via an apical foramen.

The pulp is made up of blood vessels and nerves that enter the pulp chamber through the apical foramen. The pulp also contains connective tissue, which consists of fibroblasts, intercellular substance, and tissue fluid. The blood supply is derived from branches of the dental arteries and periodontal ligament. The rich blood supply also has an important defense function in responding to a bacterial invasion of the tooth.

The nerve supply of the pulp receives and transmits pain stimuli.

1.2.3.7　Periodontium

The periodontium supports the tooth in the alveolar bone. It is composed of cementum, alveolar bone, and the periodontal ligaments. These tissues also protect and nourish the tooth. The periodontium is divided into two major units: the attachment apparatus and the gingival unit.

The attachment apparatus consists of the cementum, alveolar process, and periodontal ligament. These tissues work together to support, maintain, and retain the tooth in its functional position within the jaw.

(1) The alveolar processes: the alveolar processes are the extensions of the bone from the body of the mandible and maxilla that support the teeth in their functional positions in the jaws. Osteoblasts are responsible for resorption and remodeling of the alveolar.

The cortical plate is the dense outer covering of the spongy bone that makes up the central part of the alveolar process. The cortical plate provides strength and protection and is where the skeletal muscles attach.

The alveolar crest is the highest point of the alveolar ridge. It fuses with the cortical plates on the facial and lingual sides of the crest of the alveolar process.

In a healthy mouth, the distance between the CEJ and the alveolar crest is fairly constant. The alveolar socket is the cavity within the alveolar process that surrounds the root of a tooth.

The lamina dura is thin, compact bone that lines the alveolar socket. There are many small spaces on the lamina dura, which allow the blood vessels and nerve fibres in the bone to communicate freely with those in the periodontal ligament.

(2) Periodontal ligament: the periodontal ligament is dense connective tissue organized into fibre groups that connects the cementum covering the root with the alveolar bone of the socket wall.

1.2.3.8　The function of the periodontal ligament

(1) Supportive and protective function.

(2) Sensory function.

(3) Nutritive function.

(4) Formative and resorptive functions.

Periodontal ligament has three different types of fibre groups: periodontal fibre groups, transseptal groups, and gingival fibre groups.

1.2.4　Gingival unit

Oral mucosa almost continuously lines the oral cavity. Oralmucosa is composed of stratified squamous epithelium overlying connective tissue. The three main types of oral mucosa in the oral cavity are lining, masticatory, and specialized.

(1) Lining mucosa covers the inside of the cheeks, vestibule, lips, soft palate, and ventral surface of the tongue.

(2) Masticatory mucosa is light pink and is keratinized, which means that it has a tough, protective outer layer. Masticatory mucosa includes the attached gingiva, hard palate, and dorsum of the tongue.

(3) Specialized mucosa is presented in the form of lingual papillae. The papillae are associated with sensations of the taste.

1.2.5　Dentitions

The dentition is used to describe the natural teeth in the jawbones and their relationships. People have two dentitions throughout life. The first dentition of 20 primary teeth is called the primary dentition, commonly referred to as the deciduous dentition. The second dentition refers to the 32 permanent teeth. The permanent teeth that replace the 20 primary teeth are called succedaneous teeth.

1.2.5.1 Primary Dentition

The primary dentition, or first dentition, begins with the eruption of the primary mandibular central incisors. The period occurs between approximately 6 months and 6 years of age. The primary dentition has incisors, canines, and molars. The primary dentition usually ends when the first permanent molar erupts. The jawbones are beginning to grow during this period to accommodate the large permanent teeth. The eruption time and order of deciduous teeth see Table 1-1.

Table 1-1 Primary dentition in order of eruption

Dentition	Date of eruption(months)	Date of exfoliation(years)
Maxillary teeth		
Central incisor	6-10	6-7
Lateral incisor	9-12	7-8
First molar	12-18	9-11
Canine	16-22	10-12
Second molar	24-32	10-12
Mandibular teeth		
Central incisor	6-10	6-7
Lateral incisor	7-10	7-8
First molar	12-18	9-11
Canine	16-22	9-12
Second molar	24-32	10-12

1.2.5.2 Mixed dentition

The mixed dentition period follows the primary dentition period. This period occurs between approximately 6 and 12 years of age. Both primary and permanent teeth are present during this transitional period. During this period, both shedding of primary teeth and eruption of permanent teeth. The jawbones undergo their fastest and most noticeable growth during this period.

1.2.5.3 Permanent dentition

The permanent dentition is the final or adult dentition. This period begins with shedding of the last primary tooth(Table 1-2), after about 12 years of age. The permanent dentition is divided into four types of teeth: incisors, canines, premolars, and molars. Minimal growth of the jawbones occurs overall during this period.

Table 1-2 Permanent dentition in order of eruption

Dentition	Date of eruption(years)	Dentition	Date of eruption(years)
Maxillary teeth		Mandibular teeth	
First molar	6-7	First molar	6-7
Central incisor	6-7	Central incisor	6-7
Lateral incisor	7-8	Lateral incisor	7-8

Continue to Table 1–2

Dentition	Date of eruption(years)	Dentition	Date of eruption(years)
First premolar	9–10	Canine(Cuspid)	9–10
Second premolar	10–11	First premolar	10–11
Canine	12–13	Second premolar	12–13
Second molar	11–13	Second molar	11–13
Third molar	17–21	Third molar	17–21

1.2.6 Tooth numbering system

Numbering systems are used as a simplified means of identifying the teeth for charting and descriptive purpose. Three basic numbering systems are used: universal system, international standard organization system, and Palmer notation system(PNS). The PNS is widely used clinically(Table 1–3–Table 1–7).

Table 1–3 The palmer notation system for permanent teeth

Right maxillary	Left maxillary
8 7 6 5 4 3 2 1	1 2 3 4 5 6 7 8
8 7 6 5 4 3 2 1	1 2 3 4 5 6 7 8
Right mandibular	Left mandibular

Table 1–4 The palmer notation system for deciduous teeth

Right maxillary	Left maxillary
E(V) D(Ⅳ) C(Ⅲ) B(Ⅱ) A(Ⅰ)	A(Ⅰ) B(Ⅱ) C(Ⅲ) D(Ⅳ) E(V)
E(V) D(Ⅳ) C(Ⅲ) B(Ⅱ) A(Ⅰ)	A(Ⅰ) B(Ⅱ) C(Ⅲ) D(Ⅳ) E(V)
Right mandibular	Left mandibular

Table 1–5 The ISO system for permanent teeth

Right maxillary	Left maxillary
18 17 16 15 14 13 12 11	21 22 23 24 25 26 27 28
48 47 46 45 44 43 42 41	31 32 33 34 35 36 37 38
Right mandibular	Left mandibular

Table 1–6 The ISO system for deciduous teeth

Right maxillary	Left maxillary
55 54 53 52 51	61 62 63 64 65
85 84 83 82 81	71 72 73 74 75
Right mandibular	Left mandibular

Table 1-7   **Universal tooth numbers**

Permanent tooth letters(1-32)		Deciduous tooth letters(A-T)	
Maxillary right third molar	#1	Maxillary right second molar	A
Maxillary right second molar	#2	Maxillary right first molar	B
Maxillary right first molar	#3	Maxillary right canine	C
Maxillary right second premolar	#4	Maxillary right lateral incisor	D
Maxillary right first premolar	#5	Maxillary right central incisor	E
Maxillary right canine	#6	Maxillary left central incisor	F
Maxillary right lateral incisor	#7	Maxillary left lateral incisor	G
Maxillary right central incisor	#8	Maxillary left canine	H
Maxillary left central incisor	#9	Maxillary left first molar	I
Maxillary left lateral incisor	#10	Maxillary left second molar	J
Maxillary left canine	#11	Mandibular left second molar	K
Maxillary left first premolar	#12	Mandibular left first molar	L
Maxillary left second premolar	#13	Mandibular left canine	M
Maxillary left first molar	#14	Mandibular left lateral incisor	N
Maxillary left second molar	#15	Mandibular left central incisor	O
Maxillary left third molar	#16	Maxillary right central incisor	P
Mandibular left third molar	#17	Mandibular right lateral incisor	Q
Mandibular left second molar	#18	Mandibular right canine	R
Mandibular left first molar	#19	Mandibular right first molar	S
Mandibular left second premolar	#20	Mandibular right second molar	T
Mandibular left first premolar	#21		
Mandibular left canine	#22		
Mandibular left lateral incisor	#23		
Mandibular left central incisor	#24		
Mandibular right central incisor	#25		
Mandibular right lateral incisor	#26		
Mandibular right canine	#27		
Mandibular right first premolar	#28		
Mandibular right second premolar	#29		
Mandibular right first molar	#30		
Mandibular right second molar	#31		
Mandibular right third molar	#32		

1.3　Maxillofacial Structures

1.3.1　Marks and harmonious relationship of surface morphology

1.3.1.1　Landmarks of surface morphology

(1) surface landmarks of the palpebral region

1) Palpebral fissure: the palpebral fissure refers to the gap between the upper eyelid and lower eyelid. In adults, this measures about 10-12 mm vertically and 35 mm horizontally. It is commonly used as a symbol of facial vertical scaling.

2) Medial and lateral Palpebral commissure: respectively, the upper and lower eyelid in the medial and lateral junction.

3) Inner and outer canthus: respectively refers to the crossing angle formed by the two eyelid margins at the medial and lateral palpebral commissure. The inner canthus is blunt and round; the outer canthus is acutely angled and about 3-4 mm higher than the inner canthus.

(2) Surface landmarks of the nasal area

1) Nasal root, nasal tip, and nasal dorsum: the upper part of the nose is called the nasal root, and the anterior uplift is called the nasal tip, and nasal dorsum is between the nose root and nasal tip.

2) Nasal base (base of the nose) and nostril (anterior naris): the bottom of conical external nose is called the nasal base nose, the nasal floor has left and right oval hole, called nasal front hole.

3) Nasal columella (columella nasi) and nasal ala (alae nasi): the frontal ridge between the two nostril is called the nasal columella; the lateral ridge of the nostril is called the nasal ala.

4) Nasofacial sulcus: the nasofacial sulcus is a long indentation on the lateral side of the nose. The scar could be unobvious if the incision is along the nasofacial sulcus.

5) Nasolabial sulcus: nasofacial sulcus and labiofacial sulcus together is called nasolabial sulcus.

(3) Surface landmarks of the lip area

1) Labiofacial sulcus: it is an oblique depression of upper lip and cheek. The scar could be unobvious if the incision is along the labiofacial sulcus.

2) Oral fissure: a transverse fissure between the upper lip and the lower lip.

3) Angle of mouth: the two ends of the fissure are the angles of mouth, and their normal position is about the same between the canine teeth and the first premolar, attention should be paid to this relationship in the commissurotomy operation of opening or narrowing the commissure.

4) Vermilion: the free margin of the upper and lower lip, and the transitional area of the skin and mucosa.

5) Vermilion border: mucocutaneous junction of vermilion.

6) Labial arch (cupid's bow) and middle point of philtrum: the whole vermilion border of the upper lip are arcuate and called the labial arch (cupid's bow). The labial arch protrudes slightly in the median line, which is called the middle point of philtrum.

7) Ridge of vermilion and labial tubercle: the highest points of the labial arch on both sides of the middle point of philtrum are called the ridges of vermilion. The middle vermilion of the upper lip is protruded forward and downward like a tubercle, which is called the lip bead.

8) Philtrum: the cutaneous longitudinal shallow ditch on the upper lip from the nasal column down to

the vermilion border is known as philtrum(philtrum curved).

9) Ridge of philtrum(philtrum column) : the parallel skin ridge on each side of the philtrum, which extends from the base of nostril to the ridge of vermilion.

(4) Surface landmarks of the mandible and chin area

1) Mentolabial sulcus : the transverse depression between the lower lip and the chin.

2) Menton : the lowest point of the chin, which is often used as a landmark for measuring facial distance.

3) Mental foramen : the mental foramen is perforated by the mental nerve. It is located on the external side of the mandible, and, in the adults, mostly below the second premolar or between the first and second premolars, slightly above the midpoint between the upper and lower margin. It is about 2 – 3 cm from the midline. The mental foramen is the point of the chin nerve block anesthesia.

(5) Surface landmarks of other areas

1) Tragus : tragus is a nodular protuberance in front of the external auditory canal, below the zygomatic arch the mandibular condyle could be detected. The pulse of the superficial temporal artery can be palpated at about 1 cm in front of the tragus.

2) Infra−orbital foramen : infra−orbital foramen is located 0. 5 cm below the midpoint of the infraorbital margin, the surface landmark of which is projected in the midpoint between the tip of the nose and the outer canthus line. Orbital foramen is the injection point of the inferior orbital nerve block anesthesia.

3) Surface projection of parotid duct : the middle 1/3 segment of the line from the earlobe to the midpoint of the alare and the angle of mouth. Understanding the surface projection of the parotid duct during buccal surgery will help to avoid the injury of the parotid duct.

1. 3. 1. 2   Coordination of surface morphology

The coordination of maxillofacial surface morphology and structure refers to the relationship between the surface morphology of maxillofacial tissue and organ. The harmonious and coordinated maxillofacial relationship is the basis of normal maxillofacial morphology. The obvious correlation between maxillofacial width and height determines the aesthetic form of maxillofacial region.

(1) Horizontal proportions of maxillofacial region : it refers to the proportion of maxillofacial height. The facial area can be divided into three equal parts along the glabella point and subnasale point. From hairline to glabella is the upper 1/3. From the glabella point to subnasal point is the middle 1/3. From the subnasale point to submental point is the lower 1/3. The eyes and nose are located in the middle third of the face and the mouth is located in the lower third of the face. The deformities of the maxillofacial region can be caused by the disproportion of the upper and middle 1/3 horizontal proportion of the face ; abnormalities of middle and lower 1/3 horizontal proportion of the face can be expressed as dento−maxillofacial deformities.

(2) Transverse proportions of maxillofacial region : it refers to the proportion of the frontal maxillofacial width. Along the vertical line of the canthus, the face can be divided into five equal parts at the level of palpebral fissure. The width of each equal portion is equal to a palpebral fissure, that is, the distance between the inner canthus of the two eyes, the width of the two palpebral fissures and the distance between the left and right lateral canthus to the helix of the outer ears. The average width of the normal palpebral fissure is 3. 5 cm.

In addition, there are some reasonable proportional relationships, such as the width of the nasal alar is equal to the distance between the two inner canthus ; the ratio of the length and width of the nose is approximately 1 : 0. 7 ; the width of the oral fissure when closed is equal to the distance between the inner margin of the two corneas.

(3) The relationship between nose, eye and eyebrow: the lateral edge of the nasal alar, the medial margin of the brow and the inner canthus are in the same vertical line through the inner canthus. The outer canthus is on the line formed by the nasal alar and the lateral margin of the eyebrow. The line through the inner and lateral margin of the eyebrow is usually horizontal and constitutes a right triangle with the above two lines, which is located below the inner margin of the brow. This is the normal nose, eye, eyebrow relationship.

(4) The relationship between nose, lips and, chin: the line connecting the nose tip (pronasale point) and the most prominent point of the chin (pogonion) constitutes the ricketts aesthetic plane. By evaluating whether the upper and lower lips are located on this plane, we can judge the appearance state: if they are ahead or backward, the appearance is not beautiful. But there are racial differences. By measuring and analyzing the beautiful people in China, some scholars have found that the upper and lower lips of Chinese people are not on the aesthetic plane, and that the distance from the upper or lower lip to the aesthetic plan of varies from gender.

(5) The symmetrical relationship: the left and right symmetrical relationship with the axis of the midline of the face is one of the important marks of facial beauty. It is also used as the standard for preoperation diagnosis and postoperative evaluation in maxillofacial surgery and plastic surgery. The major maxillofacial structures such as eyes, nose, oral fissure, are highly symmetric. The six landmark points of nasal tip (pronasale point) , subnasal point, center of the lips and labial sulcus and the pogonion point are highly close to the midline. The left and right deviations from the midline are within ±0.5 mm. The nasal root point (nasion of soft tissue) is usually the closest to the midline. And closer the landmark to the lower part of the face, is the asymmetrical rate tends to increase. The deviation of pogonion point is relatively large. The asymmetrical rate of the male face is higher than that of the female. The facial structure has a high degree of symmetry, but few of them are completely symmetrical.

1.3.2　Jaws

1.3.2.1　Maxilla

(1) Anatomical features

Maxilla is the largest bone in the middle face. The maxilla is connected with the adjacent nasal bone, frontal bone, ethmoid bone, lacrimal bone, plow bone, inferior turbinate, zygomatic, palatal bone and sphenoid bone, etc. The paired maxilla form the upper jaw and the majority of the roof oral wall and lateral nasal wall and the majority of the floor of the orbit and nose. Each maxilla has one body and four processes: frontal, zygomatic, alveolar and palatine processes.

1) The maxillary body is roughly pyramidal, with anterior, posterior (infratemporal) and nasal surfaces with the orbital surface forming the "base". The maxillary sinus is contained within.

● The anterior surface of the maxilla is connected with the superior surface (orbital surface) by the inferior orbital margin. The infraorbital foramen is about 0.6−1 cm below the middle portion of the infraorbital margin, and the infraorbital nerve and blood vessels pass through therefrom. Below the infraorbital foramen, the prominent canine eminence overlying the root of the canine tooth demarcates the incisive fossa above the incisor roots medially, and the canine fossa laterally. The bone of the canine fossa is fairly thin and often chiseled to enter the maxillary sinus for operation.

● Posterior surface: also known as infratemporal surface, is often separated from the anterior surface by the zygomatical−alveolar ridge, the posterior bone of which appears to be nodular, called maxillary tuberosity. There are 2−3 small osseous foramen above the maxillary tuberosity, which are passed by the posterior superior alveolar(PSA)nerve and blood vessels. The zygomatic alveolar ridge and maxillary tuberosity are important signs of posterior superior alveolar nerve block anesthesia.

- Superior surface: also called as the orbital surface, it is triangular and forms the majority of the orbital floor. Running from the posterior of the orbital surface, the inferior orbital fissure turns to the infraorbital groove, and forms the infraorbital canal, which opens to the infraorbital foramen. The anterior and the middle superior alveolar nerve was separated from the suborbital canal and distributed through the anterior wall of maxillary sinus to the anterior teeth and premolars.

- Inner surface: also called as nasal surface, which forms anteroinferior aspect of the lateral wall of nasal cavity. The maxillary sinus opening leads to the nasal cavity by the maxillary hiatus in the posterior of the middle meatus. When performing maxillary sinus radical surgery or maxillary cyst extirpation, it can be fenestrated and drained in the nasal canal.

- Maxillary sinus: conical cavity, bottom inward, tip out into zygomatica process, maxillary sinus opens in nasal cavity. Walls of maxillary sinus are also the four walls of the maxilla body, each bone of which is thin, and the inner surface of which is lined with maxillary sinus mucous membrane. Maxillary sinus floor and maxillary posterior teeth root apexes are closely connected, sometimes only separated by the maxillary sinus mucosa. So when maxillary premolar or molar root apex gets infection, it is easy to penetrate maxillary sinus mucosa, resulting in odontogenic maxillary sinusitis. When extracting maxillary premolar and molar root, we should pay attention not to push the root into maxillary sinus.

2) Four processes of maxilla are frontal process, zygomatic process, alveolar process and palatal process.

- Frontal process: located inside and above the body of the maxilla and articulating with the frontal, nasal, and lacrimal bones.

- Zygomatic process: located laterosuperiorly on the maxillary body, articulating with the zygomatic bone, and it goes downward to the first molar to form the zygomatic alveolar ridge.

- Alveolar process: located below the maxillary body, continuous with the anterior and posterior walls of the maxillary sinus. The left and right sides are joined in the midline and become arcuate. Each side of the alveolar process has 7 – 8 alveolar fossae to accommodate the tooth roots. The labial and buccal bone plate of the alveolar process of the anterior teeth and premolars are thin and porous. This structure is beneficial to the infiltration of anesthetics into the cancellous bone and to the purpose of local infiltration anesthesia. Because the bone in the labial and buccal side is porous, the resistance is lower as the tooth is extracted in the direction of the labial and buccal direction.

- Palatine process: a horizontal plate of bone extending on the medial side of the alveolar process. The posterior portion is attached to the palatine bone. The two sides are connected in the midline forming the hard palate to separate the nasal cavity from the oral cavity. The incisive foramen is in the anterior portion of the hard palate, through which the nasopalatine nerves and vessels pass. The greater palatal foramen located in the posterior portion, through which the anterior palatine neurovascular bundles pass. There are 1 – 2 smaller palatine foramina behind the greater foramen palatine, through which the middle and posterior palatine nerves pass.

(2)Anatomical characteristics of maxilla and its clinical significance

1)Buttress structures and clinical significance: the maxilla is connected with many adjacent bones, and the central part of the bone is a cavity, thus forming a buttress structure. When it is hit by external force, the strength can be dispersed through most adjacent bones, so that fracture will not occur. If the blow force is heavy, the junction part of the maxilla and adjacent bones are more likely to fracture. When the blow force is too large and is transmitted to the adjacent skull bone, the accompanying skull base fracture and craniocerebral injury is often occurred. As there is no strong muscle attached to the maxilla, the displacement of the fracture segment is often consistent with the magnitude and direction of the external force. The maxilla is porous, abundant blood flow, and heals faster after fracture. Once the maxilla fractures, it should be reduced as soon as possible to avoid dislocation healing. In case of pyogenic infection, porous bone is beneficial to the purulent fluid penetrating through the bone to achieve the purpose of drainage. Therefore, osteomyelitis is less common in the maxilla.

2) Anatomical weak sites and clinical significance: the maxilla has some factors, such as the various dense and thickness of bone, multiple sutures, different deepness and size of alveolar fossae. It constitute some anatomically weak structures or parts. These weak sites are where fractures often occur. The main weak sites of the maxilla are the following three weak lines.

● The first weak line: from the inferior piriform foramen parallel to the alveolar process through the maxillary tuberosity to the pterygoid process of sphenoid bone. When the fracture occurs along this weak line, it is called the LeFort Ⅰ fracture of the maxilla.

● The second weak line: from nasal bone, lacrimal bone, ectad passing through the orbital floor, and downward through the zygomatic maxillary suture below the zygoma to the pterygoid process of the sphenoid bone. When the fracture occurs along this weak line, it is called LeFort Ⅱ fracture of maxilla. The middle portion of the facial fracture does not contain zygoma.

● The third weak line: through the nasal bone, the lacrimal bone, ectad passing through the orbital floor, and upward through the zygomatic frontal suture above the zygoma to the pterygoid process of the sphenoid bone. When the fracture occurs along this weak line, it is called the LeFort Ⅲ fracture of the maxilla. The middle portion of the fracture contains zygoma, referred to as "craniofacial disjunction".

1.3.2.2　Mandible

The mandible is the only movable and strongest bone in the maxillofacial region. Bilateral mandibles unite in the mid-line, horseshoe shaped. The mandible is divided into two parts: the mandibular body and the mandibular ramus.

(1) The mandibular body is divided into upper, lower margin and inner, outer surface. There are mental tubercles on the outer surface and mental spines on the inner surface separately at bilateral mandible body. The upper margin of the maxillary body is alveolar bone, with the alveolar fossae to hold roots. The bone plate of the anterior teeth region is more porous than that of the posterior teeth region, and in the posterior teeth region the buccal bone is thicker than that of the lingual side. The lower margin of the mandibular body is dense and thick, with a digastric fossa on each side of the midline, which is the attachment of the anterior belly of the digastric. Outside the mandible, equivalent to the lower part of the premolar region, there is an opening of the mental foramen. The mental nerve is perforated out of the mandible through this foramen. The linear protuberance commencing imperceptibly posterior to the mental foramen extending to the anterior border of the ramus is called the external oblique line, to which the buccinator is attached. The linear protuberance commencing on the inner surface of the mandible from the mental spine extending backwards and upwards is the mylohyoid line, to which is the attachment to the origin of mylohyoid attached. There is the genioglossus and the geniohyoid attaching to the mental spine. The sublingual fossa is above the mylohyoid line anteriorly, where the sublingual gland locates. The submandibular fossa, a concavity related to the submandibular gland, is beneath the mylohyoid line.

(2) The mandibular ramus is bilateral vertical part with two bony processes above. The former is called coronoid process, which is triangular, flat, and the temporal muscle attaches on. The latter is

called condyle, which forms temporomandibular joint with temporal fossa. The constriction beneath the condyle is called the condylar neck. The notch between the two osseous processes, called the mandibular notch or mandibular sigmoid notch, is an important marker for anaesthesia of foramen rotundum and foramen ovale via the infratemporal approach. The middle and inferior portion of the lateral side of the mandibular ramus is rough, where the masseter is attached. There is a funnel-shaped foramen in the middle of the inner(medial) side, called the mandibular foramen, which is the entrance of the inferior alveolar nerve and blood vessel. A small spur of bone on the anterior medial side of the foramen is called the lingula, to which the sphenomandibular ligament is attached. The inferior portion near the mandibular angle of the medial side is rough, to which the medial pterygoid muscle is attached.

The mandibular angle is the intersecting part between the posterior and lower borders of the mandibular ramus, where the stylomandibular ligament is attached.

(3) Anatomical characteristics of mandible and its clinical significance: the weak sites of mandible, the symphysis of mandible, the mental foramen area, the mandible angle, the neck of condyle and so on.

The blood supply of the mandible is less than that of the maxilla, so the healing of the mandibular fracture is slower than that of maxillary. There are strong and dense muscles and fascia around the mandible, as it is difficult to get drainage when inflammation suppurates, so the occurrence rate of osteomyelitis is higher than that of maxilla.

The mandible is attached and surrounded by strong masticatory muscle group, and the fracture segment is unstable when the mandible fractures. When the mouth opens and closes, the fracture segment is easy to be pulled by the contraction of masticatory muscles, and fracture dislocation occurs.

1.3.3   Muscles

Because of the different functions, the muscles of oral and maxillofacial region are divided into masticatory muscles and expression muscles. Masticatory muscles are relatively sturdy, mainly attached to the mandible and the zygomatic bone and deep in position, while the expression muscles are smaller, mainly attached to the maxilla, distributed around the mouth, nose, palpebral fissures and beneath the superficial skin of the face, connected with the skin. When contracting, the expression muscle fibers could pull the skin of frontal, palpebral, lip and buccal region to movement, showing various expressions.

1.3.3.1   Masticatory muscles

Masticatory muscles are mainly attached to the mandible, responsible for the anterior and lateral movement of the mandible, and opening and closing of the jaw, thus divided into two groups: jaw closers and jaw openers. In addition, there is the lateral pterygoid, which is related to the forward and backward movement of the mandible. Their innervation comes from the mandibular nerve of the trigeminal nerve which is mainly in charge of movement.

The masseter, temporalis and medial pterygoid are mainly attached to the mandibular ramus. The contractility of these muscles are strong, and the direction of contraction is mainly upward, accompanied by forward and backward.

The digastric, mylohyoid and geniohyoid belong to the suprahyoid muscles, mainly arising from the mandibular body to the hyoid bone, and forming the main part of the mouth floor. The direction of contraction is mainly downward and upward.

(1) Masseter

This muscle cowes from the zygomatic bone and the lower margin of the zygomatic arch, terminating on the external side of the mandibular angle and ramus. It's a short and thick muscle that serves to pull the mandible upward and forward.

(2) Temporalis

This muscle arises from the temporal fossa of the temporal bone, through the deep side of the zygomatic arch to the coronoid process of the mandibular ramus. The temporalis is a fan-shaped and powerful muscle that pulls the mandible upward, slightly to the rear.

(3) Medial pterygoid

This muscle is originated from the medial aspect of the lateral pterygoid plate of the sphenoid and the maxillary tuberosity. It is a quadrate and thick muscle which is located on the medial aspect of the mandible. It's function is to make the mandible move upward and the mouth closed, and to assist the lateral pterygoid in the the forward and lateral movement of the mandible.

(4) Lateral pterygoid

There are two heads of origin: the superior head and the inferior head. The superior head arises from the infratemporal surface and crest of the greater wing of the sphenoid. The inferior head arises from the lateral aspect of the lateral pterygoid plate. The two heads end at the anterior and medial aspect of articular disc and the front of the neck of the mandibular condyle respectively. When contracting, the mandible can be pulled forward and backward.

(5) Digastric

The anterior belly originates from the digastric fossa of the mandible and the posterior belly originates from the mastoid notch of the temporal bone, and the anterior and posterior abdomen formed intermediate tendon, which is attached by compact connective tissue to the boundary of greater cornua and the hyoid body. The action is to lift the hyoid up and pull the mandible down word. The anterior belly is innervated by the mylohyoid nerve and the posterior belly is innervated by the facial nerve.

(6) Mylohyoid

The mylohyoid originates from the mylohyoid line of the medial aspect of the mandible and ends at the body of the hyoid. It is flat triangle-shaped and interdigitated in the midline to form a mobile muscular sheet. The action is to lift the hyoid and the floor of the mouth upward, or to pull the mandible down. The innervation nerve is the mylohyoid nerve.

(7) Geniohyoid

The geniohyoid originates from the mandibular lower mental spine and ends at the hyoid body. The action is to lift the hyoid forward and pull the mandible down. The innervation nerve is the fibres from the first cervical nerve travelling alongside the hypoglossal nerve.

1.3.3.2   Expression muscles

Facial expression muscles are thin and short, weak contractility, arising from the bone or superficial fascia, ending at the skin. Muscle fibers mostly surround facial foramen, such as eyes, nose and mouth, arranged in circular or radial form. The main expression muscles are orbicularis oculi, orbicularis oris, levator labii superioris, frontalis, risorius, depressor anguli oris and buccinator. Because the facial expression muscle is closely connected with the skin, when the skin and facial expression muscle are cut off by trauma or surgery, the wound often splits up and should be sutured layer by layer so as to avoid forming the invagination scar. Facial expression muscles are innervated by the facial nerve. If the facial nerve is injured, the facial expression muscles are paralyzed, resulting in facial paralysis.

(1) Frontalis

Frontalis is located on the forehead. It starts from the galea aponeurotica and stops on the skin of the eyebrow. The muscular layer is thin but wide and quadrilateral. The main expression function is reflected by raising eyebrows and frowning.

(2)Orbicularis oculi

Orbicularis oculi is located around the orbit and consists of three parts: orbital part, palprebal part and lacrimal part. The orbital part arises from the nasal part of the frontal bone, frontal process of the maxilla, and from the medial palpebral ligament with its fibres passing around the orbit. The orbital part is the outermost part of the orbicularis oculi. Its function is to pull the eyebrow and the frontal skin. The palpebral part is subcutaneously located in the eyelid, starting from the medial palpebral ligament and the adjacent bones. The fibers of the upper and lower palpebral parts converge at the outer canthus. It is involved in closure during involuntary blinking. The lacrimal part is located on the deep side of the lacrimal sac. It rises from the posterior lacrimal crest and passes behind the lacrimal sac where the fibres bind to the palprebal part muscle. It is thought to dilate the lacrimal sac.

(3)Corrugator supercilii

It originates from the nasal part of the frontal bone and stops at the skin of the medial part of the eyebrow. It is the principal muscle in the expression of suffering, producing vertical ridges above the bridge of the nose when frowning by drawing the eyebrows downwards and inwards.

(4)Nasalis

It is divided into two parts: the transverse nasalis and the alar nasalis. The transverse nasalis muscle originates from the area above the root of the maxillary canine, and the muscle fibers converge across the back of the nose with the contralateral homonym. The alar nasalis arises from the maxilla above the lateral incisor tooth and inserts into the greater alar cartilage.

(5)Orbicularis oris

The orbicularis oris is located around the oral fissure, and composed of superficial, medium and deep muscle fibers surrounded by the oral fissure. The superficial layer is the inherent fiber of the orbicularis oris muscle, which runs from one side of the lip to the other side and forms the superficial layer of the orbicularis oris. The middle layer consists of some muscle fibers from zygomaticus, levator labii superioris, levator anguli oris, depressor anguli oris and depressor labii inferioris. The deep layer consists of a portion of muscle fibers from the buccinator. The main function of the orbicularis oris is to close the mouth and to assist in pronunciation and chewing.

(6)Zygomaticus minor, levator labii superioris and levator labii superioris alaeque nasi

These three muscles used to be called the quadratus labii superioris. The zygomaticus minor located below or deep of the orbicularis oculi, starting on the external side of the zygomatic bone behind the zygomaticomaxillary suture, and ending at the medial side of the upper lip. Its function is to draw the angle of mouth laterally and upward. The levator labii superioris starts from the infraorbital margin above the infraorbital foramen and is covered by the orbicularis oculi. It is intertwined with the orbicularis oris downward and ends at the outer half of the upper lip. Between its deep side and the levator anguli oris, the infraorbital nerve vessel is perforated through the infraorbital foramen. The main function of levator labii superioris is to pull the upper lip upward. The levator labii superioris alaeque nasi originates from the medial part of the frontal process of the maxilla. Miner fibers intertwine with the levator labii superioris and the orbicularis oris, and majar fibers insert into the greater alar cartilage and the skin. The levator labii superioris alaeque nasi pulls the upper lip upward and dilates the nostril.

(7)Zygomaticus major

It starts in front of zygomatcotiemporal suture, ends at the angle of mouth and adds to the orbicularis oris obliquely.

(8) Levator anguli oris

It arises from the maxillary canine fossa, and some of the muscle fibers stop at the mouth angle skin. Some muscle fibers are involved in the formation of orbicularis oris. And its function is to raise the angle of mouth.

(9) Depressor labii inferioris

It is located between the mental foramina and mandibular symphysis, starting from the external oblique line, running upward and inward, converging with the contralateral muscle of the same name, and ending in the skin and mucous membrane of the lower lip. The starting part is connected to the platysma. Its action is to descend the lip and the angle of mouth.

(10) Risorius

It rises from the parotideomasseteric fascia, running forward and downward across the masseter and ending at the skin of the angle of mouth.

(11) Depressor anguli oris

It is triangular, starting from the external side of the mandibular body and ending in the skin of the mouth angle. Some fibers are involved in the composition of the orbicularis oris muscle. The posterior edge of the depressor anguli oris is continuous with the upper part of the platysma.

(12) Buccinator

The buccinator is a thin, flat and quadrilateral muscle, located in the buccal region, occupying the space between maxilla and mandible, forming the buccal region. It is the deepest muscle of facial expression, and often considered an accessory muscle of mastication. It originates from the maxilla and mandible adjacent to the molar teeth and from the pterygomandibular ligament and pterygomandibular raphae posteriorly. The muscle fibers converge to the mouth angle. The central fibers originating from the pterygomandibular raphae form a chiasma, with the upper fibers passing into the lower lip and lower fibers into the upper lip, but the fibers arising from the maxilla and mandible do not decussate, passing into the orbicularis oris of respective upper and lower lips. Its function is to pull the mouth angle backward, to assist in chewing and sucking, and to aspire the air in oral cavity.

(13) Mentalis

It is conical and located deeply of the depressor labii inferioris. It arises from the buccal bone of the incisors of the mandible and ends at the chin skin. Its function is to descend the angle of mouth and lower lip, to make the lower lip close to the gingiva and to protrude it.

1.3.4 Blood vessels

1.3.4.1 arteries

The blood supply in the maxillofacial region is especially abundant, mainly from the branches of the external carotid artery, including the lingual artery, facial artery, maxillary artery and superficial temporal artery. The branches and bilateral arteries are anastomosed with each other through the peripheral vascular network, so the bleeding is more. When hemostasis by compression, you must press the proximal part of the supply artery to stop the bleeding temporarily.

(1) Lingual artery

It is separated from the lateral carotid artery at the level of the greater cornua of the hyoid bone, running inward and upward, distributed to the tongue, floor of mouth and gingiva.

(2) Facial artery

It is also called external maxillary artery, and the main artery of facial soft tissue. Slightly above the lingual artery, it separates from the external carotid artery, running inward and upward, hooking the submandibular gland and crossing the lower border of the mandible anterior to the origin of the masseter. Then it runs forward and distributes to the lip, chin, buccal and inner canthus regions. When buccal soft tissue bleeding, pressing hemostasis could be adopted by applying pressure to this vessel at the lower border of the mandible anterior to the masseter.

(3) Maxillary artery

It is also called internal maxillary artery. The maxillary artery is separated from the external carotid artery and passed forward and slightly upward behind the condylar neck, entering infratemporal fossa, and distributed to the maxilla, mandibular and masticatory muscles. The artery is vulnerable to be damaged in the operation of temporomandibular joint area, so special attention should be paid.

(4) Superficial temporal artery

It is the terminal branch of the external carotid artery, giving off the transverse artery in the parotid gland, which distributed to the pre auricular, zygomatic and buccal regions. Superficial temporal artery is distributed in frontal and temporal scalp. Subcutaneous artery pulsation could be palpated above the zygomatic arch. Applying pressure to this artery here could be used in hemostasis. Malignant tumors in maxillofacial region can be treated by arterial infusion of chemotherapeutic drugs via retrograde catheterization.

1.3.4.2   Veins

The maxillofacial venous system is complex and variable, often divided into deep and superficial venous networks. The superficial venous network consists of the facial vein and the retromandibular vein, and the deep venous network is mainly the pterygoid venous plexus. The maxillofacial veins are characterized by fewer venous flaps and are prone to regurgitate when contracted or squeezed by muscles. The triangle area from nasal root to bilateral mouth angle is called "dangerous triangle area". The infection of maxillofacial region, especially the infection of "dangerous triangle area", is easy to be retrograde into the brain if it were not handled properly, resulting in serious intracranial complications such as cavernous sinus thrombophlebitis.

(1) Facial vein

It originates from the angular vein, passing by the paranasal region, the mouth angle to the anterior and inferior region of the masseter muscle, connected with the pterygoid venous plexus by deep facial vein in buccal region. It penetrates the deep cervical fascia at the anterior inferior angle of the masseter muscle, passing by the superficial surface of the submandibular glands, merging with the anterior branch of the retromandibular vein near the mandibular angle and forming the common facial vein, which crosses the superficial side of the external carotid artery and finally joins into the internal jugular vein. Therefore, the facial vein could lead to the intracranial cavernous sinus through two ways: the angular vein and the pterygoid venous plexus.

(2) Retromandibular vein

Also called the posterior facial vein, it is formed by merging of superficial temporal vein and maxillary vein(internal maxillary vein), along the lateral side of the external carotid artery, down to the mandibular angle level, and is divided into two branches: anterior branch and posterior branch. The anterior branch merging with the facial vein forms the common facial vein, and the posterior branch merging with the posterior auricular vein forms the external jugular vein. The external jugular vein goes down on the superficial side of sternocleidomastoid muscle, penetrates into the deep at the supraclavicular fossa and flows into the subclavian vein.

(3)Pterygoid venous plexus

It is located in the infratemporal fossa, mostly in the superficial side of the lateral pterygoid muscle, and some between the temporalis and the lateral and medial pterygoid. During anaesthesia of maxillary nodules, hematoma may sometimes be formed by injury. It drainages venous blood from the jaw, masticatory muscles, nose and parotid gland, and joins into the retromandibular vein by the maxilla vein. The pterygoid plexus can also communicate with the intracranial cavernous sinus through the ovale and lacerum foramen.

1.3.5 Lymphoid tissue

The distribution of lymphatic tissue in maxillofacial region is extremely rich. Lymphatic vessels form a reticular structure, accepting lymph fluid, draining into lymph nodes, which constitute an important defense system of maxillofacial region. Normally, lymph nodes are small and soft, not palpable. When inflammation or tumor metastasis exists, the corresponding lymph nodes will be enlarged, palpable, so it has important clinical significance.

Common and important lymph nodes in the maxillofacial region are parotid lymph nodes, mandibular lymph nodes, submandibular lymph nodes, submental lymph nodes, and superficial and deep cervical lymph nodes which are located in the neck.

1.3.5.1 Parotid lymph nodes

The parotid lymph nodes are divided into two groups: superficial parotid lymph nodes and deep parotid lymph nodes. The superficial lymph nodes are located in the preauricular area and superficial to the parotid gland, receiving the lymph of the region such as nose, eyelid, frontotemporal portion, external auditory canal and auricle and draining to the superior deep cervical lymph nodes. The deep parotid lymph nodes are located deep in the parotid gland, receiving the lymph fluid in the region of the soft palate, the nasopharynx, etc, and draining to the superior deep cervical lymph nodes.

1.3.5.2 Mandibular lymph nodes

The mandibular lymph node is located in front of the masseter muscle and above the lower border of the mandible, receiving the lymph from the nasal and buccal skin and mucosa and draining to the submandibular lymph nodes.

1.3.5.3 Submandibular lymph nodes

The submandibular lymph nodes are located in the submandibular triangle, between the the submandibular gland and the lower border of the mandibular, and around the facial artery and facial vein. The lymph nodes receive lymph from the cheek, nose, upper lip, lateral lower lip, gingiva, anterior part of tongue, maxilla and mandible, and lymph from the submental lymph nodes. Lymph drains to the superior deep cervical lymph nodes.

1.3.5.4 Submental lymph nodes

The submental lymph nodes are located in the submental triangle, receiving the lymph from the middle lower lip, the lower incisors, the tip of the tongue and the mouth floor. Lymph drains to the submandibular lymph nodes and the superior deep cervical lymph nodes.

1.3.5.5 Cervical lymph nodes

The cervical lymph nodes are divided into the superficial cervical lymph nodes, the superior deep cervical lymph nodes and the inferior deep cervical lymph nodes.

(1) Superficial cervical lymph nodes

Superficial cervical lymph nodes are located on the superficial side of the sternocleidomastoid muscle, arranged along the external jugular vein, receiving lymph from the parotid gland and inferior auricle and draining to the deep cervical lymph nodes.

(2) Superior deep cervical lymph nodes

The superior cervical lymph node are located on the deep side of the sternocleidomastoid muscle, arranged along the internal jugular vein, from the skull base to the carotid bifurcation, mainly receiving lymph from the head and neck, as well as from the thyroid, nasopharynx, tonsils, etc. Lymph drains to the inferior deep cervical lymph nodes and jugular lymphatic trunk.

(3) Inferior deep cervical lymph nodes

The inferior deep cervical lymph nodes are located in the supraclavicular triangle, deep of the sternocleidomastoid muscle, below the carotid bifurcation, and along the internal jugular vein to the venous angle. They receive lymph from the superior deep cervical lymph nodes, occiput, posterior neck region and chest. Lymph drains to the jugular lymphatic trunk, then to the right lymphatic duct(right) and thoracic duct (left).

1.3.6 Nerve

The sensory nerve in oral and maxillofacial region is mainly the trigeminal nerve and the motor nerve is mainly the facial nerve.

1.3.6.1 Trigeminal nerve

The trigeminal nerve is the fifth cranial nerve(CN V). It is the largest cranial nerve. It originates from the pontine ridge and is responsible for the sensation of maxillofacial region and the movement of masticatory muscles. The larger sensory root is divided into three divisions from the trigeminal semilunar ganglion, namely, the ophthalmic division(CN V1), the maxillary division(CN V2) and the mandibular division(CN V3). The smaller motor root crosses the ganglion below the sensory root and mixes with the mandibular nerve. So the mandibular nerve belongs to mixed nerve.

(1) Ophthalmic nerve

The bulk of the ophthalmic division fibers enter the orbit from the middle cranial fossa by passing through the superior orbital fissure, distributed in the eyeball and forehead.

(2) Maxillary nerve

The maxillary nerve passes through the pterygopalatine fossa to the inferior orbital fissure from the foramen rotundum out of the cranium, and then through the infraorbital groove into the infraorbital canal. Finally, The bulk goes out of the infraorbital foramen and divides into three final branches: palpebral branch, nasal branch and superior labial branch, distributed in the skin and mucosa of the lower eyelid, the paranasal area and the upper lip. The following branches are closely related to oral and maxillofacial anesthesia.

1) The sphenopalatine nerve and the pterygopalatine ganglion: in the pterygopalatine fossa, the maxillary nerve branches into the sphenopalatine ganglion, and four branches are generated from this ganglion.

● Nasopalatine nerve: the nasopalatine nerve goes through the sphenopalatine foramen into the nasal cavity, forward and downward along the nasal septum, into the incisor canal, out of the incisor foramen in the mouth, distributed in the palatal side of mucoperiosteum and gingiva of each maxillary incisors, canines, overlapping posteriorly with the anterior palatine nerve on the palatal side of the canines.

● Anterior palatine nerve: anterior palatine nerve is the largest branch, descending through the pterygopalatine canal out of the palatal foramen, distributed forward in the palatal mucoperiosteum and gingiva of the molars, the premolars, overlapping with the nasopalatine nerve in the canine region.

● Middle and posterior palatine nerve: they descend through the pterygopalatine canal, distributed in the soft palate, uvula and tonsil.

2) Superior alveolar nerve: it is a branch of the maxillary nerve, divided into anterior, middle and posterior superior nerves according to the course and location.

● Posterior superior alveolar nerve: the maxillary nerve runs forward in the pterygopalatine fossa, and gives off several small branches near the posterior wall of the maxillary tuberosity, some of which are distributed in the buccal mucosa and gingiva of the maxillary molar region, and some enter the alveolar foramen of the maxillary tuberosity, running down the posterior wall of the maxillary sinus the maxilla body, distributed in the mucosa of maxillary sinus and the maxillary molars(except the mesial buccal root of the maxillary first molar) , overlapping with the middle superior alveolar nerve at the mesial buccal root of the maxillary first molar.

● Middle superior alveolar nerve: the maxillary nerve gives off the middle superior alveolar nerve at the place where it has just entered the infraorbital canal. It runs along the lateral wall of the maxillary sinus, distributed in the alveolar bone, the buccal gingiva and the mucosa of the maxillary sinus from the maxillary premolar to the mesial buccal root of the first molar, overlapping with the anterior and posterior superior alveolar nerves.

● Anterior superior alveolar nerve: the anterior superior alveolar nerve is divided from the infraorbital nerve before it goes out of the infraorbital foramen. The anterior superior alveolar nerve enters into the alveolar bone along the anterior wall of the maxillary sinus, distributed in the alveolar bone and labial gingiva of the maxillary incisor, canine, overlapping with the middle superior alveolar nerve and the contralateral anterior superior alveolar nerve.

3) Mandibular nerve: the mandibular nerve is the largest branch from the trigeminal semilunar ganglion. It belongs to the mixed nerve and contains sensory and motor nerve fibers. The mandibular nerve exits the skull base at foramen ovale and divides into anterior and posterior divisions in the infratemporal fossa. The smaller anterior division is motor except for the buccal nerve, and the rest motor branches innervate the masticatory muscle movement. The larger posterior division is mainly sensory apart from the motor fibres (mylohyoid nerve) of the inferior alveolar nerve. The branches of the posterior division are the auriculotemporal nerve, the inferior alveolar nerve and the lingual nerve. These branches closely related to oral and maxillofacial local anesthesia are as follows.

● Inferior alveolar nerve: the inferior alveolar nerve is the largest branch of the posterior division of the mandibular nerve. Deep to the lateral pterygoid, the inferior alveolar nerve goes descending between the sphenomandibular ligament and the mandibular ramus, enters the mandibular canal through the mandibular foramen, giving off small branches to all the teeth and alveolar bones of the ipsilateral mandible, overlapping with the contralateral inferior alveolar nerve in the midline. The inferior alveolar nerve is in the mandibular canal, giving off the mental nerve at the premolar region. The mental nerve distributs in the labial gingiva, lower lip, buccal mucosa and skin in front of the second premolars, overlapping with the contralateral mental nerve in the middle of the lower lip and chin.

● Lingual nerve: the lingual nerve arises from the posterior division of the mandibular nerve, passing between the medial pterygoid and the mandibular ramus, descending along the anterior and inner side of the inferior alveolar nerve, and entering the mouth floor on the lingual side of the bone plate of the mandibular third molar. The nerve goes forward in the mouth floor, distributed in the anterior two – thirds of the tongue, the lingual side of the mandibular gingiva and the mucosa of the mouth floor.

● (Long) buccal nerve: the buccal nerve is the only sensory nerve in the anterior division of the mandibular nerve, passing between the upper and lower heads of the lateral pterygoid and along the anterior border of the mandibular ramus, pierceing the buccinator at the level of the occlusal plane supplying the buccal mucosa, gingiva, vestibular mucosa up to the mental foramen and the skin of the cheek.

The above nerve branches are located in the pterygomandibular space, with the buccal nerve at the anterolateral side, the lingual nerve in the middle and the inferior alveolar nerve in the posterior position. Understanding this relationship is of clinical significance for mandibular block anesthesia.

1.3.6.2   Facial nerve

The facial nerve is the seventh cranial nerve, which is a mixed nerve carrying mainly motor fibers, accompanied by taste (sensory) and secretory (parasympathetic) fibers. Immediately after the facial nerve passes out of the stylomastoid foramen, it enters the parotid gland at about 2 – 3 cm deep from the skin. After running 1–1.5 cm forwards and downwards in parotid gland, it divides into temporofacial and cervicofacial divisions and then divides into five branches, namely the temporal branch, zygomatic branch, the buccal branch, the marginal mandibular branch and the cervical branch. Usually the temporofacial division goes slightly upward and ahead and divides into the temporal branch, the zygomatic branch, superior buccal branch; the cervicofacial division goes downward and divides into the inferior buccal branch, the marginal mandibular branch and the cervical branch. The branches of the facial nerve are anastomosed to form an irregular mesh. After the branches exit the parotid gland, they lie closely on the superficial surface of the masseter fascia and then fan – shaped innervate the facial expression muscles. The facial nerve damage may cause facial malformation such as incomplete eyelid closure and distortion of commissure, etc.

(1) Temporal branches

There are 1 or 2 temporal branches. The temporal branch exits the upper edge of the parotid gland and crosses the zygomatic arch in front of the joint, mainly distributed in the frontalis. When it is damaged, the frontal wrinkles disappear.

(2) Zygomatic branches

There are 1 – 4 temporal branches. After exiting the anterior superior edge of the parotid gland, the strongest zygomatic branch runs forward and upward along the zygomatic bone, distributed in the muscles of the lower part of orbicularis oculi and the upper lip muscles; 2 – 3 smaller branches pass over near the midpoint of the zygomatic arch, mainly distributed in the upper part of the orbicularis oculi and frontalis. When it is damaged, the incomplete eyelid closure will occur.

(3) Buccal branches

There are 2 – 6 buccal branches. They exit the anterior edge of the parotid gland, above and below the parotid duct, which are called the superior buccal branch and the inferior buccal branch respectively, distributed in the zygomaticus major, zygomaticus minor, levator labii superioris, levator labii superioris alaeque nasi, levator anguli oris, risorius, buccinator and orbicularis oris, etc. When it is damaged, the nasolabial sulcus will disappear and air will leak during blowing.

(4) Marginal mandibular branches

There are 2 – 4 marginal mandibular branches, which exit the anterior inferior edge of the parotid gland. It run downward and forward on the deep side of the platysma, and then upward and forward across the facial artery and facial vein, distributed in the lower lip muscles. The marginal mandibular branch is located above the lower border of the mandibular in about 80% of cases, with a lower position at the mandibular angle region. Only in about 20% of cases the marginal mandibular branch is within 1 cm below the lower border of the mandible. When the operation is performed in the submandibular area, the incision should be 1. 5-2 cm below the lower border of mandible to avoid damaging the nerve, otherwise there may be paralysis of the homolateral lower lip, showing the distortion of commissure.

（5）Cervical branch

The cervical branch is pierced from the inferior edge of the parotid gland and distributed in the platysma. Damage to this branch has little effect on function.

1.3.7　Salivary glands

The salivary glands in oral and maxillofacial region consists of three pairs of major salivary glands, namely parotid gland, submandibular gland and sublingual gland, as well as minor salivary glands scattered throughout the submucosa of the lip, cheek, palate, tongue, etc. , each with duct opening in the oral cavity.

The salivary fluid secreted by the salivary gland is a colorless and viscous liquid that enters the mouth. It moisturizes the mouth and softens food. Saliva also contains amylase and lysozyme, which can digest food and inhibit pathogenic bacteria activity.

1.3.7.1　parotid gland

The parotid gland is the largest of the paired salivary glands, and the secretion is mainly serosity. It is located anterior and lower to the earlobe and in the posterior mandibular fossa. It is irregularly pyramidal shape with the base outward. The superficial surface is covered with skin and subcutaneous fat. The gland is adjacent to the masseter, the mandibular ramus and the lateral wall of the pharynx anteriorly in deep, and to the sternocleidomastoid, the styloid process and the posterior belly of the digastric posteriorly. The superior pole reaches the zygomatic arch, between the external auditory canal and the temporomandibular joint, and the inferior pole reaches the lower border of the mandibular angle.

In the parotid gland, the facial nerve branches pass through, and the parotid gland is divided into a superficial and a deep lobe. The parotid gland superficial to the nerve is called the superficial lobe of the parotid gland, which is located superficial to the masseter, forward and downward to the ear; and the deep lobe of the parotid gland to the nerve, through the retromandibular fossa protruding to the parapharyngeal space.

Parotid gland is surrounded by dense parotid masseter fascia, and is divided into many lobules by parotid gland sheath formed from superficial layer of deep cervical fascia. The fascia sheath is incomplete in superior and deep parapharyngeal area, and even absent sometimes. Because of these characteristics, when parotid gland infection abscesses, the abscess is usually separated, and the pain is acute. When incision and drainage, attention should be paid to the thorough separation of abscess, in order to ensure the complete drainage. Abscess diffuses often to the fascia weakness, i. e. external auditory canal and parapharyngeal area.

The parotid duct is perforated from the anterior edge of the superficial lobe at one finger below the zygomatic arch, It runs forward superficial to masseter to the anterior edge of the masseter, turning medially at the anterior border of the muscle and passes through buccinator to open the buccal mucosa at the parotid papilla, in the second molar region. The parotid duct is thick and should not be damaged during buccal surgery. The surface projection of the parotid duct is the middle 1/3 segment of the line from the earlobe to the midpoint of the alare and the angle of mouth. When dissecting the facial nerve, the parotid duct can be found as a reference, and then the adjacent buccal branches are easy to be found.

1.3.7.2　Submandibular gland

The submandibular gland is located in the submandibular triangle. The secretion is mainly serosity containing a small amount of mucus. The deep lobe of the submandibular gland enters the floor of the mouth around the posterior border of the mylohyoid. The submandibular duct(Wharton's duct)starts from the deep lope and runs forward and upward from the lower rear, opening in the sublingual caruncle on both sides of the lingual frenulum. This duct is long and gentle, often blocked by salivary stones, leading to obstruction of the submandibular gland and obstructive sialadenitis.

1.3.7.3　Sublingual gland

The almond−shaped sublingual gland is located beneath the mucosa of the floor of the mouth and is the smallest pair of the major salivary glands. Secretionis mainly mucus, containing a small amount of serosity. The saliva is drained by a major duct which opens into the submandibular duct or separately at the sublingual caruncle and multiple ducts open directly into the oral mucosa in the region of the sublingual. The secretion is viscous and easily clogged, forming "retention cyst" without epithelial lining. Sublingual gland needs to be removed to treat the cyst.

1.3.8　Temporomandibular joint

The temporomandibular(TMJ) is a joint on each side of the head that allows for movement of the mandible for speech and mastication. The TMJ receives its name from the two bones that enter into its formation, the temporal bone and the mandible. The mandibular division of the fifth cranial nerve innervates the TMJ. The blood supply to the joint is from branches of the external carotid artery.

The mandible is attached to the cranium by the ligaments of the TMJ. The mandible is held in position by the muscles of mastication.

1.3.8.1　Compositions of the TMJ

(1)The glenoid fossa, which is lined with fibrous connective tissue, is an oval depression in the temporal bone just anterior to the external auditory meatus.

(2)The articular eminence is a raised portion of the temporal bone just anterior to the glenoid fossa.

(3)The condyloid process of the mandible lies in the glenoid fossa.

The above are three bony parts of the TMJ.

(4)Capsular ligament and articular space.

A fibrous joint capsule completely encloses the TMJ. The capsule wraps around the margin of the temporal bone's articular eminence and articular fossa superiorly. Inferiorly the capsule wraps around the circumference of the mandibular condyle, including the condyle neck.

The articular space is the area between the capsular ligament and the surfaces of the glenoid fossa and the condyle.

(5)Articular disc. The articular disc is a cushion of dense, specialized connective tissue that divides the articular space into upper and lower compartments. These compartments are filled with synovial fluid, which helps lubricate the joint and fills the synovial cavities.

1.3.8.2　Jaw movements

The TMJ performs two basic types of movement, a hinge action and a gliding movement. With these two types of movement, the jaws can open and close and shift from side to side.

(1)Hinge action

The hinge action is the first phase in mouth opening, and only the lower compartment of the joint is used. During hinge action the condylar head rotates around a point on the undersurface of the articular disc, and the body of the mandible drops almost passively downward and backward.

The jaw is opened by the combined actions of the external ptygoid, digastric, mylohyoid, and geniohyoid muscles. The jaw is closed by the action of the temporal, masseter, and internal pterygoid muscles.

（2）Gliding movement

The gliding movement allows the lower jaw to more forward or backward. It involves both the lower and the upper compartments of the joint. The condyle and articular disc "glide" forward and downward along the articular eminence. This movement occurs only during protrusion and lateral movements of the mandible and in combination with the hinge action during the wider opening of the mouth.

Protrusion is the forward movement of the mandible. This happens when the internal and external pterygoid muscles on both sides contract together. The reversal of this movement is the backward movement of the mandible, called retrusion.

Lateral movement, and sideway movement sideways, of the mandible occurs when the internal and external pterygoid muscles on the same side of the face contract together.

Side-to-side grinding movements result from alternating pterygoid muscles, first on one side and then on the other.

He Wei, Kang Hong

Chapter 2

Oral and Maxillofacial Examination

Oral and maxillofacial routine examinations are the basis for the diagnosis and treatment of oral and maxillofacial disease. To avoid misdiagnosis and missed diagnosis, correct diagnosis of oral and maxillofacial disease, reasonable and effective treatment must base on careful and detailed oral and maxillofacial examinations, requisite special inspection means or methods, comprehensive and thorough understand of the disease, combined with scientific analysis and judgment. Also, the oral cavity and maxillofacial region are parts of the whole body. Some oral and maxillofacial disorders can have systemic effects, and some systemic diseases can also appear features in oral cavity and maxillofacial region. Therefore, during oral and maxillofacial routine examination, in addition to focusing on the examination of teeth, periodontal, oral mucosa, and maxillofacial tissues and organs, it is necessary to have a holistic view of diseases. A systemic examination should be carried out if necessary.

2.1 Oral and Maxillofacial Routine Examination

2.1.1 Conventional oral examinations

2.1.1.1 Common inspection instruments

The most commonly used instruments for oral examination are mouth mirrors, tweezers and probes.

(1) Mouth mirror

The mouth mirror can be used for traction of soft tissues such as lips, cheeks, or tongues. The mirror can reflect the viewer's vision on observe indirect surfaces, reflect and concentrate light onto desired surfaces. The handle can be used for the percussion of the teeth.

(2) Tweezer

The tweezer is special for the oral cavity. It is used to hold dressings and medicines, removing corrupt tissue and foreign matter, holding teeth to examine the looseness, and the handle can also be used for the percussion.

(3) Probe

The tip of the probe is tapering, curved at one end and corners on the other. It is used to check the fissures, pits, defects, cavities, and sensitive areas on each surface of the teeth. It can also be used to detect the depth of the periodontal pockets and the presence of subgingival calculus, check the marginal fitness of fillings and restorations with teeth, and the sensory function of the skin or mucosa. Periodontal probe is a blunt cylindrical with scales(in millimeters) used to measure pocket depth around a tooth to evaluate the state of the periodontium.

(4) Other instruments

In addition to the three basic instruments mentioned above, the spoon excavator is commonly used in oral and dental examinations. The spoon excavator used for the oral cavity is small, with hooklike ends and a spoon-shaped head. It is used to remove foreign matter and soft carious decay in the carious cavities so that the depth of the cavities can be observed.

2.1.1.2 Preparation before examination

(1) Check position

The electronic and digital manipulation system of the modern dental chair has made the operation and control of the dental chair very convenient. At the same time, the standardization of the four-handed technique enables the physician to sit on the working chair to complete the diagnosis and treatment. The current routine oral examination method is the examiner sits on the right side of the right rear side of the patient's head, and the patient lies supine on the chair. The nurse or assistant located on the left side of the patient's head. Before starting the examination, the treatment chair should be adjusted according to the specific situation so that the patient feels comfortable and easy to operate.

(2) Check the light source

The light source must be sufficient during the examine. Modern comprehensive treatment chairs have been equipped with a good light source suitable for oral inspection, which can truly reflect the color of the crown, gums, and oral mucosa. However, the light source system can lead to insufficient brightness, which may affect the examination results. Therefore, new light sources should be replaced in time to ensure reliable examine light. Some parts of the oral cavity are away from direct light. They can be reflected in the mouth mirror.

2.1.1.3 Routine inspection methods

(1) Inquiry

Before the examination, the doctor should first understand the occurrence, development, examination, and treatment of the disease, the past health status, and the health status of the family members. The purpose of the inquiry is mainly to find out the patient's chief complaint, current medical and family history.

The inquiry should include the following.

1) Chief complaint: it is the painful problem that the patient needs to solve most urgently. It is also the main reason for the patient's visit. The main symptoms, sites, and time of illness should be asked.

2) Current medical history: it refers to the whole process of the occurrence, development, and evolution of the disease before the visit: ①Onset time, incentives, causes, and symptoms. As for toothache, you should ask when did the pain start and what cause the pain, the site of the toothache, the character (sharp, dull, spontaneous, provocative, etc.), time (day, night, paroxysmal, persistent, etc.) and degree (severe or slight). ②The evolution of the disease. It is initial or recurrent episode, aggravation or remission, etc., and whether there are complications. ③The inspections and treatments have been performed. The results and effectiveness of the treatment.

3) Past medical history: in addition to the past situation related to the diagnosis and treatment of current diseases, it is also important to understand the systemic diseases that patients have suffered in the

past, such as heart disease, hypertension, diabetes, hemophilia, etc. , which may affect the treatment for oral diseases. It also includes infectious diseases such as hepatitis, syphilis, and allergies to medications, especially anesthetics.

4) Family history: the health status of the patient's family members and whether someone had a similar illness should be inquired. For family history of cleft lip and palate, at least three generations of family history should be documented.

(2) Visual examination

Oral cavity visual examination includes teeth, gums, tongue, oral mucosa, salivary glands, and other organs.

1) Teeth: it is important to examine whether teeth arrangement, occlusal relationship, number, shape, and color are normal. Whether there are caries, cracks, residual crown, residual root, and dental calculus.

2) Gingival: the gingival tissues are checked for morphology color and character, including swelling, hyperplasia, atrophy, disappearing of gingival stippling, abscess formation, bleeding, and pyorrhea.

3) Mucosa: it should be noted whether the mucosa color is normal and the epithelium coverage is complete, without herpes, papule, erosion, ulcers, hyperkeratosis, scars, lumps or pigmentation.

4) Tongue: pay attention to the surface of the tongue, including color, furrow or ulcer, whether there is swelling or disappearance of tongue papilla, abnormal movement or sensation, swelling or malformation. Squamous cell carcinoma is most common on the lateral border of the tongue.

5) Salivary glands: always palpate salivary glands bimanually. In suspected inflammatory disease, see if clear saliva can be secreted from the duct orifice or, alternatively, whether turbid, mucopurulent secretion indicative of infection is presented.

(3) Probing

Use a dental probe to examine and determine the location, extent, and response of the lesion. Including the check of tooth decay, determine its location, depth, presence of the pain and the exposure of pulp. Examine marginal integrity and structural integrity of the existing restoration. Detailed periodontal probing around suspect teeth may reveal a sulcus within normal limits. Periodontal probing should be undertaken systematically on each tooth to determine the probing depth, bleeding after probing and the extent of attachment loss. The probe can also be used to identify the sinus tract pathway.

(4) Percussion

Percussion refers to gently tapping or pressing the occlusal or lateral surface of a tooth. A painful response indicates periapical inflammation. The percussion should not be overexertion, first percuss the adjacent normal tooth, then objective tooth, to make a comparison.

(5) Palpation

Palpate with your finger or with forceps between cotton ball, press the gingival margin or apical gingival, observe whether there is pyorrhea, tenderness, or mobility. This helps to diagnose periodontal disease and periapical disease. Press and hold the buccal side of two adjacent teeth with fingers, ask the patient to make various occlusal movements, in order to check the existence of traumatic occlusion. Check the movement of teeth using the dental tweezers. For the anterior teeth, hold the crown with tweezer; for the molar teeth, close the tweezer tips, place the tweezer on the occlusal surface of the teeth, shake tweezers to find out the loose condition of the teeth.

Tooth mobility is scored according to a simple index:

0 normal, physiological mobility (<0. 3 mm).

Ⅰ°horizontal mobility >0. 3 mm to 1. 0 mm.

Ⅱ°moderate horizontal mobility of 1. 0-2. 0 mm.

Ⅲ°severe mobility >2. 0 mm in horizontaland vertical movements.

(6)Olfactory examination

Use the physician's sense of smell to help diagnose, for instance, pulp gangrene has a special putrefactive odor and necrotizing ulcerative gingivitis(NUG)has a more peculiar smell of corruption.

(7)Bite test

Ask the patient to bite or bites down on a cotton roll. Typically, the pain occurs on the release of biting pressure. The use of a piece of cotton bud or a cotton roll between the teeth may aid diagnose of periapical disease or the primary occlusal contacts. Occlusal contacts can also be checked by the use of articulating paper.

2.1.2 Maxillofacial routine examination

The routine examination of the maxillofacial region mainly includes inquisition, inspection, palpation, and auscultation. Method and contents of the consultation are the same as routine oral examination. Palpation is the process of using physician's finger or instrument to touch or press lesion locations, in order to detect the range, size, shape, firmness, mobility, presence and extent of tenderness, fluctuation and warmth of lesions.

The examination of the maxillofacial region should include the following aspects.

2.1.2.1 Expression and consciousness

Changes in maxillofacial expressions can be both a representation of certain oral and maxillofacial surgical diseases and a reflection of various systemic diseases. Based on facial expressions, you can understand the patient's state of consciousness, personality, physical condition and severity of illness.

2.1.2.2 Shape and color

Observe and check whether the shape of the maxillofacial facial contour is symmetrical, whether the upper, middle and lower proportions are coordinated, whether there are protrusions or dimples. Changes in the color, texture, and elasticity of the skin have clinical significance for the diagnosis of certain diseases.

2.1.2.3 Maxillofacial organs

(1)Observe the presence, location, the extent of defects of the eyelids, external ear and nose, the size of the palpebral fissure, the interorbital distance, and eyelids mobility.

(2)For patients with maxillofacial injuries, special attention should be paid to the shape, size, and light reflex of the bilateral pupil to clarify whether there is a brain injury. Pay attention to check for cerebrospinal fluid otorrhea or rhinorrhea. Otorrhea indicates the middle cranial fossa fractures and rhinorrhea indicates the anterior cranial fossa fractures. If the external auditory canal only appears as hemorrhage, it can be the rupture of external auditory canal due to condylar fracture.

(3)For patients with maxillary sinus cancer, one of the early symptoms are nasal obstruction or hemorrhagic secretion at the affected side. Exophthalmos, dyskinesia, and diplopia may occur in the late stage. For inflammation and tumor in the vicinity of the ear (such as the temporomandibular joint and parotid gland), audition should be checked.

2.1.2.4 Lesion location and characters

For the discovered lesions, further palpation examination should be performed to pay attention to the temperature, moisture, firmness, and elasticity of the skin lesions; the extent, depth, shape, size of the lesions and their relationship betwen deep tissues, skin and mucous membranes; the mobility of the lesion and signs of fluctuation, subcutaneous crepitus or haphalgesia, etc. For maxillofacial deformity and bilateral asymmetry, attention should be paid to distinguish the difference between bony or soft tissue malformation. Whether there is swelling, distention, or atrophy and defect of the other side. Probing can be used for detecting the fistula and sinus tract of the oral and maxillofacial region; coloring agent or radiocontrast agent can be used to check for the direction and depth of the lesion if necessary.

2.1.2.5 Maxillofacial bone examination

Including orbit, zygoma, zygomatic arch, maxilla, nasal bone, mandibular ramus, mandibular angle and mandibular body examination. Attention should be paid to their size and symmetry, the continuity of bone, complete or defects, the presence of tenderness, fricative or abnormal movements. For bone distention, it is necessary to check for crepitus or fluctuation.

2.1.2.6 Pronunciation and auscultation examination

Pronunciation examination has special significance for the diagnosis of certain diseases, such as children with cleft palate have an obvious nasal voice, known as cleft palate speech. Lump at the base of the tongue can appear slurred speech. A blowout murmur can be heard from the arteriovenous malformation. Patients with temporomandibular joint disorder can hear joint clicking with different characters in the joint area, which helps make a definite diagnosis and classification for the disease.

2.1.2.7 Maxillofacial and cervical lymph nodes examination

The percussion of the maxillofacial and cervical lymph nodes is of great significance in the diagnosis and treatment of maxillofacial inflammation and tumors. During the examination, the patient should maintain a seated position. The examiner should stand in front of patient's right side or behind his right side. Patient's head should be slightly lower and tilted to the area being examined so that the skin and muscles can be relaxed. The examiner's fingers are close to the checking site and sliding palpation. Starting from the occipital region, followed by front and behind of the ear, parotid gland, cheek, submandibular, submental area, along the anterior and posterior borders of sternocleidomastoid muscle, anterior and posterior cervical triangle until the supraclavicular fossa. Check carefully for the deep and shallow lymph nodes for swelling, location, size, number, stiffness, mobility, tenderness, fluctuation and adhesion to the skin or basement.

2.1.2.8 Temporomandibular joint examination

The examination of the temporomandibular joint should contain the following.

(1) Shape and joint motion

Whether the face is symmetrical, the size and length of joint area, mandibular angle, ramus, and mandible body are normal; whether the two sides are consistent. Pay attention to abnormal tenderness and condylar activity. There are two ways to check the temporomandibular motion: ① Place index fingers or middle finger on both sides of tragus(lateral condylar), feel the movement of the condylar process when the patient doing an opening and closing movement. ② Insert two little fingers into the external auditory canal, palpate forward to feel the movement and impact of the condyle. In addition, it should be noticed that whether the mentum is in facial midline and whether there is a significant increase or decrease in the lower 1/3 part of the face.

(2) Masticatory muscles

Examine the contraction force of the chewing muscles, press the muscles, in turn to check for tender points. Ask the patient to do occlusion at the same time to feel whether the bilateral muscle movements are symmetrical and coordinated. The anatomical sites of the chewing muscles in the oral contact pressure are as follows: anterior part of the ramus reflect the anterior part of the temporalis; upper part of the maxillary tuberosity reflect the outer head of the lateral pterygoid muscle; behind and below the mandibular molar lingual side and the inner side of the ramus reflect the lower part of medial pterygoid.

(3) Mandibular movement

Opening and closing jaw movements: ① Check whether the opening degree is normal, whether the opening type is skewed, whether there is an abnormal phenomenon such as joint locking, etc. ② Protrusive movement: check the distance of mandibular extension and whether there is a deflection of the facial midline. ③ Lateral movements: check the symmetry of the left and right side lateral movement, whether the condyle movement is consistent and compare the function during masticatory movement. While doing the above movements, you should also pay attention to the joint pain, sound or noise. Notice the time, character, frequency and loudness of the sound. If there is an obvious sound, you can generally feel it with the finger palpation, use a stethoscope to assist if necessary.

(4) Occlusion relationship

The temporomandibular joint disease is closely related to the condition of teeth and occlusion. Therefore, attention should be paid to checking whether the occlusal relationship is normal and whether there is any malocclusion; whether the overjet, overbite, Spee's curve are normal; whether the degree of abrasion is uniform. In addition, pay attention to the absence of teeth, the time of missing and whether molar teeth is leaned or embedded.

2.1.2.9 Salivary gland examination

The key point of salivary glands examination is the three pairs of salivary glands, but for some diseases, the examination of small salivary glands can not be ignored.

(1) Facial symmetry: first, it should be noted whether the face is symmetrical. Observe the presence of anatomical signs of each gland. Patients with parotid gland lesions or malignant tumors should check for the functions of facial nerve branches. For patients with sublingual glands and submandibular gland malignancies, attention should be paid to tongue motions, such as biased side or lingual muscle tremor on the affected side, indicating the lingual nerve is paralyzed.

(2) Saliva secretion: pay attention to the catheter mouth redness, swelling and pyorrhea; whether the saliva secretion is unobstructed when massage and squeeze the gland; whether the saliva is clear, sticky or purulent.

(3) Patients with parotid gland tumors should also check the pharyngeal and soft palate bulges, if so, it may be due to a deep parotid gland tumor.

(4) Pay attention to the lump during the palpation of the gland. If the lump exists, check for its location, size, character, mobility, and the relationship with the surrounding tissue.

(5) Palpation of the salivary gland duct should check for the presence of calculus, also pay attention to the thickness and character of catheter. Examine should start from the proximal to the direction of catheter mouth with sliding palpation, in order to avoid pushing the calculus into the deep.

(6) Palpation of salivary glands: parotid gland palpation is generally with the index finger, middle finger and ring finger only. Avoid pulling the glands. The palpation of submandibular, sublingual and deep parotid glands is applied with bimanual examination.

2.2   Oral and Maxillofacial Special Examination

2.2.1   Periodontal probing and measurement of periodontal pocket

2.2.1.1   Periodontal probing

Using a calibrated and blunt periodontal probe to detect the relationship between gums and attached tendons, understanding the extent, depth, and attachment of gums to teeth. During the examination, keep the fulcrum stable. The probe should be placed on the tooth surface as much as possible in the same direction with the long axis of the tooth. The strength should be slight to avoid pain.

2.2.1.2   Periodontal pocket measurement

Measurement of periodontal pocket means measurement and examination of periodontal pocket depth. Three sites including buccal, middle, lingual side of the teeth were measured and recorded. The depth from the gingival margin to the bottom of periodontal pocket was examined. Check for the loss of attachment to confirm the severity of periodontal destruction. The loss of attachment should be measured after the measurement of the periodontal pocket depth and the distance from the gingival margin to the enamel cementum boundary. If the gingival margin is located in the root surface below the cementum boundary, the measurement record is negative.

Attachment level is periodontal pocket depth minus the distance from the gingival margin to the enamel cemental boundary.

2.2.2   Dental pulp vitality tests

The normal dental pulp has a certain tolerance to the stimulation of temperature and electric current. When there are lesions in the pulp, the stimulus threshold will change. The pulp will be sensitive to the originally tolerable stimulus, conversely, it will be torpid or even irresponsive to the strong stimulus. Therefore, according to the response to temperature or electric current, dental pulp vitality tests are commonly used in clinics to help diagnose the health of the dental pulp, the stage of lesions, and the vitality of dental pulp.

In normal conditions, the dental pulp does not respond to the temperature stimulation at 20 – 50 ℃. Sensitive response to temperature stimulation indicates inflammation in dental pulp. Lingering or even no response to temperature stimulation indicates the pulp disturbance or necrotic pulp.

The temperature examination including cold and heat tests. There are several methods are generally used for cold testing: cold water, chloride, anhydrous ethanol, popsicle, etc. The simplest method in clinic is to use cold water which sprayed out of three way syringes. During the test, we should remember one principle: when the teeth are difficult to be determined, test the mandibular teeth first and then measure the maxillary teeth. The teeth should be checked one by one to avoid misdiagnosis. Spray hot water or place the heated gutta-percha on the tooth surface to observe patient's reaction to make a heat test. The test results should be compared with the adjacent teeth or the homonymous teeth on the opposite side.

The electric current examination is tested with electrical pulp vitality tester(also called as electrical pulp vitality dynamometer). The dynamometer categories are massive, so the doctors should be familiar with their performance and operation methods. Explain the purpose to the patients to achieve their cooperation. During the test, operators should dry the teeth and strictly isolate the teeth from saliva. Apply the toothpaste on the tester probe and placed it on the measured tooth surface. Adjusting the tester's electric potential gradually from the "0" until the teeth have tingling. Operators should inform the patient to raise their hands. Finally, record the results of the tester as a reference for diagnosis. It is also essential to test the adjacent teeth or the homonymous teeth on the opposite side as a comparision. The response of the dental pulp to the stimulation can gradually decrease with aging. On the contrary, during the period of menstruation, pregnancy, and mental stress, the reaction can be enhanced. Therefore, operators should give attention to these conditions.

2.2.3 Salivary glands secretory function test

Including the qualitative and quantitative examination of salivary secretion and composition analysis of saliva. Salivary glands secretory function test is essential for the diagnosis of salivary gland disease and several metabolic diseases.

2.2.3.1 Qualitative examination

The patient is treated with acidic substances, such as 2% sodium citrate, vitamin C or 1% citric acid, etc. Placed the substances on the back edge of the tongue to increase the reflexes of the glands. The secretory function and degree of patency of the catheter are judged according to the changes and secretion of the glands.

2.2.3.2 Quantitative examination

The total amount of saliva in the normal person is 1,000–1,500 mL in 24 h, 90% is from the parotid gland and submandibular gland, sublingual gland is account for only 3% – 5%, and the small salivary gland secretes even less. Therefore, the quantitative examination of the secretory function of the salivary glands is based on the detection of salivary secretion of salivary glands. The diagnosis of certain salivary gland diseases is through the measurement of the salivary secretion within a certain period. For example, saliva secretion increases when acute oral inflammation or heavy metal poisoning occurs, whereas decreases when chronic salivary gland inflammation, salivary gland stone disease, and lymphoepithelial disease.

2.2.3.3 Composition analysis of saliva

Saliva contains endogenous substances and exogenous substances, including electrolytes, proteins, enzymes, trioxypurine, urea, immunoglobulins, and drugs. Endogenous substances have a certain range of normal values. However, under pathological conditions, the composition changes to a certain extent, and it has certain auxiliary value for the diagnosis of certain diseases.

2.3 Oral and Maxillofacial Imaging Examinations

Oral and maxillofacial radiology, also known as dental and maxillofacial radiology, is that specialty of dentistry concerned with performance and interpretation of diagnostic imaging used for examining the craniofacial, dental and adjacent structures. Oral and maxillofacial imaging includes dental film, panoramic X-ray film, cephalometric roentgenography, X-ray contrast examination, multislice CT, cone beam CT, MRI, radionuclide imaging examination, ultrasonography, in addition to special tests like sialographs.

2.3.1 Dental film

Dental film, also known as periapical film, has become the most commonly used dental imaging exam in clinic. It mainly displays the tooth, dental pulp cavity, root canal, and periapical tissue. A dental film, 3 cm × 4 cm in size, displays the periapical tissue, root canal, and crown of 1 – 3 teeth.

The most common technique for positioning the beam head in dental radiography is the bisecting angle technique. For this technique, place the film as parallel as possible to the tooth root. Then measure or approximate the angle between the long axis of the tooth root and film. Finally, divide this angle in half(bisect the angle) and direct the incident X–ray beam perpendicular to this imaginary angle.

2.3.1.1　Positioning the patient

In radiography of the maxilla, the head should be positioned so that the occlusal surfaces of the maxillary teeth are in a horizontal plane. This is done by adjusting the headrest so that the median plane(sagittal plane) is vertical and a line from the ala of the nose to the tragus of the ear is horizontal. In periapical radiography of the mandible, the head should be positioned so that the occlusal surfaces of the mandibular teeth horizontal when the mouth is opened to the position the radiographs are to be made. This is done by adjusting the headrest so the median plane is vertical and a line from the corner of the mouth to the tragus of the ear is horizontal.

2.3.1.2　Placement of film packets

Center the film lingual to the tooth/teeth(except the bicuspid) being radiographed. Front teeth in vertical position. Back teeth in a horizontal position. Instructing the patient to breathe deeply through the nose also aids in controlling the gag reflex. Maxillary teeth is immobilized with the thumb in opposite side. Mandibular teeth is immobilized with index finger in opposite side. Sometimes teeth images get stretched, shortened or overlapped image. By comparing the tooth length in dental film to the actual (the magnification of the image), the actual tooth length is calculated.

Digital X–ray, which replace the film with an electronic sensor, address some of these issues, and are becoming widely used in dentistry as the technology evolves. It may require less radiation(10% of conventional radiographic films) and are processed much more quickly than conventional radiographic films, often instantly viewable on a computer.

2.3.2　Panoramic X–ray film

Panoramic X–ray film is a distinctive examination method of oral and maxillofacial imaging. A panoramic viewis produced by rotating an external synchronized X–ray beam and film cassette. Panoramic techniques in oral radiography have the capability of making radiographs of the entire upper and lower dental arches, the bilateral mandible and maxilla, the anterolateral aspects of both maxillary sinuses, and the temporo–mandibular joint on one film. It is used most frequently in oral and maxillofacial oncology, trauma, inflammation and jaw deformity exams. A good comparative analysis of left–right structures. Digital pantomography makes the image clearer after computer processing.

2.3.3　Cephalometric roentgenography

Cephalometric roentgenography is used in dentistry, and especially in orthodontic and orthognathic, to gauge the size and spatial relationships of the teeth, jaws, and cranium. This analysis informs treatment planning, quantifies changes during treatment, and provides data for clinical research. The patient is taken frontal and lateral cephalometric radiographs. Cephalometry focuses on linear and angular dimensions established by bone, teeth, and facial measurements. It has also been used for measurements of hard and soft tissues of the craniofacial complex.

Cephalometer is an equipment indispensable to take cephalometric radiograph. It accurately positions a patient's head with reference to the X-ray source to ensure good repetition and reliability during the treatments of orthodontic and orthognathic.

2.3.4 X-ray contrast examination

Radiocontrast agents are substances used to enhance the visibility of internal structures in X-ray-based imaging techniques. Radiocontrast agents with intraluminal injection are typically iodine, barium-sulphate or gadolinium based compounds. They absorb external X-rays, resulting in decreased exposure on the X-ray detector. Contrast agents, enhance the radiodensity in a target tissue or structure. It is used most frequently in salivary glands, temporal mandibular joint, blood vessel, nasopharyal meatus, cyst, sinus cavity, fistulas exams and so on. The most common contrast exams are parotid, submandibular gland and temporal-mandibular joint contrast.

2.3.5 Computerized tomography(CT)

The advantages of CT exam is avoiding image overlapping, having high image definition and density resolution, and displaying the location, size of tumor in oral and maxillofacial deep regions and the relationship with the surrounding tissues. Contrast media used for CT is useful to highlight structures such as blood vessels and tumor. 3D reconstruction makes image display clearer and more directed on the diagnosis and treatment of oral and maxillofacial factures.

2.3.5.1 Indication

(1) Benign and malignant tumors, especially located in oral and maxillofacial deep region.

(2) Complicated fracture and dislocation of joint in oral and maxillofacial region.

(3) Infection in oral and maxillofacial deep region.

(4) Diagnosis and differential diagnosis on congenital malformation in oral and maxillofacial region, diseases of temporo mandibular joint and salivary gland.

(5) To evaluate the post-operative outcomes of oral and maxillofacial tumor.

(6) Computer-aided preoperative planning and post-operative evaluation on oral implantology.

2.3.5.2 Contraindication

(1) Contrast - enhanced CT must be forbidden in the case of hypersensitivity to iodinated contrast media.

(2) Contrast CT on duct of salivary gland is inadvisable in the case of acute infection.

2.3.6 Cone Beam CT(CBCT)

Cone beam computed tomography(CBCT) is a medical imaging technique consisting of X-ray computed tomography where the X-rays are divergent, forming a cone. Cone beam technology was first introduced in the European market in 1996 and into the US market in 2001. CBCT has become increasingly important in treatment planning and diagnosis in implant dentistry, endodontics, orthodontics and orthopedics, among other things. During dental/orthopedic imaging, the CBCT scanner rotates around the patient's head, obtaining up to nearly 600 distinct images in 10s. For interventional radiology, the patient is positioned offset to the table so that the region of interest is centered in the field of view for the cone beam. A single 200 degree rotation over the region of interest acquires a volumetric data set. The scanning software collects the data and reconstructs it, producing what is termed a digital volume composed of three-dimensional voxels of anatomical data that can then be manipulated and visualized with specialized software. CBCT shares many similarities with traditional(fan beam) CT however there are important differences, particularly for lower resolution of reconstruction and soft tissue anatomy determination.

Radiation dose of CBCT will be one-forty to one-thirty of conventional CT. CBCT measures on average 0.15 mm, however 64-slice CT measures on average 0.325 mm. In high resolution region (root canal system, mandible, mandibular canal, subtle hard tissue structure of temporo mandibular joint) , CBCT provides better imaging quality. Dental professionals build 3D reconstruction image according to the need for oral and maxillofacial disease diagnosis. Compared to conventional CT, CBCT has many advantages: ①hard tissues(jawbone, tooth and temporo mandibular joint) display clearly; ②shorter scanning time; ③lower radiation dose; ④lower cost of equipment and exam. However, CBCT lacks appropriate soft tissue anatomy determination, especially soft tissue lesion.

2.3.7　Magnetic resonance image(MRI)

Generally applied to the patient with a wide range of tumor invading surrounding tissues or organs, an allergy to iodic agent, cardiovascular diseases, administration of intravenous contrast at risk. To display the relationship of tumor and internal jugular artery and vein directly.

2.3.7.1　Indication

(1)Space occupying and vascular lesions in oral and maxillofacial region.

(2)Craniomaxillofacial junction lesion(to know the origin, development and communication relationship).

(3)Complications of craniofacial trauma, such as location estimation of traumatic cerebrospinal fluid rhinorrhea.

(4)Diseases of temporo mandibular joint.

2.3.7.2　Contraindication

(1) Patients implanted with cardiac pacemakers, silver clip of postoperative intracranial aneurysm or metal denture.

(2)Critically ill patient, noncooperationist or patient breathing with ventilator.

(3)Claustrophobic.

2.3.8　Radionuclide imaging examination

In oral and maxillofacial regions, radionuclide imaging examination is mainly used in salivary gland imaging and function test, jaw bone imaging, cervical lymphoscintigraphy, head-neck tumors imaging and so on. The short half-life and low-energy radionuclides are the most clinically used, such as 99 mTc(V) - DMSA, which has a good effect in the treatment for oral and maxillofacial tumors.

2.3.9　Ultrasonography

Ultrasonography is typically used to detect the deep-seated tumors in mouth floor, parotid gland, and cervical region. There are two equipments: type-B ultrasonic diagnostic unit and color ultrasonic diagnostic unit. Color doppler flow imaging(CDFI) can show whether the blood supply of tumor is abundance or not. It is very significant in the diagnosis of vascular tumors.

2.4　Additional Examinations

2.4.1　Examination by centesis and cell smear

There are two kinds of aspiration cytology—fine needle and coarse needle. Fine needle aspiration cytology is used in the examination of oral and maxillofacial masses. Coarse needle aspiration cytology is used in the examination of oral and maxillofacial infection and cyst to distinguish the essence of the tumor contents, observe whether it's pus, cyst fluid or blood. Except the visual inspection, the contents can be examined in a smear test for cytological examination. When the mass is suspected as carotid body tumor or aneurysm, centesis is forbidden.

2.4.1.1　Fine needle aspiration cytology

Fine needle aspiration cytology is a diagnostic procedure used to investigate masses. In this technique, a thin(size 5,7, or dedicated puncture device), hollow needle is inserted into the mass for sampling of cells, after being stained, will be examined under a microscope(biopsy).

2.4.1.2　Coarse needle aspiration cytology

A hollow needle(size 8 or 9) is inserted into the abscess or cyst for sampling of liquids which will be examined under a bacterial culture and drug sensitive test to provide assistance to the reasonable use of antibiotics clinically. Once the liquids are withdrawn, stop the aspiration. After the needles placed into the mass, cells are withdrawn by aspiration with a syringe and spread on a glass slide.

2.4.2　Biopsy

A biopsy is a medical test commonly performed by a surgeon, involving extraction of sample cells or tissues for examination to determine the presence, character, degree of differentiation or extent of a disease. Biopsies are most commonly performed for insight into possible cancerous and inflammatory conditions. The tissue is generally examined under a microscope by a pathologist, and can also be analyzed chemically. When an entire lump or suspicious area is removed, the procedure is called an excisional biopsy. An incisional biopsy or core biopsy samples a portion of the abnormal tissue without attempting to remove the entire lesion or tumor. A small lesion should be recommended for an excisional biopsy and an intraoperative frozen section diagnosis, which have become a decisive factor for diagnosis and treatment of patients with cancer. It is widely acknowledged as the gold standard for clinical oncologists. A deep lesion should be recommended for intraoperative frozen section biopsy combined the biopsy and radical surgery, while avoiding those important tissue structure. When a disease fails to be diagnosed definitely at its first biopsy, more biopsies are needed. Important tissue structures should be avoided.

A routine intraoperative frozen section diagnosis is performed in parotid gland and submandibular gland tumors. While malignant melanoma is highly suspected, the interval time between biopsy and radical surgery should be minimised. Biopsy is prohibited in patients with hemangioma and carotid body tumor.

2.4.3　Laboratory examination

Laboratory tests on blood, urine, saliva, cytological examination, bacterial smear test or culture, and so on. Laboratory, biochemistry, serological test and bacteriologic test are routine examinations in patients undergoing oral maxillofacial surgery.

2.5 Dental Records and Writing Specifications

2.5.1 Contents of dental records

Comprehensive and accurate records are a vital part of dental practice. Good record keeping is fundamental for good clinical practice and is an essential skill for practitioners. The primary purpose of maintaining dental records is to deliver quality patient care and follow-up. Dental records can also be used for forensic purposes and have an important role in teaching and researching, as well as in legal matters. A dental record is the detailed document of identification data (name, date of birth, phone numbers, and emergency contact information), chief complaint, history of the illness, physical examination, diagnosis, treatment, management of a patient, and signature of doctor. Inpatient record should describe the elemental oral and maxillofacial examinations in detail.

2.5.2 Writing specifications

The most common clinical dental site record in China is dental site record. Dentition is divided into four quadrants with+. A, B, C, D represent four sites respectively. Arabic numerals represent the teeth. For example, the right mandibular permanent first molar is recorded as 6C. Another dental site record is double figures record recommended by the International Association for Dental Research. Double figures represent the teeth. Ten digits represents the quadrant, and single digits represents the teeth. 1, 2, 3, 4 represent four sites of permanent teeth respectively. 5, 6, 7, 8 represent four sites of deciduous teeth respectively. The teeth is sorted from the mesial to the distal. Sequence numbers of permanent and deciduous teeth are both Arabic numerals.

Dental site record:

A(permanent tooth 1 quadrant) (deciduous tooth 5 quadrant)	B(permanent tooth 2 quadrant) (permanent tooth 6 quadrant)
C(permanent tooth 4 quadrant) (permanent tooth 8 quadrant)	D(permanent tooth 3 quadrant) (permanent tooth 7 quadrant)

For example, the right mandibular permanent first molar is known as 46, and 85 represents the right mandibular deciduou first molar.

2.5.2.1 Out-patient record

Name: Zhang ××, Gender: female, Age: 25, Professional: teacher, Nationality: han, Marriage: married, Domicile of origin:×× province ×× city, Address:×× city ×× road ×× number, Medical date: 2017-10-26.

Subjective: patient, reported sensitivity to cold and hot drink, severe pain on upper left side for two months.

Objective: $\overline{}|6$ meiso-occlusal deep caries, palpation(-), percussion(++), cold test: no response.

Assessment: $\dfrac{6}{}$ pulpal necrosis

symptomatic apical periodontis

Plan: $\dfrac{6}{}$ caries clean out, root canal treatment(RCT) if restorable, onlay or crown restoration.

Treatment: caries clean out, restorability checked with operative faculty. Anesthesia achieved by buccal infiltration and posterior suprior alveolar nerve(PSA) blocking with 2 mL of 2% lidocaine with 1 : 100k epinephrine.

Isolation with rubber dam.

Access opening done from occlusal, four canals identified.

Coronal fare done with orifice opener and gates Glidden bur.

Working length determined using apex locater and verified with periapical X-ray. Working length established with file #15, MB 17 mm, MB2 17 mm, DB 18 mm, P 20.5 mm, with cavity margin as reference point.

Canals irrgated with sodium hypochlorite. Canals filled with calcium hydroxide. 1 cotton pellet placed on orifice. Temporized with pink GC Fuji. Occlusion checked.

Post operation instruction given. Patient responded well to the treatment, Dismissed in good condition.

Next visit: $\dfrac{6}{}$ continues RCT.

Signature: Dr. Luo ×

2.5.2.2   Inpatient record

Writing specifications of oral and maxillofacial inpatient medical records is the same as outpatiend record. Essential information, disease development, clinical manifestation and general physical check-up are needed in detail. Especially focus on elemental oral and maxillofacial exams, special checking methods and results.

Liu Bin, Luo Wen

Chapter 3

Oral Healthcare

Oral cavity serves as a reservoir of more than 300 microorganisms, an access of many chronic diseases risk factors and infectious diseases, such as hepatitis B, AIDS. Oral diseases induce pathophysiological changes and poor oral hygiene which endangers human health.

3.1 Oral Hygiene

Oral hygiene is the practice of keeping one's mouth clean and free of disease and other problems (e.g. ,bad breath) by regular brushing and cleaning between the teeth. It is important that oral hygiene be carried out on a regular basis to enable prevention of dental disease. It is up to each individual to choose which tool he or she prefers to use. The main approaches include as follows.

3.1.1 Mouthwash

3.1.1.1 Over-the-counter mouthrinses

The most common use of mouthwash is commercial antiseptics, which are used at home as part of an oral hygiene routine. Commercial mouthwashes companies include Colgate, Listerine, Oral-B, and so on. Mouthwashes combine ingredients(essential oil, cetyl pyridinium chloride and so on) to treat a variety of oral conditions. Variations are common, and mouthwash has no standard formulation so its utilize and recommendation involves concerns about patient safety. Some manufacturers of mouthwash state that antiseptic and anti-plaque mouth rinse kill the bacterial plaque that causes cavities, gingivitis, and bad breath. It is, however, generally agreed that the use of mouthwash does not eliminate the need for both brushing and flossing. The American Dental Association asserts that regular brushing and proper flossing are enough in most cases, in addition to regular dental check-ups, although they approve many mouthwashes. For many patients, however, the mechanical methods could be tedious and time-consuming and additionally some local conditions may render them especially difficult. Chemotherapeutic agents, including mouthrinses, could play a key role as adjuncts to daily home care, preventing and controlling supragingival plaque, gingivitis and oral malodor.

Common use involves rinsing the mouth with about 20-50 mL(2/3 fl oz) of mouthwash. The wash is typically swished or gargled for about half a minute and then spat out. Most companies suggest not drinking-water immediately after using mouthwash. Mouthwash should not be used immediately after brushing the teeth so as not to wash away the beneficial fluoride residue left from the toothpaste. Similarly, the mouth should not be rinsed out with water after using mouthwash.

Minor and transient side effects of mouthwashes are very common, such as taste disturbance, tooth staining, sensation of a dry mouth, etc. Alcohol–containing mouthwashes may make dry mouth and halitosis worse since it dries out the mouth. Soreness, ulceration and redness may sometimes occur if the person is allergic or sensitive to mouthwash ingredients such as preservatives, coloring, flavors and fragrances. Such effects might be reduced or eliminated by diluting the mouthwash with water, using a different mouthwash (e. g. , salt water), or foregoing mouthwash entirely.

3.1.1.2　Hibitane

Hibitane, also called chlorhexidine gluconate, is an antiseptic mouthrinse that should only be used in two–week time periods due to brown staining on the teeth and tongue. Use of a 0. 12% or 0. 2% chlorhexidine–based mouthwash in combination with normal tooth care can help reduce the build–up of plaque and improve mild gingivitis. Twice a day, 10 mL and 1 minute at a time. Oral epithelium and teeth surface adsorb about 30% medicine, which will be released in 8–12 hours. Such mouthwash also has a number of adverse effects including damage to the mouth lining, tooth discoloration, tartar build–up, and impaired taste.

3.1.1.3　Metronidazole

An antimicrobial effective against some protozoa and strict anaerobes. It has effective use in dentistry as it is the primary drug prescribed for periodontal diseases. It is also sometimes used either alongside penicillin or alone against dentoalveolar infections with the advantage of having a low allergenicity. When the concentration of metronidazole mouthwash reaches about 0. 025 mg, the most common periodontal anaerobe will be inhibited. Twice a day the metronidazole mouthwash is a good treatment for gingivitis, bleeding gums, bad breath and periodontitis, showing no stimulating effects on oral mucosa.

3.1.2　Tooth brushing

3.1.2.1　Toothbrush

A soft bristle brush is the most beneficial. Hard and medium texture tooth brushes can abrade the gum and cause recession. Additionally, soft bristles can flex into hard to reach areas. If the bristles of any toothbrush are worn, bent or frayed, replace the brush. A worn out brush will not clean the teeth properly. If the gums are inflamed some bleeding may result, but this usually stops after 2 weeks of brushing and flossing.

There are two types of toothbrush as follows.

(1) Manual tooth brush(Figure 3–1):the modern manual tooth brush is a dental tool which consists of a head of nylon bristles attached to a long handle to help facilitate the manual action of tooth brushing. Furthermore, the handle aids in reaching as far back as teeth erupt in the oral cavity. The tooth brush is arguably a person's best tool for removing dental plaque from teeth, thus capable of preventing all plaque–related diseases if used routinely, correctly and effectively.

(2) Electric tooth brush(Figure 3–2):electric toothbrushes are toothbrushes with replaceable moving or vibrating bristle heads. The two main types of electric toothbrushes are the sonictype which has a vibrating head, and the oscillating – rotating type in which the bristle head makes constant clockwise and anti–clockwise movements. Sonic or ultrasonic toothbrushes vibrate at a high frequency with a small amplitude, and a fluid turbulent activity that aids in plaque removal. The rotating type might reduce plaque

and gingivitis compared to manual brushing, though it is currently uncertain whether this is of clinical signif-icance. The movements of the bristles and their vibrations help break up chains of bacteria up to 5 mm be-low the gum line. The oscillating—rotating electric toothbrush on the other hand uses the same mechanical action as produced by manual tooth brushing, removing plaque via mechanical disturbance of the biofilm, however at a higher frequency. Using electric tooth brushes is less complex in regards to brushing technique, making it a viable option for children and adults. The bristle head should be guided from tooth to tooth slowly, following the contour of the gums and crowns of the tooth. The motion of the toothbrush head replaces the need to manually oscillate the brush or make circles.

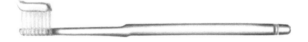

Figure 3–1 **Manual tooth brush**

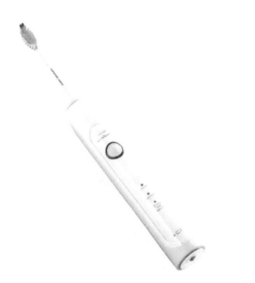

Figure 3–2 **Electric tooth brush**

3.1.2.2 Toothpastes

Toothpaste is a paste or gel dentifrice used with a toothbrush as an accessory to clean and maintain the aesthetics and health of teeth. Toothpaste is used to promote oral hygiene; it serves as an abrasive that aids in removing dental plaque and food from the teeth, assists in suppressing halitosis, and delivers active ingre-dients(most commonly fluoride) to help prevent tooth decay(dental caries) and gum disease(gingivitis). Salt and sodium bicarbonate(baking soda) are among materials that can be substituted for commercial tooth-paste. Toothpaste is not intended to be swallowed due to the fluoride content, but is generally not very harm-ful if accidentally swallowed in small amounts. Toothpastes are derived from a variety of components, the three main ones being abrasives, fluoride, and detergents.

3.1.2.3 Toothbrushing techniques

The right way is known as the modified bass technique, shown in Figure 3–3. Brush in circles and up and down, but when it comes to the gum line, you should tip the toothbrush at a 45–degree angle, and ap-ply gentle pressure so it blanches just under the gums, then vibrate there and flick away. Your brush shouldn't travel across the gums. It's important to get just underneath the gum because a lot of food and bacteria get trapped there. Brush the outer surfaces of each tooth, upper and lower, keeping the bristles angled against the gum line. Use the same method on the inside surfaces of all your teeth. Brush the biting surfaces of both upper and lower teeth. To clean the inside surfaces of the front teeth, tilt the brush vertically and make several small circular strokes with the front part of the brush. Brushing your tongue will help freshen your breath and clean your mouth by removing bacteria. Don't brush in half an hour after eating, as giving your saliva to do its job and neutralise the acid caused by eating and drinking. Before this, your teeth are at their weakest and brushing can damage the enamel.

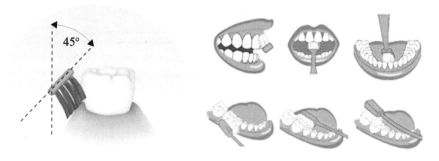

Figure 3–3   **Bass method of tooth brushing**

3.1.2.4   Frequency and time

Regular brushing consists of brushing twice a day: after breakfast and before going to bed. Cleaning between the teeth is called interdental cleaning and is as important as tooth brushing. This is because a toothbrush can not reach between the teeth and therefore only cleans 50% of the surfaces. There are many tools to clean between the teeth, including floss, toothpick, and interdental brush. It should take 2 – 3 minutes to do a thoroughful job.

3.1.3   Diastema cleaning

3.1.3.1   Toothpick

A toothpick is a small stick of wood, plastic, bamboo or other substance used to remove detritus from the teeth, usually after a meal. A toothpick usually has one or two sharp ends to insert between teeth. The correct technique to use a toothpick is as follows: find a toothpick. Hold the end that is not pointy as the pointy end goes inside the mouth. Locate the unwanted object stuck in the teeth. Dislodge the unwanted object between the teeth. Push too hard, and the toothpick buries itself in your gum. Do it slowly and gently in case of hurting the gum, as shown in Figure 3–4.

Figure 3–4   **Toothpick**

3.1.3.2   Flossing

The most vulnerable area of the gum to periodontal disease resides between the teeth and below the gumline. Even the best brush designs can not clean these areas. Tooth brushing alone will not remove plaque from all surfaces of the tooth as 40% of the surfaces are interdental. One technique that can be used to access these areas is dental floss. When the proper technique is used, flossing can remove plaque and food particles from the teeth and below the gums. The American Dental Association (ADA) reports that up to 80% of plaque may be removed by this method. The ADA recommends cleaning between the teeth as part of one's daily oral hygiene regime. There are different types of floss available. ①Unwaxed floss: unbound nylon filaments that spread across the tooth. Plaque and debris get trapped for easy removal. ②Waxed floss: less susceptible to tearing or shredding when used between tight contacts or areas with overhanging restorations. ③Polytetrafluoroethylene (Teflon): slides easily through tight contacts and does not fray.

Flossing is the most effective way to reach these areas. Technically, flossing may be difficult to master, but repetition will soon make flossing a secondary habit that can be done easily. The type of floss used is a personal preference, however without proper technique it may not be effective. The correct technique to ensure maximum plaque removal is as follows: begin with a piece of floss that is 15 – 25 inches long. Lightly wrap most of the floss around the middle fingers of each hand, then grasp a length of about one inch between your thumb and index fingers. Gently insert the floss between the teeth. A slight "sawing" motion may be necessary to pass the floss between the tight contacts. Curve the floss into a tight "C" shape, pulling it against one tooth until you feel tight resistance. Move the floss up and down against the side of the tooth, extending 2 to 3 millimeters below the gumline. Remember that there are two tooth surfaces that need to be cleaned in each space. Continue to floss each side of all teeth. Be careful not to cut the gum tissue between the teeth. Do not forget the back side of the last tooth on both sides, upper and lower. As the floss becomes frayed or soiled, a turn from one middle finger to the other will bring up a fresh section. When you are done, rinse vigorously with water to remove plaque and food particles. Do not be alarmed if during the first week of flossing your gums or are a little sore. If your gums hurt while flossing, you could be doing it too hard or pinching the gum. As you floss daily and remove the plaque, your gums will heal and the bleeding should stop. Do this at least once a day.

If it's hard to manipulate the floss, use a floss holder or an interdental cleaner—such as a floss pick or stick designed to clean between the teeth, as shown in Figure 3 – 5.

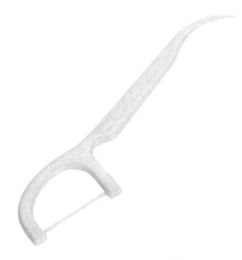

Figure 3 – 5　**Floss stick**

3.1.4　Gum massaging

After brushing the teeth or rinsing, get the thumb and index finger on the lingual and buccal sides of gums massaging gently for 5 minutes. Massaging the gum properly promotes the blood circulation and makes it healthy. For gingival papilla and gingiva in roots furcation, gum stimulator/rubber tip could be considered. The usage is as follows. Place rubber tip between teeth and apply light pressure in a circular motion to massage the gums. This may also remove plaque in between tooth surfaces. Repeat from tooth to tooth.

3.1.5　Supragingival scaling

Supragingival scaling, nonoperative treatment, is provided by professionals. The local stimulations (dental plaque, tartar, calculus and so on) are removed by professionals with mechanical means to restore the periodontal health. Supragingival scaling is the procedure where dental calculus and plaque are removed from the supragingival surfaces of the teeth to prevent and cure periodontal disease. Polish the tooth surface and prevent the dental calculus and plaque redeposition. Scaling may be performed using a combination of mechanical and hand instruments. Whilst hand scaling is sometimes more precise and allows a better tactile feel, mechanical instruments require less time to remove the deposits and result in less operator fatigue.

3.1.5.1　Ultrasonic supragingival scaling

Ultrasonic scalers are the most commonly used scaler in dental practice. It allows easy removal of calculus, are more time efficient, and require less training to use effectively. A regular cleaning, which is called prophylaxis by dental professionals, is what most people think of when they think of going to the dentist for a checkup. A dental hygienist or a dentist uses a specialized cleaning device, called an ultrasonic scaler, to remove plaque and calculus. This cleaning occurs only on the visible part of the tooth, known as a the crown. Regular cleaning is only recommended for patients who have generally good oral health and do not suffer from bone loss or gum problems (bleeding, recession, infection, etc.).

Ultrasonic scaling is an excellent procedure to help keep the oral cavity in good health and also halt the progression of gum disease. It is recommended once annually as a preventative measure visiting to the general dentist.

3.1.5.2　Hand instrument supragingival scaling

Each hand instrument has a handle, a shank and a working tip. A proper grasp is essential for precise control of movements made during periodontal instrumentation. The most effective and stable grasp for all periodontal instruments is the modified pen grasp. Scalers should be used by gently pulling away from the gingival margin towards the tip of the crown.

3.2　Oral Health Care

Oral health care is a component of overall health care. In 1965, WHO pointed out: "The health of teeth is that there are no abnormalities in the structure and function of the teeth, periodontal tissues, adjacent parts of the mouth, and maxillofacial regions." The oral health standard set by the WHO in 1981 was "clean, no cavities, no pain, normal color of gums, no bleeding". Although the definitions of oral health vary from each other, the following three aspects are indispensably included in all the definitions, that is, good oral hygiene, healthyoral function and no oral disease. To achieve this goal, people shall put prevention first, creating favorable conditions for oral prevention and oral healthcare, breaking bad habits that are detrimental to our oral hygiene and eliminate all possible pathogenic factors, thereby strengthening the resistance of the oral cavity and improving the level of oral hygiene. To prevent and control oral diseases, proper preventive measures should be taken before the diseases are found or once the diseases occur.

3.2.1   Oral health care for the general population

3.2.1.1   Regular oral health examination

Regular health examination is conducted to find out the oral health status of the inspected person and the prevalence state of common oral diseases, thus achieving the purpose of "early treatment and prevention of disease". The frequency of inspection can be decided based on the individual needs and objective conditions.

In terms of oral cancer, the purpose of regular examination is to detect it earlier and increase the early treatment rate, which generally will contribute to longer survival time and better life quality. If the found tumor has a diameter of 2 cm and there is no metastasis, the 5-year survival rate will be greatly improved. If the tumor is of 2 cm or less in diameter, the 5-year survival rate can be increased by 2 times. If it is of 1 cm or less, the rate can be increased by 3 times. Therefore, early detection and early treatment are significantly meaningful in reducing the mortality rate of oral cancer.

For people over the age of 40 who have long terus smoking history, smoking more than 20 cigarettes per day, those who have both smoking and drinking habits, those who have had white spot in the oral cavity due to stimulation of alcohol and tobacco, and those who have long-term habits of chewing betel nuts, it would be better for them to learn self-examination method other than receiving regular oral care from doctors.

The methods and steps for self-examination are as follows: the patient faces the mirror under adequate lightning.

(1) Observe the symmetry of the head and neck, and pay attention to changes in skin color.

(2) Touch the face with both index fingers, and if there appear any changes in color, tenderness, lump or growth in volume of verruca and nevus, seek medical help immediately.

(3) Touch the neck from behind the ear to the clavicle. Pay attention to the pain and lumps. Check both left and right sides of the neck.

(4) The lowerlip. Open the lowerlip and observe the vermilion and the inner mucosa. Use the index finger and thumb to touch the lowerlip from the inside out and left to right. Examine the upper lip in the same way. Check if there are lumps or wounds.

(5) The gums and buccal mucosa. Pull the cheeks open with index finger to observe the gingiva, and hold and check the buccalmucosa with index finger and thumb.

(6) The tongue and the floor of mouth. Extend the tongue to observe its color and texture, wrap the tip of the tongue with sterile gauze, and then pull the tongue left or right side to observe the edges. Touch the tongue with index finger and thumb and note if there is an abnormal lump. To check the floor of the mouth, lick the upper palatewith the tongue to observe the changes in color and shape at the floor of mouth, and then touch it with the index finger.

(7) The palate. To check the palate, at times we need to use a toothbrush to suppress the tongue. Bend the head slightly backwards to observe the color and pattern of the soft and hard palate.

It is necessary to raise public awareness of warning signs of the oral cancer, so that they can be vigilant and seek medical help as early as possible. The warning signs are as follows.

(1) Unhealed ulcers in oral cavity lasting more than 2 weeks.

(2) White, red or dark spots on oral mucosa.

(3) Abnormal swelling in the mouth, neck and lymphadenectasis.

(4) Repeated bleeding inside the oral cavity for unknown reason.

(5) Numbness and pain in the face, oral cavity, throat and neck for unknown reasons.

3.2.1.2   Fix oral habits

Oral habits are also one of the important factors that affect oral health. There are various types of them, and each generates different impact, such as affecting the normal alignment of the teeth and the normal development of the jaw, or resulting in the loss of physiological stimulation. The normal physiological state is the tongue pushes outwards, and the lips and cheeks draw back, the three together form a balanced pattern, which allows the teeth and jaws developing normally under this condition. If a bad habit destroys this balance, abnormal development of the dental jaw system will occur. The following listed habits are particularly harmful and should be corrected before it is too late.

(1) In appropriate feeding position. Breastfeeding from one side can cause unbalanced jaw development for babiesin the long term.

(2) Asymmetrical chewing. In the long run, chewing food on one side only could result in tissue degeneration and dysplasiain the non-functional side due to the unbalanced physiological stimuli on both sides. Besides, the lack of self-cleaning action and the accumulation of calculus would result in periodontal diseases.

(3) Mouth Breathing. Long-term mouth breathing will result in narrow upper arch, high upper palate, protrusion of the upper anterior teeth, flaccidity of the lip muscles, and inability to close the upper lip and lower lip, which are responsible for the "incompetent lips" leads to oral mucosal dryness and gingival hyperplasia.

(4) Lip sucking, tongue biting and cheek biting. Frequent upper lip sucking may cause deep anterior overbite, while upper lip sucking may cause reverse occlusion. Tongue biting may lead to crossbite. Cheek biting can affect the distance between posterior teeth and upper and lower jaws. All of these can lead to malocclusion.

(5) Habits such as pen biting, chopsticks biting, and finger licking will drive the upper anterior teeth to move towards the labial side, and the lower anterior teeth to the lingual side, which is a cause for malposition and malocclusion.

(6) Other habits. Sleeping on one side for the long run, sleeping on hard objects and children eating candy and biscuits before sleeping all can cause negative effects, therefore should be corrected at an early date.

3.2.1.3   Eliminate negative factors affecting oral hygiene

The pit and fissure of the tooth surface are the predilection sites for caries. Hence the pit and fissure sealant should be applied timely to prevent caries from appearing supernumerary teeth(also known as extra teeth), impacted teeth and malposed teeth can cause oral malocclusion and other lesions, therefore should be removed or corrected as the circumstances may require. The gap left by the premature loss of deciduous teeth should be filled in time with space maintainer to keep the distance, so as to prevent the displacement of the adjacent teeth and the excessive extension of the paired jaw teeth from causing the permanent teeth to dislocate or impact. Missing teeth should be repaired in time, and residual root and crown should be promptly removed in order to avoid chronic adverse stimulation.

3.2.1.4   Adequate nutrition

From the perspective of keeping oral health and preventing oral diseases, the following points merit attention.

(1) Enhance the nutrition during the growth and development period of the dentognathic system. During the fetal period, infancy and childhood, special attention should be paid to the intake of calcium, phos-

phorus, vitamins, fluorine, and microelement.

(2) Mind the physical nature of food. Eat rough and comparatively harder food ingredients to strengthen the self-cleaning function of oral cavity and the massage effect to the gums, as well as to increase the physiological stimulation produced by chewing, thus enhancing the decease resistance ability of periodontal tissue.

(3) Control the daily intake of sugar and refined carbohydrates. Both responsible for the occurrence of caries, excessive intake of these two elements is detrimental for preventing caries. Instruct the children to limit or give up sweets and cakes between meals, and more importantly, sweets should be for bidden before going to bed.

3.2.1.5　Improving the labor environment

For workers exposed to toxic substances such as acid mist, lead, and mercury, it is a must to improve their working environmentby measures like increasing sealing equipment, directional ventilation, wearing protective gowns, masks and gloves, etc. The purpose is to avoid or reduce the contacts of harmful substances on human body, ensuring oral and systemic hygiene of the body.

3.2.2　Oral hygiene for special groups

Everyone is a particular individual. They have distinct problems with their body health and oral hygiene, and also their own personal needs. Considering from the perspective of epidemiological pattern, diverse social groups vary on the oral diseases they might suffer from, and on their demand for oral healthcare. For example, pregnant women are prone to gingivitis; disabled people are unable to use dental care products due to the lack of self – care ability; infants have strong imitative ability but poor manual dexterity, therefore need parental education, guidance and supervision for tooth-brushing; preschoolers and pupils are prone to caries; periodontal problems are common among adolescents and middle school students. As a result, oral health care must be tailored to the needs of each specific group of people. Only when oral healthcare, whether preventive or rehabilitation, are operated on the basis of their own characteristics and troubles, can the formulated plan be fruitful.

3.2.2.1　Oral health care for pregnant women

(1) The purpose and importance of oral health care for pregnant women. The difficulty of oral health care for pregnant women can be divided into two aspects. First is the special status of pregnancy and childbirth, which requires the oral health care to be customized for the physiological changes of the mother. Second is the fetus growing in the mother's body, which needs nutrition for the normal growth and development of the oral cavity.

(2) Regular oral health examination. Oral diseases should be detected and treated timely. Attention should be paid to the prevention and treatment of gingivitis during pregnancy, thus promoting the oral hygiene of pregnant women.

Once pregnant, it is necessary to do oral examination and to treat the found diseases, if any, as soon as possible. The first 3 months of pregnancy is the high – risk period of miscarriage. Generally, oral medical treatment is limited to handling emergencies, and X – ray irradiation should be particularly avoided. The 4 – 6 months is an appropriate period for the treatment of oral diseases, so dental treatment is best to finish at this stage. But protective measures are still necessary when X–ray is used, avoiding irradiation to the pelvic cavity or abdomen. During the last 3 months of pregnancy, it is necessary to avoid general anesthesia, and only local anesthesia is optional when urgent treatment is required.

(3) Nutrition of pregnant women and the oral health of fetus. Nutrition is the material basis of physical

and mental health of human beings. The nutritional status of pregnant women is directly related to the growth and development of the embryo. Lack of nutrition of the mother will lead to the malnutrition of embryo, affecting the development of their body, cerebrum and intelligence, and also changing the oral tissue.

A normal pregnancy lasts about 40 weeks, and is usually divided into three stages according to the growth and development of fetus, each lasts 3 months:

(1) First trimester(the first 1－3 months): adequate nutrition and balanced diet are vital both for the health of pregnant women and for the growth offetus. During this period, the germ of deciduous teeth is forming. The deciduous tooth germ matrixis developed 35 days after the embryogenesis. Therefore, mothers need to intake high－quality protein, sufficient calcium, phosphorus and vitamin A in the first 2 months of pregnancy, otherwise it may affect the resistance of deciduous teeth in the future. Besides, it is also necessary to be careful about virus infections such as rubella, and to avoid using hypnotics and tranquilizer. These stimulation may not only affect the development of tooth germs, but also cause deformities such as cleft lip or cleft palate.

(2) Second trimester(4－6 months): increase the uptake of inorganic salts, vitamin A, and vitamin D under instruction. During this period, most of the deciduous teeth are in the process of mineralization, so the intake of inorganic substances such as calcium and phosphorus, as well as vitamins A and D, which related to calcium metabolism, must be fully guaranteed.

(3) Third trimester(8－9 months): this period includes the perinatal period(28 weeks from pregnancy to 1 week after birth), and is the period when babies' deciduous teeth and some of the permanent tooth germs is forming. Certain types of drugs might have impacts.

3.2.2.2　Oral health care for infants and toddlers

Infancy and toddlerhood. The goal of oral health for infants and toddlers is zero caries and completely healthy gums. Parents should be aware of the importance of oral health for infants. Establishing good habits in the early stages of life can affect future health. In the first 6 months after birth, we should help parents to understand that it is possible for infants to suffer from caries and oral mucosal infections. After birth, the baby should be provided with an appropriate amount of fluoride everyday to promote the mineralization of teeth and bones. Within 6 months, the first tooth will erupt. Parents should bring the baby to the first oral examination between 6 and 12 months after birth, in order to discover, suspend and change any possible parental practices that may be harmful to the baby's oral hygiene. Proactive preventive measures should be taken, such as fluoride supplement, appropriate feeding methods and plaque removal.

Fluoride drop is the appropriate manner for fluoride supplement for infants, which should begin since 6 months after the birth. To ensure the medicine take effects in both local body parts and all over the body, carefully apply the fluoride drops into the infant's mouth and instruct the infant to stir with tongue in the mouth, so that the droplets reach each tooth surface. We may also add fluoride drops to the baby's daily food or let the fluoride tablet melt in drinking water.

After the baby's first oral examination, it shall be done regularly every 6 months. Observe the eruption of the teeth, the dentition, the occlusion, and the condition of caries and soft tissues.

3.2.2.3　Oral health care for preschoolers

During the growth and development of the dentognathic system, infants experience periods of pre－eruption of deciduous teeth, eruption of deciduous teeth, and completion of primary dentition. Oral health care in each period of has different emphasis. As children grow up, attention should be paid to the care of the erupted deciduous teeth, especially to preventing caries, providing proper instruction on oral cleaning. After the primary dentition is completed, it is important to stress the prevention of caries and to maintain the integrity of deciduous dentition. At the end of the preschool years, as permanent teeth start to erupt, the incidence of deciduous teeth caries increases, so regularly examination is necessary to treat caries at early stage.

(1) Home oral health care. Due to the young age, children tend to have short attention span. Oral physicians should instruct the parents on how to teach and help the children to brush their own teeth. Soft and small-headed nylon toothbrush is helpful to clean and massage the gums. Children over 2 years old are keen on brushing teeth on their own, but at this time they still have less flexible hands, and therefore need parental help and guidance.

The prevention program of children between 3 and 6 years lies on cultivating their oral hygiene habits and mastering the technique of brushing teeth methods. A small amount of tooth paste with fluoride can be used to remove plaque and brush the teeth effectively.

Children around 6 years old begin to lose deciduous teeth, and their permanent teeth gradually erupt. At this time they may experience pain, gingival edema and other uncomfortable symptoms, therefore should seek medical treatment. Parents ought to help children maintain the established oral hygiene habits, protecting the newly erupted permanent teeth.

(2) The use of fluoride. Fluoride is a kind of microelement necessary for the normal metabolism of the human body and for the natural growth and development of teeth and bones. Proper supplementation of fluoride is a vital preventive measure in childhood. A large number of studies have confirmed that supplementing fluoride is beneficial for preventing caries during the period of enamel formation and mineralization. Since human milk, same as cow milk, contains only a very small amount of fluorine, children living in low-fluorine and under high caries risk should be supplemented with fluoride since 6 months old.

The best way for children aged 3 - 6 years to get fluoride supplement is fluoride tablets. At this time, the amount of fluoride in food shall be noted, especially in low-fluorine areas. Local use of fluoride plays an important role in this age group, including toothpastes with low fluoride concentrations, fluoridated coatings and mouthwashes. The fluoride droplets and tablets should be prescribed by a dental professional or used collectively in kindergartens, under direction and supervision by experts on oral health care to ensure their safety.

3.2.2.4 Oral health care of primary and middle school students

Oral health care for primary and middle school students is also known as oral health care in schools.

(1) Contents of oral health care for primary and middle school students

1) Monitor the health status of students, including regular oral health examinations and monitoring.

2) Health education for students, including oral health education.

3) Cultivate good sanitary habits, including tooth brushing and dietary habits.

4) The prevention of common diseases, including the prevention and treatment of oral diseases.

5) Prevention of physical accidents, including anterior teeth trauma and jaw fractures.

(2) Oral health instruction

Oral health education in school curriculum should be gradual and progressive, and its content should include the following aspects.

1) Oral health knowledge, including the morphology and function of teeth, the eruption and structure of deciduous teeth and permanent teeth.

2) Common oral diseases, such as caries, periodontal disease, malocclusion, and anterior teeth trauma.

3) Prevention and treatment of oral diseases, including clearing dental plaque and calculus with toothbrush, toothpaste and correct brushing methods; food, eating habits and oral health; fluoride and fissure seal-

ing;other oral hygiene products.

4)Oral health care facilities,including oral physicians,oral health services in schools,and oral health services in communities.

Through instruction,students are able to understand the following facts:pit and fissure sealant and the use of fluoride can best control the occurrence of dental caries;to prevent periodontal disease means to continuously remove plaque in a lifetime;regular oral examination and health care is necessary to maintain oral health;smoking and drinking are the major risk factors for oral cancer and periodontitis.

Promoting oral health care in schools is one of the major ways to build future oral health and lay foundation for enhanced oral health level of the whole nation.

3.2.2.5　Oral health care for the disabled people

Oral health problems for the physically disable people are mainly caries and periodontal diseases,as well as congenital defects of children with disabilities,such as malocclusion and maxillofacial trauma,etc. It is common for the disabled to have poor oral hygiene,mainly due to the total or partial loss of self-care capabilities,and lack of necessary preventive measures or appropriate treatment. Therefore,based on the specific conditions of our country,oral health care for disabled people should be advanced in the following aspects.

(1)Early oral hygiene instruction. The degree of limb movement disorders in children varies from mild to severe,and those with mild degree are completely free of mental disorders,thus can clean the oral cavity by themselves as normal children. Critically ill children can not take care of themselves and must rely on the help of the guardian. In order to enable the child patients to maintain their oral hygiene and to participate in social activities in the future,it is important to start functional training and instruction in the early stage.

(2)Selection of oral health products. The oral hygiene products necessary for disabled children are basically the same as normal children. Mostly,the appropriate method of cleaning the mouth is chosen based on the degree of actual capacity of the child,including plaque display fluid,toothbrush,dental floss,dental floss gripper,toothpick,mouth-gag,etc. If available,electric toothbrushes and water rinsing devices can also be used.

1)Individually modified toothbrush:commercially available toothbrush modified into a special shape that is easy to be used by children with disabilities. The handgripis changed into a ball or added with a rubber handle for easier handling,and the toothbrush has two rows of bristle. The modified toothbrush is also useful for cleaning some dentitions out of reach for an ordinary toothbrush,or for those people who do not have brushing habits since childhood,those who have not received instruction on tooth-brushing until teenage,and those who have difficulties on holding toothbrushes. The modification of toothbrushes should be combined with the oral hygiene management of the children,being designed in accordance with the children's exercise performance and capacity of acceptance.

2)Electric toothbrushes:for disabled children who have difficulty in maintaining oral hygiene using ordinary toothbrushes,electric toothbrushes is recommendable. It can help to clean the mouth and massage the gums,relieving the fatigue of children with disabilities when brushing the teeth.

3)For those who have trouble holding toothbrushes,there are several solutions to help them:① the toothbrush can be wrapped with a wide elastic or nylon belt,and the handle can be thickened using sponge,foam or rubber,so that patients can easily grasp it without dropping;② in order to limit the range of motion of patient's shoulder,a wooden or plastic bar can be used to extend the handle;③ if the patient can stand or lean,but has disability on hands and shoulders,then the electric toothbrush can be fixed on a low table or behind a chair.

(3) Special dental care for disabled patients: dental plaque removal. For disabled people who are unable to take care of themselves, they should be helped to to brush their teeth thoroughly or floss their teeth once a day at least to effectively remove plaques. If necessary, use electric toothbrushes.

(4) Appropriate use of fluoride supplement. If possible, choose a systemic method of supplementing fluoride(especially for disabled children), such as water fluoridation, fluoride salt, fluoride tablets, or fluoride milk. It should be combined with another topical fluoride: such as toothpaste with fluoride, gargle with fluoride water, or fluoride gel used by professionals. All these will have good anti−caries effect.

(5) Regular oral health examination. Another aspect of dental care for people with disabilities is regular inspections, scaling, topical fluoride, health instruction and appropriate treatment services provided by oral professionals. The examination should be done at least once every half year to one year, and the problem found must be dealt with promptly.

Luo Wen, Xu Yingying

Chapter 4

Endodontic Disease

4.1 Dental Caries

Dental caries is a multifactorial and chronic bacterial disease that involves the destruction of tooth hard tissue structure. It directly results from acid dissolution of the mineral phase of the teeth, the acid being produced by metabolism of dietary carbohydrates by oral bacteria in dental plaque. The disease can affect enamel, dentin, and cementum. The disease is seldom selflimiting and, in the absence of treatment, caries progresses until the tooth is destroyed. The localized destruction of the hard tissues, often referred to as the "lesion", is the sign of the disease.

Dental caries is one of the most prevalent infectious diseases to afflict mankind. The proportion of the world's population affected by dental caries increased dramatically once refined carbohydrates became available to those within developed and developing countries. Dental caries is the key factor responsible for dental pain and tooth loss in populations throughout the world.

4.1.1 Etiology

Dental caries is a multifactoria disease. This can probably best be understood by looking at a diagrammatic representation of the way the essential factors in caries etiology were considered in their most simplistic pattern(Figure 4 – 1). The four circles represent the parameters involved the carious process, including microorganisms, host and teeth, sugar or diet and time.

4.1.1.1 Bacteria

Normal flora of the oral cavity contains abundance of bacteria, streptococcus mutans are the primary cariogenic agents, and bacterium lacticum and actinomyces are also believed to have close relationship with human caries. The cariogenic ability of cariogenic bacteria is related not only with coherence, and acidogenic ability, but also closely with acid resistance. Formation of oral biofilm is a prerequisite factor contributing to dental caries.

4.1.1.2 Diet

Diet plays a significant role in the carious process because the bacteria are capable of fermenting carbohydrate substrate such as the sugars sucrose to produce acid to cause the pH to fall.

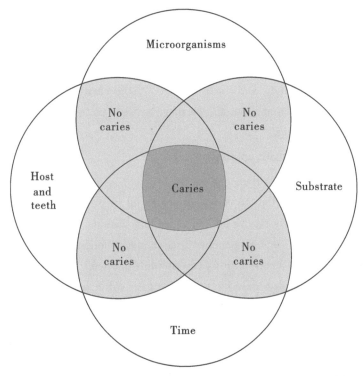

Figure 4-1   The four circles represent the parameters involed in
the caries process

4.1.1.3   Host

Host susceptibility to dental caries is mainly affected by tooth and saliva.

4.1.1.4   Time

Dental caries is a chronic progressive disease, and each process of the occurrence needs some time.

4.1.2   Clinical features

Caries lesion may be classified in a number of ways according to the clinical features. It can be classified according to the rate of progress of lesions, anatomic site and the depth of the lesion.

4.1.2.1   Classify according to the rate of progress of lesions

(1) Acute caries

Acute caries is ususlly present among children or young people. It is characterized by the presence of a white halo around the cavity and soft light brown dentine. It's also called wet caries.

(2) Rampant caries

Rampant caries is the name given to multiple active carious lesions occurring in the same patient. It is a rapid process involving a large number of teeth. Rampant caries is most commonly observed in the patient who are given radiation therapy in the region of the salivary glands. It is also seen in people who is a poor oral hygiene and a sudden marked reduction in salivary flow such as severe xerostomia.

(3) Chronic caries

The decalcified lesion is dark brown and leathery.

Arrested caries is a lesion that has become inactive and stopped progressing. It is one of the chronic caries. As the oral environment has changed from conditions predisposing to caries to conditions that tend to slow the lesion down, lesion stop and maintain the present status. A proximal caries probably stopped after extraction of the adjacent teeth as the environment change easier to clean.

(4) Secondary caries

Secondary caries is a lesion at the margin or under an existing restoration. The common locations of secondary caries are the rough margin and fracture places of the cavity where plaques are most likely to stagnate. It may be also caused by a marginal microleakage between materials and tooth tissue or a failure to remove all caries lesion in treatment.

4.1.2.2　Classify according to their anatomical site

(1) Occlusal caries and smooth surface caries

Occlusal caries is used to describe the caries lesions found in pits and fissures. Occlusal pits and fissures vary in shape but are generally narrow and irregular that bacteria and food are mechanically retained but can not be properly cleaned. As enamel demineralization always follows the rods, it is natural that the lesion initiated in a fossa is shape of a cone with its base towards the dentin. It is wider at the base than at the top. Undermining caries is also used to describe the lesion that with a relatively complete enamel surface.

Smooth surface caries is most commonly located on the mesial and distal surfaces at the point of contact with the adjacent tooth. It is also common around the buccal and lingual surface near the cemento-enamel junction. On a smooth surface the lesion is classically triangular in shape. As the sloping fissure walls and the direction of the enamel prisms, the lesion assumes an undermining character, which explains why something apparently so small on the surface can be so large when entered.

(2) Root caries

Dentine caries on the root of a tooth is called root-surface caries. It is predominantly a disease of older people as gingival margin recedes and roots exposed is more common.

(3) Linear enamel caries

Linear enamel caries is seen to occur in the region of the neonatal line of the maxillary anterior teeth. It is an atypical caries often occur in children of Latin America and Asia.

(4) Hidden caries

Hidden caries is a term used to describe lesions that has been missed on visual examination but could be found on radiograph. It is most commonly located under molar pits and fissures or the adjacent teeth.

4.1.2.3　Classify according to the depth of the lesion

According to the depth of the lesion it can be classified as superficial caries, inter mediate caries and deep caries.

(1) Superficial caries

Caries has affected the enamel layer, but has not yet penetrated the dentin. It can be divided into occlusal caries and smooth surface caries. Non-cavitated lesions often present as darkly stained pits and fissures on occlusal caries. It feels rough to a sharp probe. A white or brown spot lesion can be seen on smooth surface caries. The patients is asymptomatic, and do not have significantly respond to cold or hot stimulus. It is difficult to see a hide lesions, even with careful training and examine. At this time, radiography is extremely useful in diagnosing these caries. Flourescent display and argon ion laser can be used as a auxiliary diagnosis.

(2) Inter mediate caries

Caries has penetrated up to the dentin and cavitation has occurred. The patient may feel a hole in a tooth with the tongue, yellowish-brown or dark brown cavities may be seen. The patient will usually complain of sensitivity to hot, cold, and sweet food and drink, especially to the cold. The symptom resolves immediately after the stimulus removed. It is more obvious in a dentin caries of the neck.

(3) Deep caries

Caries has penetrated up to the dentin layers of the tooth close to the pulp. A deep approximal caries lesion may be seen just in the outer enamel with a small cave, but actually it have already throughout the depth of the enamel or reaching right through the dentine. The patient present as a pain with heat or cold things or chemical stimulation and especially when food impaction into the cavity. The pain resolves immediately after the stimulus removed. There is no spontaneous pain in deep caries.

4.1.3　Treatment

4.1.3.1　Chemical therapy

Chemical therapy is a method that by using chemical medicine such as 75% sodium fluoride and glycerol paste, 10% silver nitrate or silver ammoniacal nitrate to terminate or eliminate dental caries. It is applicable to early enamel caries of permanent teeth, approximal caries of deciduous anterior teeth, superficial and arrested occlusal caries of primary molar.

4.1.3.2　Remineralization therapy

Caries remineralization therapy can effectively arrest or reverse the progression of incipient demineralized caries lesions by promoting ion deposition into crystal voids caused by demineralization. Remineralized solution contains different proportions of calcium, phosphorus and fluorine. Applying topical fluoride such as a daily rinse of mineral mouthwashes or utilike of remineralized solution by a cotton ball is effective in reversing the progression of early enamel lesions.

4.1.3.3　Preventive resin restoration

The preventive resin restoration was born out of the use of pit and fissure sealants. It is suitable for occlusal caries where a microcavity or suspicious decay is present. The fissure sealants is made of the composition of resin, diluent, initiator, and some auxiliary element (such as filler, fluoride and dyestuff). Clinical procedure of the therapy are as follow: the tooth is cleaned with a bristle brush in a slow – speed handpiece, then the surface is etched with phosphoric acid solution, rinsed, and dried, and then the sealant is applied and light-cured for 20 seconds.

4.1.3.4　Restorative treatment

The role of operative restorative treatment in the management of dental caries is to facilitate plaque control and restore the appearance, form and function of the tooth. It is done by repair material after removing the caries and making a cavity preparation.

(1) Cavity preparation

Cavity preparation is usually carried out to remove dental caries and make a cavity with a certain shape to accommodate and support the repair material.

1) Cavity classification

G. V. Black's classification

• Class I: Cavities on caries affecting pits and fissures, including occlusal surface of molars and premolars, occusal 2/3 of buccal and lingual surfaces of molars or premolars and lingual surfaces of anterior tooth.

• Class II: Cavities on caries affecting the approximal surfaces of posterior teeth, including proximal cavity, meiso-occlusal cavity, meiso-buccal cavity and meiso-lingual cavity of molar or premolar teeth.

● Class Ⅲ：Cavities on caries affecting the approximal surfaces but do not involve the incisal angle of anterior teeth, including proximal cavity, meiso-lingual cavity and meiso-labial cavity of anterior teeth.

● Class Ⅳ：Cavities on caries affecting the approximal surfaces of anterior teeth and involving the incisal angle, including meiso-incisal cavity of incisor and canine teeth.

● Class Ⅴ：Cavities on caries affecting the cervical surfaces, including cervical third of the buccal and lingual surfaces of anterior and posterior teeth.

After that, some scholars put forward class Ⅵ that cavities on caries affecting self-cleaning area involving cuspal of posterior teeth and incisal edges of anterior teeth.

According to the number of surfaces involved in the cavity to classify, it can be divided into simple cavity, double-sided cavity and complex cavity.

2）The name of the cavity：the name of the cavity is named after the tooth surface in which it is located, such as cavity on the occlusal surface is called occlusal cavity. In order to facilitate clinical records, it often records in the form of upper case of the first letter of each tooth surface's english word, such as "I" represent incisal.

3）Structure of the cavity：the cavity consists of cavity wall, cavity angle and cavity margin and the cavity wall is divided into lateral walls and pulpal walls.

● lateral walls：cavity wall perpendicular to the tooth surface is called lateral walls. It is named after the tooth surface.

● pulpal walls：cavity wall vertical with the lateral walls and located in the cavity bottom covering with pulp is called pulpal walls. The pulpal walls which parallel to the long axis is also called axial walls.

● cavity angle：cavity angle formed by the intersection of the cavity wall is divided into line angle and point angle. The two walls intersect to form a line angle and three walls intersect to form a point angle.

● cavity margin：the lateral walls of the cavity intersects with the tooth surface to form the edge of the cavity, which is called cavity margin.

4）Basic principles of the cavity preparation：as much as possible to remove dental caries lesions, try to keep healthy tooth tissue and make a resistance form and retention form. Resistance form was used to describe a shape that making the restorations and remaining tooth tissue get enough resistance to avoid breaking under normal occlusal force. Retention form was a term used to describe the design features of a cavity which prevents movement of the restoration under forces directed in an apical or oblique direction.

（2）Tooth isolation

In dentistry, a good isolation from saliva is an essential part of the clinical technique, even for a simple filling. This makes it easier to prevent bacterial contamination from saliva. Without a good isolation, the restorations will be a failure as properties of materials is very susceptible to saliva contamination while being placed.

1）Cotton rolls isolation：isolation of teeth can be achieved with the help of a disinfected cotton rolls.

2）Saliva pump：saliva pump is taking advantage of the negative pressure created by water flow and aspiration to suction out saliva in the mouth. It is often used with cotton rolls isolation.

3）Rubber dam isolation：the method which gives the most complete control over moisture in the mouth is the rubber dam. A rubber dam is placed on the tooth after holes have been punched. After it is positioned the teeth is isolated by stretching and forcing of the dam between the interproximal contacts. A rubber dam clamps is used for fitting the neck of the tooth and holding the rubber dam in position.

（3）Cavity sealing, lining and basing

In order to protect the pulp from external stimulus and to restore the internal form of a cavity to produce a flat pulpal floor and a smooth axial wall, it need to do some proper treatment of the cavity according to depth of the cavity and properties of repair material before filling

1) Cavity sealing: cavity sealing is placing a sealant in the cavity wall. The effect of cavity sealing is to close dentinal tubule to prevent bacterial invasion and shield chemical stimulation of the repair material. It can also increase the close adaptation of the repair material to the cavity wall to reduce microleakage to avoid a secondary caries and a discolored teeth. The cavity varnish and resinoid bond are commonly used in cavity sealing.

2) Cavity lining: in a deep cavity a sublining of a therapeutic cement may be used to act as an insulator. The thickness is general less than 0.5 mm. The commonly used of cavity liner are calcium hydroxide-containing cement, glass ionomer cement and zinc oxide eugenol cement.

3) Cavity basing: basing a base is applied to the pulpal floor during a restoration, when it approached the pulp. It is used as a dentin replacement and as a pulpal protection to isolate external stimuli for the pulp. The material should have a sufficient thickness to restore the internal form of a cavity to produce a flat pulpal floor to bear filling pressure and chewing force. The commonly used of basing material are zinc oxide eugenol cement, zinc phosphate cement, zinc polycarboxylate cement paste and glass ionomer cement.

(4) Filling

The cavity is filled with the appropriate filler material to restore the shape and function of the affected teeth.

4.2　Tetracycline Stained Teeth

Tetracycline is an effective antibiotic, but it can also produce untoward side effects, including the dark staining of teeth which is called tetracycline stained teeth.

4.2.1　Etiology

Tetracycline, when consumed during the developmental period of the teeth, will result in a discoloration of the dentin. The character of the staining changes with time; the yellow coloration darkens and transforms to a brownish staining. The affected teeth will fluoresce bright yellow under UV light in a dark room. Tetracycline can also stain the primary teeth through the mother's placenta. The incisors tend to be more affected than the molars. Permanent teeth show a less intense but more diffuse staining than deciduous teeth.

Tetracyclines can cause discoloration and enamel hypoplasia of both the primary and permanent dentitions if administered during the period of tooth development.

The major factors Tetracycline impacting discoloration and enamel hypoplasia are as follows: ①the color of the tetracyclines itself(e. g. ,demeclocycline is copper yellow, terramycin is lemon yellow). ②Likely the result of an oxidation product of tetracycline, which is light induced. Prolonged exposure of the teeth to direct sunlight hastens the discoloration. ③When the drug is given to a child during the time of tooth formation, it binds with the hydroxyapatite crystals which are deposited in the forming dentin. As a consequence, the tetracycline molecule imparts its color to the tooth. Apparently the tetracycline molecule, and therefore the discoloration, is most concentrated in the dentin. The closer to enamel-dentinal junction, the easier the colored band is to coloring. ④ The enamel hypoplasia may also be the result of the childhood disease, hereditary defects in enamel formation or prematurity of the child; all of which are known to cause enamel defects. The color of the dentin is more obvious.

Therefore, the administration of TCN to pregnant women must be avoided during the 2nd or 3rd trimester of gestation and to children up to 8 years of age because it may result in discoloration and enamel hypoplasia.

4.2.2   Treatment

Clinical management of TST includes the following methods to improve the aesthetic appearance.

(1) Composite resins.

(2) Porcelain laminate veneers or full coverage metalceramic/all ceramic crowns.

(3) The use of bleaching.

Bleaching is the most conservative treatment option without sacrifice of sound tooth substances patients' satisfaction and oral health related quality of life has been improved after bleaching. Two approaches have been used to treat tetracycline discoloration.

1) bleaching the external enamel surface: the crown surface is cleaned and polished for removing the organic substances, coating the surfaces of gingiva and soft tissue with vaseline. Cotton pellets or a cotton roll cut in half longitudinally are moistened with 30% hydrogen peroxide solution and placed on the labial surface of anterior teeth. Hydrogen peroxide can easily damage soft tissues, so there should be a little distance from the margin of the gingiva. Infrared or incandescent lamp is irradiated for 30 seconds for each tooth, and the sessions can be repeated up to 5-8 times. The gel also can be applied on the surface of the teeth.

2) intracoronal bleaching following intentional root canal therapy: finishing the routine preparation of root canal, remove of root canal filling to the 2-3 mm below root canal orifice. 30% hydrogen peroxide or a thick paste of sodium perborate mixed with 30% hydrogen peroxide is placed in the pulp chamber and sealed. During the treatment, the pulp chamber is refilled with fresh bleaching paste once three days, a total of 4-6 times. When satisfied with the color and lustre, the hole is filled with the composite resins.

4.3   Wedge-shaped Defect

Wedge-shaped defect, a common dental disease, is dental hard tissues of the neck in some chemical and physical factors in the formation of the slow progressive loss that compose of two defects, lip and buccal common.

4.3.1   Etiology

Enamel-cement border structure is a weak area where is more vulnerable to mechanic abrasion than other sections of the enamel-covered dental crown. The habit of tooth-brushing had significant relation to wedge-shape defects of tooth, and acidic corrosive or the stress fatigue due to occlusal force also had relations to the formation of wedge-shaped defects. The tensile stress due to lateral forces may disrupt the chemical bonds of the crystalline structure of enamel and dentin.

4.3.2   Clinical features

There are two or three defects compose of the typical wedge-shaped defect. The surface of the defects looks smoothly polished and hard. It has a wedged shape with a regular edges and/or a color change. It is believed that the initial stage of a wedge-shaped defect almost does not manifest itself or only in a tooth sensitivity. But this is not applied to the cases when the defect area is deeply affected, in particular, reach the pulp tissue. It happens together with symptom of pulposis or periapical disease, or even crow breaks off at the point of the penetration. Wedge-shaped defects most often observe on premolars, especially on the first premolars, always with gingival recession. Such types of defects are more frequently observed in aging people and the older the more serious.

4.3.3   Treatment

It requires a modification of the tooth brushing technique to prevent a further progression. No special treatment required in the initial stage, but when dentinal hypersensitivity is present, desensitization treatment is suggested. There are many composite resins, glass ionomer and other fixes available to repair a deep wedge-shaped defect. Fillings near the pulp must first be covered with a basing cement. Once lesions of symptomatic pulposis or apical periodontitis emerge, endodontic treatment is needed. If the lesions move toward the deep stage to make the crown breaks off. It can select a crown restoration after root canal treatment or removal the teeth according to the situation.

4.4   Dentine Hypersensitivity

Dentine hypersensitivity is a pain condition that develops followed by exposing of dentin surfaces. It is most often located in the cervical area of the tooth. Patients often complain of transience sharp or shooting pain that is induced by a stimulation within the range of physiology. Patients often complain of a transient and sharp pain that is induced by a stimulation within the range of physiology.

4.4.1   Etiology

It may also occur in response to dentin exposure that cause by diseases such as attrition, wedge-shaped defect, caries, odontagma, periodontal disease.

4.4.2   Clinical features

Patient presents with a sudden onset of sharp pain provoked by cold drinks, tooth cleaning, especially mechanical stimulation. The pain lasts only a few moments and resolves immediately after the stimulus is removed. Most of the patients can localize the diseased tooth.

4.4.3   Diagnosis

4.4.3.1   Probe test

A sensitivity point can be located by probing the exposed dentin surface. It usually locate in enamel-dentinal junction or enamelo-cemenal junction.

4.4.3.2   Thermal tests

Cold air from the three ways syringe of dental unit may elicit a pain response when blow over a sensitive surface.

4.4.3.3   Subjective assessment

The patient had a symptoms of dentine hypersensitivitys and ask the patient to evaluate the level of sensitivit, including the digital and three-level pain assessment methods.

4.4.4 Treatment

4.4.4.1 Desensitization treatment

Various of fluorides are used in the clinic for the treatment of dentin hypersensitivity. It usually smear locally and the curative effect vary from person to person.

4.4.4.2 Prosthodontic treatment

Patient who fail to respond to desensitization treatment or the exposure area near the pulp, endodontic treatment and a full crown are suggested.

4.5 Cracked Tooth

Cracked tooth refers to a non-physiological crack of the tooth surface which involves the enamel and dentin without a perceptible separation. If the crack affects only the enamel, there are no obvious symptoms, but if it reaches the dentin is a veritable highway for bacteria headed for the pulp which is one of the causes of toothache. It is hardly possible to wedge this line or to demonstrate the crack radiographically. "Crack" most occur in maxillary molar, mandibular molar and maxillary premolar is followed by. The maxillary molar was the tooth demonstrating the highest number of cracked. The mandibular molar and maxillary premolar came in second place.

4.5.1 Etiology

The exact etiology of the phenomena is unknown. Most authors concur that it mainly because of occlusal force. Weaken tooth structure is main predisposing factor. Big cusps accompanied by deep grooves and fossae always lead to the increase occurrence rate of the crack as it resulting in greater horizontal component. Pathologic abrasion which with a high-steep cusp is the main factor for the crack. The force exerted on the fossa by the high-steep cusp caused a greater horizontal component.

4.5.2 Clinical features

Cracks occur in crowns surface, superimposing with some of physiologic sulcus or extending along either or both marginal ridges. If the crack affects only the enamel, there are no outward symptoms. The patient will complain of discomfort to chewing and sensitivity to heat and cold, when a crack reaches the dentin. If the crack has already reached the deep dentin, there are symptoms of chronic pulpitis or a acute attack. It always couple with a pain when chewing certain food on the affected side.

4.5.3 Diagnosis

①The patient has a fixed point pain on chewing and symptoms resemble those of an endodontic problem, but without a deep caries or a deep periodontal pockets or a hypersensitive point. ②Coloring agents such as iodine tincture or methylene blue seep into the crack. ③Probe press along the crack line cause a pain. ④A sharp, lacerating pain of short duration when doing bite test with a cotton swab place on cusp of the suspicions tooth is pathognomonic of an cracked tooth.

4.5.4　Treatment

4.5.4.1　Occlusal adjustment

Occlusal adjustment should be applied to eliminate occlusal interference and reduce the inclination of cusp to relieve the lateral forces subjected by tooth so as to ease the stress burden of the tooth.

4.5.4.2　Balancing burden of bite force

Extracte the tooth with no reservation value and recover function of the full dentition.

4.5.4.3　Dealing with the cracked tooth

If the crack affects only the enamel without a secondary, advise using acid etching and enamel bonding agents to eliminate the smear layer and residues from the crack. If it has already reached dentin or with a secondary caries or a deep staining line, advise preparing a cavity along the crack. And then, use calcium hydroxide as a base and glass ionomer cements as a temporary restoration. If no further symptoms are manifested, a final restora tion can be undertaken after 2 weeks.

A deeper crack or affects the pulp, endodontic treatment is often needed, following by a full crow to bind the cracked segments and protect the cusps. At the same time of endodontic treatment, it need to remove the tooth from occlusion to decrease crack force. As it is extremely to fracture along the crack, authors suggest to place a well fitting cop per band or orthodontic band to prevent propagation of the crack during the endodontic treatment.

4.6　Endodontology

Endodontology includes pulp and periapical biology and pathology. The pulp communicates with the periodontium via the apical foramen. Endodontic disease concerns structures and processes within the pulp tissue, whereas apical periodontitis is an inflammatory reaction process of the tissues surrounding the root apex of a tooth. Most apical periodontitis is a sequel to a primary infection of the pulp space as the bacteria with their toxins, immunological agents, and the products of pulp degeneration invade the periodontal tissues via the apical foramen. So, treatment in such cases is essential to eliminate the pulp infection. Generally, once the endodontic disease is cure, the periapical inflammatory tissue lesions can remedy.

4.6.1　Etiology

4.6.1.1　Bacterial factors

Bacterial etiology has been confirmed for main factors for periodontal and endodontic infections. When enamel and cementum are damaged from dental caries, trauma, attrition from mastication or iatrogenic injury, the exposed of dentinal tubules, pulp, periodontal pocket or the hematogenic infection serve as pathways to the pulp for entry of bacterial macromolecules. These ways provoke pulp inflammation, while the periapical infection is a sequel to pulp inflammation (when enamel and cementum are damaged from dental caries, trauma, attrition from mastication or iatrogenic factors. The exposed of dentinal tubules, pulp, periodontal pocket or blood-borne infections serve as pathways to the pulp for entry of bacterial macromolecules, which may provoke pulp inflammation, while the periapical infection is a sequel to pulp inflammation).

4.6.1.2　Physical factors

(1) No matter an acute dental trauma or a chronic injury can frequently threaten the vital functions of the pulp as neurovascular bundles are often torn at this time. This may cause temporary is chemic injury of the pulp, or even cause immediate, avascular necrosis of pulp tissue lying peripheral to the neurovascular tear.

(2) Thermal insults, including overheating from insufficiently cooled dental drills and heat generated by polishing of the restorations, or a deep cavity filling directly with silver amalgam. All this may cause pulp hyperemia or even pulpitis.

(3) Dissimilar metal restorations between two contact surface, or an inappropriate operative procedure such as vtality testing, electrosurgery or iontophoresis can threaten the health of the pulp.

(4) Laser may cause various degrees damage to the pulp tissue.

4.6.1.3　Chemical factors

(1) Dental materials in common use such as acid-etching primer, binder or filling matterial is more or less has some chemical stimulation which that can cause inflammation of the pulp.

(2) Toxic components in disinfectant can causes severe dental pulp disease when use in deep cavity. Inappropriate use of these materials can cause periapical periodontitis. It is also called medicinal apical periodontitis.

4.6.1.4　Immune factors

Antigen substance come from pulp tissue or periapical tissue can induce body-specific immune response to pulp and periodontal injury.

4.6.2　Reversible pulpitis

Reversible pulpitis is pulp tissue to vascular expansion and congestion as the main pathological changes of the initial inflammation. It is equivalent to pulp hyperemia of classification in endodontic histopathological.

4.6.2.1　Clinical manifestations

(1) Reversible pulpitis is characterized by pain initiated by hot and cold stimulation lasting for a few seconds and disappearing when the stimulus is removed. It is simply a mild inflammation of the dental pulp that without spontaneous pain.

(2) Commonly, there may be some very close to the pulpal cavity exist in the tooth, such as dental hard tissue lesions, deep periodontal pockets, or traumatism.

4.6.2.2　Diagnosis

(1) Diagnosis depends upon an exhaustive dental history and to reproduce the symptoms with endodontic tests. With chief complaint for transient sensitivity to temperature stimulus, especially the cold, without spontaneously pain.

(2) There may be some evidence of the cause of the endodontic lesions.

(3) The diagnosis of reversible pulpitis must be considered as a provisional diagnosis which needs to be confilmed after the pulp recovers which requires at least 6-8 weeks.

4.6.3　Irreversible pulpitis

Irreversible pulpitis is a severe inflammation of the pulp which usually progressing from reversible pulpitis. It would ending with total pulp necrosis that can only choose to remove the pulp to eliminate the lesions. According to the clinical features and duration of disease it can divided into acute pulpitis(including the acute exacerbation of chronic pulpitis), chronic pulpitis, residual pulpitis and retrograde pulpitis.

4.6.3.1   Acute pulpitis

The symptoms of acute pulpitis is a sudden onset of spontaneous pain and can be very sensitive to the slightest temperature change. The clinical symptoms of pulpitis are poorly correlated with the histological appearance of the pulp. Most of the acute pulpitis is an acute attack of the chronic pulpitis. A case without a chronic course, it occurs more often in the cases of an acute injured and stimulating of the pulp such as excessive heat production from cutting dental tissues and chemical stimulation of filling material.

(1)Clinical features

Acute pulpitis is very painful and the nature of the pain has the following characteristics: ①spontaneous, intermittent pain that lingers; ②increased pain when lying down; ③thermal stimulation can exacerbate the pain; ④poorly localized to the affected tooth.

There may be some very close to the pulpal cavity exist, such as deep caries ora heavily restored tooth, deep periodontal pockets, or traumatism.

Probing for affected tooth can cause a severe pain, sometimes with a small perforation.

A severe pain being initiated by thermal tests and the pain lingers even after withdrawal of the stimulus. The pulp was sensitive to vitality testing in the early stage, but unresponsive in the late stage.

Teeth in the late stage of inflammation, there may be a slight pain when percuss in the vertical direction.

(2)Diagnosis

①With typical pain symptoms. ② There may be some evidence of the cause of the pulpitis, such as caries or a heavily restored tooth. ③Thermal tests can help to locate the affected tooth.

4.6.3.2   Chronic pulpitis

In clinical practice chronic pulpitis is the most common type of pulpitis. With absence of positive signs, it is one of the most difficult conditions to diagnose.

(1)Clinical features

Pain with chronic pulpitis is much more tolerable than with acute pulpitis. Generally, there is no severe spontaneous pain and sometimes may be a intermittent or a dull pain. Chronic pulpitis is a longer course that the patient can have a long history of cold or hot stimulative pain. The tooth will usually respond to vitality tests and the patient may feel a very mild pain on biting or mild pain on percussion.

1)Chronic closed pulpitis: there is no obvious spontaneous pain, but with a long history of cold or hot stimulative pain. The teeth can be found a deep caries or a heavily restored tooth or other dental hard tissue lesions that are very close to the pulp. After removing all carious lesion, the pulp tissue do not expose and sensitive to probing. The response of the teeth to the temperature test and the electrical test is mostly delayed and pain on percussion.

2)Chronic ulcerative pulpitis: there is no spontaneous pain, but the patient will present a severe pain when food impaction into the cavity. A characteristic sign of this form of the disease is that a cold or hot stimuli will induce a sharp pain. There may be some pulpal lesions exist such as a deep caries. As long-term disuse of the affected tooth there can see a large number of material alba or dental calculus accumulate. A small perforation can find after remove the caries lesions. With sharp probe to explore the pulp through the perforation, there is not pain in superficial layer exploration but a sharp pain in deep exploration. At the same time there can see a small amount of dark blood bleeding in deep exploration. It show sensitive to the temperature test and will not be tender to percussion.

3) Chronic hypertrophic pulpitis: chronic hypertrophic pulpitis is common in children and young people. Generally there is no obvious spontaneous pain, but the patients will complain of pain and bleeding from the carious cavity when chewing food. Therefore, they are afraid to use the affected side to chew food.

When examined in a carious cavity, an overgrown, hypertrophied pulp is visible. Probing is slightly painful, but causes bleeding from pathological formations. As long – term disuse of the affected tooth there can see a large number of dental calculus accumulate.

(2) Diagnosis

① A long history of cold or hot stimulative pain with or without spontaneous pain history. The patient can locate the affected tooth. ② There may be some evidence of the cause of the pulpitis, such as a dental hard tissue lesions. ③ Abnormal reaction to temperature test. ④ There is a reaction on percussion.

4.6.3.3　Residual pulpitis

Aninflammation of the radicular pulp which is remain after the root canal therapy is called residual pulpitis. It belongs to the category of chronic pulpitis.

(1) Clinical features

Pain characteristics is similar to chronic pulpitis. It often show a spontaneous dull pain, or a radiation pain, or a temperature stimulative pain. Most of the patient may feel a very mild pain on biting as the inflammation exist near the apical foramen.

Crowns of the affected tooth can be fond some traces of the endodontic treatment, such as a temporary materials. Note that a deep root canal exploration may cause pain, but do not respond in the upper part. The response of the teeth to the temperature test is mostly delayed. Percussion of the affected tooth is often produce a mild pain or discomfort.

(2) Diagnosis

① A history of endodontic treatment. ② With symptoms of pulpitis. ③ Slow pain initiated by strong temperature stimuli. The tooth is painful on percussion. ④ Residual pulpitis can be diagnosed when pain cause by a deep root canal exploration.

4.6.3.4　Retrograde pulpitis

Retrograde pulpitis is a type of endodontic–periodontal lesions. It is a primary periodontal lesion with secondary endodontic involvement. The infection arising from a deep periodontal pocket. Progression of the periodontal disease and the pocket leads to pulpal involvement via either a lateral canal foramen or the main apical foramen. The pulp subsequently being infected. Lindhe also reported that bacteria coming from the periodontal pockets may reach the pulp when there is accessory canal exposure, through apical foramens and canaliculi of the furcation area.

(1) Clinical features

1) The affected tooth presents a typical symptoms of acute or chronic pulpitis. All the affected tooth has a long medical history of periodontitis that with a series of uncomfortable symptoms such as bad oral breath, looseness of teeth, or feel powerless or painful on biting.

2) A deep periodontal pockets or severe furcation involvement is observed in the affected tooth. The gums is swelling, hyperaemic and purulent discharge of pocket. There can not find any hard tissue lesions that can cause the dental pulp lesions in the tooth.

3) Temperature test on different parts of multirooted teeth, the reaction is different.

4) Percussion of the affected tooth is often produce a mild or moderate pain.

5) X–ray images show extensive destruction of the periapical tissue or root bifurcate.

(2) Diagnosis

①A long medical history of periodontitis. ②Recently appears a typical symptoms of pulpitis. ③The affected tooth do not find any hard tissue lesions that can cause the dental pulp lesions. ④The affected tooth has severe periodontitis symptoms.

4.6.4　Pulp necrosis

Pulp necrosis, a death of the pulp tissue, is thus the direct consequence of pulpitis, but it may also arise immediately after other reasons such as trauma, iatrogenic injury that damages the vascular peduncle.

(1) The tooth with a necrotic pulp is completely asymptomatic.

(2) There may be some very close to the pulpal cavity exist, such as deep caries or a heavily restored tooth, or deep periodontal pockets.

(3) The crown is discolored(grayish).

(4) The pulp is insensitive to vitality testing.

(5) The radiographic findings are normal.

Diagnosis: ①Without subjective symptom. ②The crown is discolored and insensitive to vitality testing. ③X-ray images show no abnormity in the root tip.

4.6.5　Pulp calcification

Dental pulp calcification occurs in all age groups with an increase in frequency in older age groups and in those teeth there is an injure of the pulp. It is presents as masses of calcified tissue present on the level of the pulp chamber and roots of the teeth. Pulp calcification has two types, one is nodular calcification which also called pulp stone and the other is called diffuse calcification.

4.6.5.1　Clinical features

(1) Generally pulp calcification does not cause clinical symptoms. In individual cases it may appears a spontaneous pain which is associated with body position. It can also spread along the trigeminal nerve area.

(2) The affected tooth is sensitive or dull to vitality testing.

(3) X-ray images show radiodensity of calcium compound in pulp chamber, or even a diffuse radiodensity to make the radiolucent area of the pulp chamber disappeared.

4.6.5.2　Diagnosis

(1) X-ray examination results can be used as an important basis for diagnosis.

(2) A history of trauma and calcium hydroxide treatment can be used as a reference.

4.6.6　Acute apical periodontitis

Acute apical periodontitis is an acute inflammation at the level of the periodontal ligament. It may be caused by the extension of pulp disease into the periapical tissues. The lesion typically develops near the tips of roots, as it communicates with the periodontium via the apical foramen. It is a series of reaction process which starts from serous inflammation in periodontal membrane of root apex to suppurative inflammation in the periapical tissue. Although very rare, when the inflammation spread through the medullary spaces it would develop into a osteomyelitis of alveolar bone or even the jaw.

4.6.6.1　Acute serous apical periodontitis

(1) Clinical features

1) The symptoms of acute serous apical periodontitis are pain on biting or percussion. It also can be a

spontaneous or persistent dull pain the patient can localize the tooth. The patient is afraid to eat as the affected tooth is extreme sensitivity to chewing.

2)The affected tooth is often having a large decay area, a filling, a deep periodontal pockets or other dental hard tissue lesions.

3)The crown is discolored and there is non-responsiveness to vitality testing, but primary tooth or young permanent teeth can respond to it.

4)There may be a discomfortable or painful feeling when palpate the root tip and pain on percussion is (+)-(++).

5)Tooth mobility degree(I°).

(2)Diagnosis

①Typical pain on biting. ②There is a reaction on percussion and palpation. ③Non-responsiveness to vitality testing. ④A history of pulpitis or trauma or endodontic treatment.

4.6.6.2　Acute suppurative apical periodontitis

(1)Clinical features

1)Periapical abscess:the affected tooth appears a spontaneous and throbbing pain and the pain is violent and usually persists for long periods of time. Patients feel that the tooth has become elongated or like it is coming out and is very sensitive to occlude. The gum over the root of the affected tooth is red but without significant swelling. Pain on percussion reach to(++)-(+++)and a slight sore on palpation. Tooth mobility degree(III°). The corresponding submandibular or submenta lymph nodes may have a swelling and a pressing pain.

2)Subperiosteal abscess:once the exudate causes erosion of the bony cortical plate, the purulent exudate causes detachment of the periostium, the moment of greatest pain. At this stage patients feel extremely painful as pressure builds up in the restricted periosteum. The tooth feels more "high" and the tooth mobility degree reach three degrees. The tooth will be very tender to touch, let alone percuss, and there may be some tenderness over the apex in the buccal sulcus. Percussion pain reached the most serious stage (+++). The gum is red and the migration ditch become flat as swelling of apical mucosa and when palpate the deep may feel a sense of fluctuations. It sometimes connect with fever or body discomfort and affect sleeping and eating. Severe case may spread the infection to the relevant maxillofacial areas.

3)Submucosal abscess:once the periostium is eroded, the pus can be able to drain and allow pain to subside. At this stage, a tender local swelling which is easily to rupture will appear. The sense of fluctuations is obviously and pain on biting or percussion is relieved. Pain on percussion reduced to(+)-(++)and the tooth mobility degree return to I°. Systemic symptoms is relieved.

(2)Diagnosis

Mainly based on the typical clinical symptoms and signs of teeth and through the degree of pain and swelling to distinguish the stage of inflammation of the tooth.

4.6.7　Chronic apical periodontitis

Chronic apical periodontitis:chronic apical periodontitis is usually a low-grade infection following an acute infection that has not completely healed or was inadequately treated. A slow inflammatory process begins in the periapical tissue as the products of cellular degeneration and bacterial toxins in root canal spread through the apical foramen or the various lateral foramina into the surrounding periradicular tissue. The important histopathologic feature is tomplied with the formation of inflamed granulation tissue and absorption of the alveolar bone. On a microscopic level, different structural frameworks of chronic apical periodontitis can be identified. These forms include periapical granuloma, chronic periapical abscess, apical cyst and periapical condense osteitis.

4.6.7.1　Clinical features

(1)Chronic apical periodontitis is generally asymptomatic or only a slight of symptomatic on chewing and the patient may often be unaware of its presence. Sometimes, a fistula may be present, through which the patients have noticed an intermittent discharge of pus. The patients may relate a history of acute(pulpitic)pain or a history of trauma or a history of endodontic treatment.

(2)The affected tooth is often having a large cavity, a filling or other dental hard tissue lesions.

(3)The crown is discolored and there is no responsiveness to vitality testing.

(4)No obvious abnormality on percussion and the tooth is firmer.

(5)A sinus tract is a typical feature of the chronic apical abscess, which allows continuous discharge of pus form in the periapical lesion.

(6)Apical cyst is an epithelium-lined cavity that contains fluid or semi-solid material. The cyst can be sized from pea to egg size. When it reaches a significant size, it may present as a soft and hemispherical swelling in gingival tissue of the affected tooth. It may cause loosening of the affected tooth or even the adjacent tooth and those roots may also be subjected to external resorption.

(7)Radiographic features: ①circular radiolucent area surrounding the root tip also appear in periapical granuloma. The radiolucency is defined and the surrounding sclerotin is normal or only a slight dense. Generally, the diameter of the lesion is less than 1 cm. ② Chronic periapical abscess, the radiolucency is ill-defined and irregular-shape. The surrounding sclerotin become loose. ③ The radiographic image of a round, sharply-demarcated radiolucency 1 cm or greater in diameter suggests a cyst. There is also a obvious border between the cyst and surrounding bone. ④Condense osteitis causes more bone production rather than bone destruction in the area, so the radiolucent imaging appears that the sclerotin become denser.

4.6.7.2　Diagnosis

Bone destruction in the radiographic image is the basis of diagnosis. Pulp vitality testing, clinical history and whether the crown discolored or not can as auxiliary diagnosis markers. There is no practical need to distinguish the pathological types and can be collectively called chronic apical periodontitis in clinical diagnosis.

4.6.8　Commonly used treatments

4.6.8.1　Emergency treatment

(1)Open pulp drainage

1)Acute pulpitis: quickly and effectively to resolve the pain is the first principle of treatment of acute pulpitis, therefore, open pulp drainage is the most effective emergency treatment method. It is necessary to remove all the pulp tissue under local anesthesia and an aseptic cotton pellets is being put in the access opening.

2)Acute apical periodontitis: opening the root canal(s)gives an opportunity to obtain drainage of exudate or pus. Leave root canals open with an aseptic cotton pellet for 1-2 days, and return to visit.

(2)An incision and drainage procedure

With a localized, fluctuant, soft-tissue swelling indicating a submucosal abscess, surgical incision can be attempted to drain off an abscess under local anesthesia.

(3) Remove of stimulation

The apical periodontitis patient may relate a history of trauma, or the pulp may have become necrotic from chemical or mechanical irritation. The stimulus needs to be removed. It is particularly important to perform prolonged irrigations with sodium hypochlorite. In order to avoid reinfection and to prevent surviving microbes from growing, the canal is sealed with an intracanal dressing or aseptic cotton twisting.

(4) Adjust the occlusal contacts

In treating acute apical periodontitis by trauma, one must never forget to relieve the tooth from the occlusion.

(5) Anti-inflammatory pain

The general approach can be given orally or by injection of antibiotics or painkillers.

4.6.8.2   Methods of treatment

Many authors agree that because of poor correlation between the histological appearance of the pulp tissue and the clinical situation, it is impossible in practice for the dentist to classify the various clinical situations. Bacause the patient may present in accordance with any histological system and from there draw the treatment of choice. Therefore, we will adopt a therapeutic method based on the symptoms and clinical diagnosis.

If the diagnosis of pulpal lesions are limited or reversible, one approach is conservative and aims to preserve the vital pulp, like direct capping, indirect pulp capping or pulpotomy.

If the pulp disease is large or irreversible, the approach is a procedure whereby the entire tissue is radically removed and replaced with a root canal filling, aiming to preserve the teeth; in the case of immature teeth with pulp necrosis or apical periodontitis, apexification and apical barrier technique can be chosen.

(1) Pulp capping

Pulp capping is aimed to preserve the vital pulp. An appropriate wound dressing which can promote soft-tissue healing and hard-tissue repair is placed onto the surface of exposed pulp or the dentin where near the pulp to protect the pulp and eliminate lesions. Pulp capping can be divided into direct pulp capping and indirect pulp capping.

Direct pulp capping: direct pulp capping is placement of a protective dressing directly over the exposed pulp to maintain the vitality pulp.

1) Indication

● Mechanical or traumatic exposure of a clinical or asymptomatic pulp in young permanent molar tooth with a immaturity apex.

● Small pinpoint mechanical or traumatic exposure of < 0.5 mm diameter of a clinical vital or asymptomatic pulp in permanent molar tooth with a maturity apex.

2) Common pulp-capping materials

● Calcium hydroxide: it is a commonly used dressing for treatment in direct pulp capping. When applied to an exposed pulp, cauterizes the tissue and causes superficial necrosis. "Dentin bridge" may be formed when calcium hydroxide is used as a pulp-capping agent and placed in the contact with healthy pulpal. There will be a layer of coagulation necrosis and inflammatory cell infiltrates. Repair by hard tissue of a pulpal wound is a multifactorial process. Stem cells located in the pulp differentiate into elongated and polarized odontoblast-like cells that secrete dentinal matrix. Reparative dentin may form as calcium enter into dentinal matrix via pulp blood supply. Calcium hydroxide has a high pH 9–12. The alkaline PH induced not only neutralizes lactic acid from the inflammatory reaction, but also activate alkaline phosphatases which play an important role in hard tissue formation. It also has a anti-bacterial effect.

● Mineral trioxide aggregate(MTA): MTA is a recent development of the 1990s. It use as a direct pulp capping or pulpotomy material. MTA is different from other materials currently in use because of its biocompatibility, antibacterial properties, sealing properties and radiopaque properties. MTA maintains an extended duration of high pH that provides beneficial irritancy and stimulates dentine repair and regeneration which similar to calcium hydroxide. Comparing to calcium hydroxide, MTA cause a lighter inflammation and a more normal "dentin bridge". MTA also widely use to repair perforations, to close open apices, or in apexification.

3)Treatment procedures

● Cavity should be preparation to remove dental caries lesion.

● Place the pulp capping material such as calcium hydroxide on the exposed pulp with application of minimal pressure so as to avoid forcing the material into pulp chamber. And then, a zinc oxide eugenol cement is used as to temporarily restore the teeth.

● permanent filling: final restoration is done after determining the success of pulp capping which is determination by pulp vitality testing and asymptomatic in affected tooth after 1－2 weeks. With 1－2 mm was kept as the first basing, removing most of the zinc oxied eugenol cement. And then, glass ionomer cement or zinc polycarbonoxylate cement or zinc phosphate cement use for a second basing. Silver amalgam or compound resins is used for final filling.

(2)Indirect pulp capping

Indirect pulp capping is placement of a dressing over residual dentine where near the pulp. It is in an attempt to stimulate secondary dentine formation within the pulp chamber to continue pulp vitality.

1)Indication

● Deep carious lesion or traumatism, which the dentin is close to the pulp.

● Reversible pulpitis cause by deep carious lesion but with a normal pulp vitality and without clinical and/or radiographic signs of pathology.

● It can use as a diagnostic treatment when it is difficult to judge whether it is a chronic pulpitis or a reversible pulpitis.

2)Common pulp－capping materials

Calcium hydroxide: the greatest benefit of calcium hydroxide when use as an indirect pulp－capping material is the stimulation and induction of reparative dentin bridge. This is due to its high alkalinity, which is beneficial to differentiation of odontoblast－like cells to form reparative dentin.

Zinc oxide eugenol: it is usually used in indirect pulp capping. Acting as a derivative of phenol, eugenol has analgesic action to soothe the pulp pain. It providing a high marginal adaptation and sealing properties as it fit closely with dentin and it also has a antibacterial properties.

3)Treatment procedures

● After local anesthesia, as far as possible to remove all peripheral caries but avoid to expose the pulp.

● A layer of calcium hydroxide is placed on the remaining carious dentin and covered with a zinc oxide eugenol cement to temporarily restore the teeth.

● After 1－2 weeks, a layer of setting zinc oxide eugenol cement is kept and then the cavity is permanently restored.

(3)Pulpotomy

Pulpotomy, a vital pulp therapy, is a term used for partial removal of pulp tissue and the remaining dental pulp is covered with a suitable material that protects the pulp from further injury and promotes healing.

1)Indication: in young individuals with incompletely developed roots, no matter what cause the pulp expose, it can use pulpotomy to maintain the pulp of the root portion vital and allow continued development of the tooth structure.

2)Treatment procedures

● Local anesthesia and a rubber dam are applied. In the whole process of treatment must under strict aseptic conditions to prevent reinfection of pulp tissue.

● Remove caries dentine with a sharp excavator and irrigate cavity with 3% hydrogen peroxide prepare access opening to the pulp chamber with high-speed turbine tooth drill.

● Prepare access opening to the pulp and remove the coronal pulp with a bur in an air-rotor.

● Remove the coronal pulp with a spherical bur and high-speed equipment and remove the small tissue fibers in pulp chamber as much as possible to make a neat section in root canal orifice.

● Place pulp capping material such as calcium hydroxide on the section pulp. The thickness of the material is about 1 mm. And then, restore the cavity with a zinc oxide eugenol cement.

● After 1 - 2 weeks, surface layer of setting zinc oxide eugenol cement is removed, and zinc phosphate cement basing. Silver amalgam or compound resins is used for final filling. It can also permanent filling as soon as pulp capping finish.

(4)Apexification

The completion of root development and closure of the apex occurs up to 3 years after eruption of the tooth. The treatment of pulpal injury during this period provides a significant challenge for the clinician. Apexification is defined as "a method to induce a calcified barrier in a root with an open apex or the continued apical development of an incomplete root in teeth with necrotic pulp". This technique is by placement of an intracanal medicament after cleaning of the root canal to permit deposition of periodontal tissues to continue root development to create a natural apical constriction for root canal filling.

1)Indications

● Immature teeth with pulp lesions that have spread to root pulp.

● Immature teeth with necrotic or periapical inflammation of the pulp.

2)Treatment procedures

● Prepare the canal. The preliminary step is the preparation of the access cavity, the opening in the dental crown. To facilitate complete removal of infected tissue in the root canal, it is necessary to irrigate by the alternative use of normal saline and 3% hydrogen peroxide. And the depth to which the tissue is removed should be determined by clinical judgment to avoid damaging the dental papilla and the residual vital pulp in root tips.

● Disinfect the canal. After drying with sterile paper points, a dressing of intracanal medications with strong sterilizing and little stimulation[e. g. ,$Ca(OH)_2$] and temporary cement(e. g. ,Cavit,zinc oxide-eugenol)are used to close the canals up. Change once a week until no exudative or asymptomatic.

● Medications induction. Although a variety of materials have been proposed for induction of apical barrier formation, calcium hydroxide(e. g. , Vitapex) has gained the widest acceptance. Removing medications and previous root canal filling, the Vitapex paste is injected into the root canal until it's filled and contact the apical tissue. The Vitapex placement is radiographically examined to determine the degree.

● Temporarily fill and recall. The cavity is filled with zinc oxide or glassionomer liner material. The patient should be recalled at 3-6 monthly intervals in order to determine the vitality of the pulp and the extent of apical maturation.

● Fill the canal. Filling the root canal is undertaken normally when the apical calcific barrier is formed

(5)Apical barrier technique

MTA has been popularly employed as a suitable material in apical barrier technique. It is used to create an apical stop or constriction in order to achieve a hermetically sealed root canal filling, also called MTA apical barrier technique.

1)Indications: MTA apical barrier technique is indicated for following pathological situations: pulp necrosis and apical periodontitis occur in permanent teeth with an immature apical foramen, or experiencing long apical induction but failure to form the root tip barrier. Common to the conditions is the absence of conical shape of the root canal, a feature that causes difficulties in conventional obturation.

2)Treatment procedures

● Clean the root canal. A round diamond burr is used to prepare an appropriate access cavity to allow removal of all necrotic tissue. After the necrotic pulp is extirpated, measure the working length and confirm it by a radiograph taken with a film holder.

● Prepare the canal: Canals are prepared and copious irrigation with chlorhexidine or sodium hypochlorite is used for maximum cleaning and minimal dentin removal. After biomechanical preparation, Calcium hydroxide paste may be used for affected tooth with periapical disease to control the apical inflammation.

● Put MTA into the canal: patients are recalled for a second appointment after 7 days, at which time the root canal are reaccessed, the $Ca(OH)_2$ dressing is removed with reamers and the canal is irrigated with ethylenediaminetetraacetic acid follow by 2. 5% sodium hypochlorite. After minor instrumentation, canals are irrigated with sterile saline solution and dried with sterile paper points. MTA is mixed in line with the manufacturers' instructions and inserted into the apical using a carrier until the third of the root canal filled dense. A conventional periapical radiograph is taken to confirm the appropriate placement of the material. And then a cotton pellet moistened with sterile water is placed over the apical plug, followed by a dry cotton pellet, and the endodontic access cavity is sealed with temporary sealing materials.

● Fill the canal. After 1−2 days, patients are recalled for a third appointment. The cotton pellets are removed, and a reamer is used to check the apical plug for set and hardness. Once MTA is been completely hardened, thermoplasticized gutta−percha technique is used to tightly fill the root canal.

● Regular follow−up. Review every 3−6 months after treatment.

(6)Root canal therapy(RCT)

Root canal treatment for the infected pulp of a tooth aims to eradicate pathological microbiota and prevent future infection within the root canals. The procedure includes several phases, of which mechanical instrumentation to clean the inflammatory pulp and necrotic substances in the root canal, shape, irrigation and proper disinfection are critical elements. Then a filling is placed in the instrumented root canal(s) to remove the undesirable stimulation of the root canal content to the periapical tissue, thereby eliminating a root canal infection and remedying periapical inflammatory tissue lesions

1)Indications

● Irreversible pulpitis.

● Pulp necrosis.

● Endodontic absorption.

● Internal resorption.

● Apical periodontitis.

● Traumatic tooth; transplanted tooth; replanted tooth.

● Other non−carious dental hard tissue diseases, like severe enamel hypoplasia, severe attrition and cracked tooth.

Normal dental pulp for other treatment needs, like a tooth that needs to be treated because of maxillofacial surgery or denture repair.

2) Treatment procedures

● Root canal preparation: access opening, removing sources of substrate for bacterial regrowth and multiplication, including necrotic tissue and tissue – breakdown products, establishing working length, initial root canal preparation, irrigating the canal system, expanding and shaping.

Access opening: aligning the direction of the bur to the long axis of the tooth facilitates the procedure. Initial penetration into the pulp chamber should be on the lingual surfaces of the anterior teeth or the occlusal surface of the posterior teeth. Removed the entire roof of the pulp chamber, the outline of the access cavity is dictated by the number and position of the root canal orifice(s). All cavity walls are then smoothed and connected with the orifice(s) of the respective canal(s). Care should be taken to avoid forming ledges on its walls as the root canal orifices are to be sought along the groove system.

Measure working length. Establishing and maintaining adequate working lengths is critical for root canal treatment. Working length is equal to the distance from cusps tip or incisal edges to the apical foramen. Instrumentation and root canal obturation stops at the cemento dentinal junction, where it has been recorded as far as 0. 5−1 mm from the anatomical apex. Therefore, the actual length of the instrument to the root tip should be about 1 mm shorter than the length of the tooth.

Accurate determination of working length during a root canal preparation is a challenge. The ways of measuring root canal working length: ① root canal instruments detection; ② digital radiographs; ③ electronic apex locators.

Clean the canal. Root canal treatment should obtain proper root canal shape, so an efficient cleaning can be performed before three−dimensional filling. Cleaning is the significant reduction of tissue as well as micro−organisms and their by−products from the pulp system, of which, removing all intracanal material and irrigating are intimately related. In sufficiently wide and straight canals, broaches are recommended to withdrawn the pulp tissue all in one piece. Pulp tissue that is necrotic or in an advanced state of degeneration can not be removed with a broach. The complete elimination of root canal contents is achieved by the use of irrigating solutions and the mechanical action of the endodontic instruments. The irrigating solution is absolutely necessary between the use of one endodontic instrument and the next, to prevent the suspension of dentin mud from becoming too concentrated, which would increase the risk of blocking the canal.

Enlarge and shape the canal. The "biological" and "mechanical" objectives of shaping of the root canal to receive the gutta−percha obturation have been listed. The infected contents of its canal system have been extracted, which can obtain a successful outcome and healing of the lesion. Limit the instrumentation to within the root canal and don't force necrotic material beyond the foramen. Make consequently greater penetration of the intracanal medications into the dentinal tubules and better adaptation of the canal obturation material to the walls to assure a tight apical seal and a good control of the material. Files and reamers are utilized in sequence from the smallest instruments to the largest to enlarge the canal.

Prepare root canal: ① Standardized technique. It can be used in straight canals, but not curved. ② Step−back technique. The preparation of straight canals and those with curves of the apical and middle third can be performed. ③ Step−down technique. This method addresses the canal by expanding the preparation coronally before an attempt is made to reach the apex. ④ Crown−down technique. The instruments are used in sequence from largest to smallest and the sequence must be repeated at least twice. ⑤ Balanced force technique. The technique is a variation of reaming, but purportedly maintains the contour of the canal and does not transport, or zip the apical foramen. ⑥ Anticurvature filing. It is suitable for moderate to severe curving. In round but more or less straight roots, in which the canal is in a central position, the wall thicknesses are approximately the same, buccolingually and mesiodistally. Consequently, the circumferential filing, which requires concentric enlargement of the original canal, can be used confidently. In curved roots, on the other hand, but particularly in the molars, the canal is not in a central position. Rather, it is displaced closer to the internal zone of the curve, that is, toward the bifurcation. Therefore, enlargement and flaring of these canals must take into consideration these anatomical peculiarities. ⑦ Chemical root canal preparation. It is an auxiliary method of mechanical preparation. ⑧ Ultrasonic root canal preparation. The ultrasonics in combination with NaClO has been shown to be extremely effective in the removal of organic substrate even in the areas where the instruments were unable to have contact with the canal walls such as cavities, depressions, internal resorption, apical deltas and lateral canal.

- Intracanal antisepsis

Medications disinfection: put a cotton pellet dipping the medication, a paper point infiltrated with medication into the root canal orifice, or the paste with a lentulo spiral into the deep root canal.

Medications for endodontic use must meet precise requirements: ① They must be able to digest proteins and dissolve necrotic tissue. ② They must have a low surface tension to reach the apical delta and all the areas that can not be reached by the instruments. ③ They must have germicidal and antibacterial properties. ④ They must be non-toxic and non-irritating to the periapical tissues. ⑤ They must keep the dentinal debris in suspension. ⑥ They must lubricate the canal instruments. ⑦ They must prevent discoloration of the tooth; indeed, they should bleach the tooth. ⑧ They must be relatively harmless to the patient and dentist. ⑨ They must be readily available and inexpensive.

Chlorhexidine and calcium hydroxide are the intracanal medications most used today.

Electrolysis therapy: the drug ions are introduced into the root canal so as to achieve the effect of disinfection. The most common one is iodine solution.

Microwave therapy: through the joint action of electric field, magnetic field, microwave field and heat effect, the protein of necrotic tissue is solidified to reduce exudation.

Laser therapy: the mechanism of action of lasers on the biological tissue is mediated via transient high intensity photothermal effects, photochemical action, photoelectromagnetis. Photochemical effects occur when the laser is used to stimulate chemical reactions, such as the curing of composite resin. The breaking of chemical bonds, such as using photosensitive compounds exposed to laser energy, can produce a singlet oxygen radical for disinfection of periodontal pockets and endodontic canals. Certain biologic pigments, when absorbing laser light of a specific wavelength, can fluoresce, which can be used for caries detection on occlusal surfaces of teeth. A laser can be used in a nonsurgical mode for biostimulation for more rapid wound healing, pain relief, increased collagen growth, and a general antiinflammatory effect. The pulse of laser energy on hard dentinal tissues can produce a shock wave, which is an example of the photo-acoustic effect of laser light. This process is often called spallation.

Ultrasonic therapy: ultrasonic high frequency oscillation can activate the irrigation within the root canal, causing the acoustic flow effect, cavitation effect, chemical effect and thermal effect, to kill bacteria and remove the organism within the root canal.

Temporary sealing: after putting the medications into the root canal, the root canal is closed temporarily and the disinfectant effect of the drug is played. Those commonly used are glass ionomer cement, zinc oxide and eugenol(ZnOE), epoxy resin, methacrylate resins and so on.

- Root canal obturation. The prime objective of the root filling is to prevent microbial organisms from entering, growing and multiplying in the empty space that resulted from the instrumentation procedure. A hermetic and permanent seal of the wound surface is essential to allow proper healing after pulpectomy and to prevent bacterial elements from later accessing the periapical tissue if, for any reason, the coronal restoration breaks down. Permanent root filling of teeth with an infected necrotic pulp should not be carried out unless the biomechanical preparation is complete and no exudation exists in the canal that prevents adherence of the filling to the root canal walls. It is also regarded good clinical practice to postpone permanent root filling until the tooth is free from pain and other clinical symptoms of root canal infection. An objective means which helps the clinician to decide when bacterial elimination is complete is not readily available. It was once believed that a bacterial sample would be able to provide guidance in this respect.

Root canal filling materials may be divided into three types: ① cones; ② sealers; ③ combinations of the two.

Cones are prefabricated root canal filling materials of a given size and shape (taper), like gutta-percha points and Thermafil.

Sealers are pastes and cements that are mixed and hardened by a chemical setting reaction after a given amount of time. Sealers commonly used are based on; polyketone; glass ionomer cement; zinc oxide and eugenol (ZnOE); epoxy resin; calcium hydroxide; methacrylate resins; mineral trioxide aggregate (MTA); silicone.

Lateral condensation technique: as the most basic and most commonly used root canal filling technology, this technique requires the introduction of a gutta-percha cone that fits well to the apical preparation (master cone), together with a small amount of sealer. The appropriate metallic, rigid, conical and smooth instrument (spreader) is used cold to compress the cone against the canal wall, introducing this instrument between the dentin and gutta-percha. In this way, one creates the space into which the first auxiliary cone is to be introduced. The spreader is then re-introduced vertically. It pushes aside the gutta-percha placed previously, so as to make space for a second auxiliary cone, and so on, until one obtains a dense, well-adapted filling.

Vertical condensation technique: it consists of injecting gutta-percha heated by an electrical device into the prepared root canal. The gutta-percha cone is cut off using the special gauge for gutta-percha points or by selective removal of varying amounts of the apical tip, until it enters the canal comfortably and binds. This must happen at the working length and the depth is marked on the cone with a notch made by the cotton pliers at the reference point of the stop. Then the heat-carrier is handed to remove the portion of gutta-percha extruding into the pulp chamber and soften the remainders. A plugger (whose tip is powdered with left-over sealer so that the gutta-percha cone does not attach to it) begins the vertical compaction of the gutta-percha just heated by the preceding heat carrier, so as to achieve close filling in the apical one third. One proceeds by adding pieces of gradually increasing size and being re-heated by the heat-carrier and re-compacted, until the entire canal is completely filled.

Continuous wave condensation technique: the continuous wave of condensation obturation technique was born out of the desire to simplify vertical condensation technique. Through the use of specially designed instruments and devices can achieve filling of primary and lateral canals in one step. The heat-carrier descends to a depth of about 5 mm from the apical foramen. Plugger end condenses the apical mass of filling material and then is withdrawn with the surplus gutta-percha. Backfilling with a warm gutta-percha syringe is the least important part of the continuous wave technique.

Thermaplasticized injectable technique: injectable gutta-percha obturation technique delivers either high- or low-temperature thermoplasticized gutta-percha inside the root canal system with the use of a cannula. It is to be preferred in some certain cases, when there is a ledge formation, perforation, or unusual canal curvatures, internal resorptions, or large lateral canals. The risk of overfilling is the limitation of the technique. Combining thermoplastic gutta-percha with vertical condensation technique can prevent overfilling in a similarly effective manner and with a significant saving of time.

Solid-core carrier insertion technique: core carrier techniques are unique among the various root canal filling techniques for delivering and compacting gutta-percha in the prepared root canal system. Thermafil (TF), considered the major core carrier device, is provided as an obturator consisting of a master core coated with thermoplasticized gutta-percha. Advantages of the core carrier technique include ease and speed of placement and the potential for the plasticized gutta-percha to flow into canal irregularities. Potential problems include stripping the gutta-percha from the core carrier and overfilling.

3) Microscopic root canal therapy: microscopic root canal therapy is a method of root canal therapy with the aid of the root canal microscope and microscopic instruments. Its application in endodontics started from the end of 1980s to the beginning of 1990s. Now it has been applied in every field of dental pulp treatment, including diagnosis, routine root canal therapy, root canal retreatment and apical surgery. The microscope intended for dental operations consists of two key components: the illumination system and the mechanical system. The total magnification values suitable for endodontics range from $3\times$ to $30\times$, offering a stereoscopic, three-dimensional, enlarged image under bright illumination at a comfortable working position that will greatly enhance the precision of endodontics. Thereby root canal orifices can be more easily found, cracks and fractures revealed. Root canal microscopy can be used in the whole process of root canal therapy: ① locating canal orifices and searching for supernumerary, hidden or malformed canals, like in maxillary molars for MB2. ② Finding and negotiating calcified root canals. ③ Dealing atypical root canals, like root canal C type. ④ Removing of root filling material and intracanal obstacles, such as broken instruments and insoluble sealers. ⑤ Handling intracanal ledge and canal deviation. ⑥ Aiding in the detection of untreated root canals, perforations of the pulp chamber floor and stripping of the canal walls.

4) Surgical endodontics: Surgical endodontics combines root canal therapy with a surgical approach for the treatment of the endodontic and periapical disease, of which periapical surgery is the most common. The indications for periapical surgery are the failure of root canal therapy or retreatment, serious variation of root canal anatomy, or needing a definite diagnosis by exploration. General outline of the procedure includes local anesthesia, incisions and flap designing, raising the flap, bone removing, curettage of the soft-tissue lesion, root-end resection, root-end preparation, retrofilling, flap closure and suturing.

Chu Jinpu

Chapter 5

Periodontal Diseases

Periodontal disease is a term that describes a serious of disorders that occur on periodontium, which is composed of gingival, periodontal ligament, alveolar bone and cementum. These diseases comprise two principal groups, namely gingival diseases and periodontitis. Gingival disease a group of diseases that occur only on the gingival tissues, while periodontitis are inflammatory destructive periodontal diseases involving all the four kinds of tooth supporting tissues. In this chapter, the etiology, clinical manifestation, diagnosis and treatment about different types of gingival diseases and periodontitis are discussed.

5.1 Gingival Diseases

Gingival diseases are a group of diseases that occur on the gingival tissues, including dental plaque induced gingival diseases such as chronic gingivitis, puberty gingivitis, pregnancy gingivitis and drug−induced gingival leision and non plaque induced gingival lesions such as gingival diseases of viral origin, gingival diseases of fungal origin, gingival diseases of genetic origin and gingival manifestations of systemic conditions.

5.1.1 Chronic gingivitis

Chronic gingivitis, also called marginal gingivitis or simple gingivitis, is the most common plaque induced gingival diseases. It is characterized by the presence of clinical signs of inflammation that are usually confined to the marginal gingiva and interdental papillae.

5.1.1.1 Etiology

The primary etiological factor of chronic gingivitis is the bacterial plaque cumulated on the tooth surface adjacent to the gingival margin. Other predisposing factors including calculus, faulty restorations, tooth misalignment or crowding, food impaction and mouth breathing. These factors are contributory for their ability to retain plaque microorganisms and inhibit their removal by patient−initiated plaque control techniques, may cause and exacerbate the gingival inflammation. When gingivitis happens, more dental plaques can be seen near the gingival margin. The quantity and variety of bacteria in the plaque are higher than that adjacent to the healthy gingiva.

5.1.1.2   Epidemiology

Chronic gingivitis is a very common gingival disease, especially among children and adolescents, and its incidence has been reported as 60% – 90%. Children may suffer from chronic gingivitis from 3 – 5 years old, and the prevalence and severity increase along with the growth of age, peaking at puberty. However, a gradual decline can be seen after the age of 17.

5.1.1.3   Pathogenesis and pathology

Chronic gingivitis is the result of an interaction between the microorganisms in the dental plaque biofilm attached to the tooth and the tissues of the host. Microscopically, some classic changes of acute inflammation can be seen in the gingival tissue. The chronic inflammation shows the exudative and proliferative feature. Some lesions have a preponderance of in flammatory cells and fluid, with vascular engorgement, new capillary formation, and associated degenerative changes related to enzyme collagenase produced by some oral bacteria and by polymorphonuclear neutrophils, while others have a greater fibrotic component with an abundance of fibroblasts and collagen fibers.

5.1.1.4   Clinical manifestation

The lesions generally start in the marginal and papillary areas and sometimes spread to the attached gingivae, often localized to the anterior region, especially in the lower jaw. Bleeding provoked by tooth brushing, toothpicks, or food impaction or by biting into solid foods such as apples is the main reason for the patients to ask for treatment, while spontaneous bleeding is rare. Swelling and loss of stippling occur when in flammatory exudate and edema are the predominant microscopic changes. The gingiva is soft and friable and bleeds easily, and its surface is smooth and shiny, its color changes from pink to deep or bluish red. When fibrosis predominates in the in flammatory process, gingival enlargement can be seen, and the gingival surface is firm, resilient and nodular, the color is pink.

5.1.1.5   Diagnosis

Chronic gingivitis can be diagnosed by the clinical manifestation the presence of local factors.

5.1.1.6   Differential diagnosis

(1)Priodontitis

Chronic gingivitis is diagnosed by the menifestation of redness, swelling, and increased edema of the gingival tissues. There may be increased pocket depth caused by gingival enlargement. All of these changes may occur in periodontitis, and bleeding on probing is a hallmark of gingivitis and periodontitis. Furthermore, chronic gingivitis may progress to periodontitis. The key point to differentiate chronic gingivitis from periodontitis is that the former has no periodontal bone loss, which can be distinguished by X – ray. It is noteworthy that chronic gingivitis also may occur on a periodontium with previous attachment loss that is stable and not progressing. Longitudinal records of periodontal status, including clinical attachment levels is very important for the diagnosis to be made.

(2)Gingival bleeding associated with blood discase

Gingival bleeding is easily encountered in some blood diseases including leukemia, thrombocytopenic purpura, hemophilia and aplastic anemia, gingival hemorrhage. A patient whose main complaint is gingival bleeding should be paid more attention. Related blood system examination is needed for accurate diagnosis.

5.1.1.7   Treatment

The objective of the treatment is eliminating the microbial etiology and factors that contribute to gingival inflammation. The therapies include complete removal of calculus and microbial plaque, correction of defective restorations and other factors favoring plaque accumulation. Flushing the gingival sulcus with 1% – 3% hydrogen peroxide and rinse with 0.12% chlorhexidine solution twice daily can be adopted. The enlarged gingivae in some patients could not return to normal after the inflammation subsides, while gingivectomy or gingivoplasty should be performed.

5.1.1.8 Prophylaxis

The most important prophylactic measure of chronic gingivitis is effective daily plaque removal at home. Extensive oral hygiene instruction including teaching proper use of toothbrush, tooth floss and tooth stick can effectively prevent gingivitis.

5.1.2 Puberty gingivitis

Puberty gingivitis is a kind of gingivitis affected by endocrine which refers to the chronic nonspecific inflammation that occurs in adolescents. It can be encountered both in males and females, but slightly more in females.

5.1.2.1 Etiology

Dental plaque is still the primary cause of puberty gingivitis. During adolescency, crowding in the mixed dentition, the presence of fixed orthodontic appliances or mouth breathing can often make plaque and food removing more difficult, and poor oral hygiene leads to an increased incidence of gingivitis; despite little calculus can be found. Furthermore, hormonal changes magnify the vascular and in flammatory response to dental plaque and modify reactions of dental plaque microbes.

5.1.2.2 Clinical manifestation

Puberty gingivitis often occurs interproximally and marginally at the anterior region. The facial gingivae are enlarged with prominent bulbous interproximal papillae, red or deep red, shinny, soft, and easily bleeding on probing. Gingival pocket is formed by gingival enlargement without attachment loss. The patient has scarcely any overt symptoms, occasional breath malodor or bleeding on tooth brushing or biting into solid foods.

5.1.2.3 Diagnosis

Puberty gingivitis is easily diagnosed by the special period of its onset. Another character of this disease is that the size of the gingival inflammation greatly exceeds that usually seen in association with comparable local factors. After puberty the gingivitis undergoes spontaneous reduction but does not disappear completely until plaque and calculus are removed.

5.1.2.4 Treatment

The key of the treatment of puberty gingivitis is still removal of the local factors. Scaling coupled with topical use of adjunctive agents such as chlorhexidine mouthwash can reduce the inflammation effectively.

5.1.3 Pregnancy gingivitis

Pregnancy gingivitis refers to the previous gingivitis that aggravated due to the endocrine changes during pregnancy. The swollen gingiva and tumor–like gingival enlargement can reduce spontaneously after the termination of pregnancy.

5.1.3.1 Etiology

Dental plaque is still the direct etiological factor. If the pregnant women fail to keep good oral hygiene, plaque and calculus accumulated on the marginal tooth surface, resulting in gingivitis. The increase in levels of both progesterone and estrogen induce changes in vascular permeability, leading to gingival edema and an increased in flammatory response to dental plaque.

5.1.3.2　Clinical manifestation

Chronic gingivitis initiates before pregnancy, and the inflammation increases from the 2nd to 3rd month, peaks at the 8th month of pregnancy, and reduces to the previous level 2 months after delivery. Pregnancy gingivitis may involve gingivae locally or generally, more often the anterior areas. The painlessly enlarged gingiva, which is bright red or deep red, soft, and friable and has a smooth, shiny surface, may form gingival pocket, with no attachment loss. Bleeding often occurs spontaneously or on slight provocation. Tumor-like gingival enlargement usually appears after the 3rd month of pregnancy but may occur earlier. The single or multiple discrete, mushroom-like, flattened spherical masses often protrude from the interproximal space of crowding teeth or teeth with occlusal trauma, especially the mandibular incisors. They may be smooth or lobulated, attached by a sessile or pedunculated base, normally less than 2 mm in diameter. After the termination of pregnancy, the size of gingival enlargement may spontaneously reduce, but complete elimination of the in flammatory lesion requires the removal of all plaque deposits and factors that favor its accumulation.

5.1.3.3　Diagnosis

Women of childbearing age, whose gingiva is red, swollen, and hypertrophic or enlarged like tumor, with increased tendency for bleeding, should be asked about the menstruation. The diagnosis can be confirmed when pregnancy is identified.

5.1.3.4　Treatment

Treatment principle of this disease is similar to chronic gingivitis. Dental plaque and all the local factors favorite plaque retention should be eliminated. When severe inflammation results in overt gingival hypertrophic and exudation from gingival pocket, irrigating with 3% hydrogen peroxide and physiological saline can be used. As to some large tumor-like gingival enlargement interfering with occlusion, beside a thorough removal of the local factors, resection should be considered. The surgery should be done during the 4th to 6th month of pregnancy, in order to avoid premature birth or abortion.

5.1.3.5　Prophylaxis

Rigorous plaque control and good oral hygiene is very important for the women of childbearing age to prevent pregnancy gingivitis. Comprehensive oral examination is recommended before pregnancy.

5.1.4　Drug-induced gingival enlargements

Drug-induced gingival enlargements refer to the gingival fibrous hyperplasia and enlargement as a consequence of the long-term administration of some drugs.

5.1.4.1　Etiology

The inflammatory gingiva may overgrow fibrously after prolonged administration of anticonvulsant phenytoin. The gingival overgrowth occurs 40%-50% in patients receiving this drug, and affects children more frequently than adults. Drug-induced gingival enlargements can also be caused by immunosuppresant cyclosporine and calcium channel blockers such as nifedipine and verapamil.

5.1.4.2　Clinical manifestation

The gingival overgrowth induced by phenytoin generally occurs 1-6 months after the beginning of continuous administration. The growth starts as a beadlike enlargement of the interdental papilla and extends to the facial and lingual gingival margins. As the condition progresses, the marginal and papillary enlargements unite and may develop into a massive tissue fold covering a considerable portion of the crowns; they may interfere with occlusion. The lesion is mulberry shaped, firm, pale pink, resilient, with a lobulated surface and no tendency to bleed. The enlargement characteristically appears to project from beneath the gingival margin, from which it is separated by a linear groove. The enlargement is usually generalized throughout the mouth but is more severe in the maxillary and mandibular anterior regions. It occurs in areas in which teeth are present, not in edentulous spaces, and the enlargement disappears in areas from which teeth are extracted.

5.1.4.3 Diagnosis

It is easy to make the diagnosis according to the parenchyma hyperplasia and prolonged administration of the drugs. The history of systemic disease should be enquired.

5.1.4.4 Treatment

With the physicians' assistance, discontinuation of the drug or substitution of drugs that do not induce gingival overgrowth is the utterly treatment for drug-induced gingival enlargements. Alternate use of different drugs can be adopted to alleviate the side effects. Removal the local stimulating factors by scaling, irrigating the gingival pockets with 3% hydrogen peroxide, putting antimicrobial agents into the gingival pockets, and the usage of antimicrobial mouth rinse may reduce the gingival inflammation. Gingivectomy and gingival plastic procedures can be adopted when general condition is stable. However, the gingival enlargement would recur after the surgery with poor oral hygiene or continuation of the drugs.

5.1.5 Hereditary gingival fibromatosis

Hereditary gingival fibromatosis, which is also called familial or idiopathic gingival fibromatosis, is a kind of diffuse fibrous connective tissue hyperplasia in gingiva. It is a rare disease.

5.1.5.1 Etiology

The cause of disease is undetermined. Some with family history may be autosomal recessive or dominant inheritance.

5.1.5.2 Clinical manifestation

This disease may occur on primary dentition, while generally begins with the eruption of permanent teeth. The extensive enlargement affects full mouth gingivae including gingival margin, interdental papillae and attached gingivae, even arrives at the mucogingival junction. It's more serious on the maxillary molar palatal gingiva. The teeth which are partially or completely covered by the enlarged gingivae may be displaced. The enlarged gingiva is pink, firm and smoothly, with obvious stippling and no tendency of bleeding.

5.1.5.3 Diagnosis

Diagnosis of this disease can be made according to the characteristic manifestation or the family history, while the patients with no family history should be included absolutely.

5.1.5.4 Treatment

The therapy of this disease is mainly gingivoplasty, respecting and remolding the enlarged gingiva. The internal bevel incision for flap surgery can be adopted to the gingivectomy to preserve the attached gingiva. The surgery should be performed after puberty.

5.1.6 Epulis

Epulis, a kind of inflammatory tumor-like mass, generally occurs on the gingival papilla or on the gingival margin. It arises from the periodontal ligament or the gingival connective tissue. Epulis isn't true neoplasm because it has no biological features and structures of neoplasm. However, a recurrence after resection of the mass is possible.

5.1.6.1   Etiology

Local factors such as dental plaque, calculus, food impaction and defective restoration lead to prolonged inflammation on the gingival, which cause reactive puffiness of gingival connective tissue. Epulis may occur on the gingiva of pregnant woman affected by the hormonal changes. It may diminish or stop growing after delivery.

5.1.6.2   Clinical manifestation

This disease is more common in female, especially in young and middle-aged woman. In terms of histopathology, there are three general types of epulis: fibroma, granuloma, angeioma. The labial or buccal gingival papilla is affected more often. The solitary tumor-like mass is round or oval in shape, from several millimeters to 1-2 cm in diameter. The mass protrudes from the interproximal space and is attached by a sessile or pedunculated base. It's slow - growing. A large mass may be injured by occlusion, resulting in bleeding, ulcer or infection. In some cases, alveolar bone breakdown and widening periodontal ligament space can be seen by X-ray. The teeth involved may become mobile or displaced.

5.1.6.3   Diagnosis

It's easy to make a diagnosis according to the clinical manifestation, while the pathological examination contributes to definite the type of the epulis.

5.1.6.4   Treatment

The lesion should be surgically removed. Excision must be complete to prevent recurrence. During the operation, the lump and the adjacent periostum should be resected entirely, exposing the bone surface, and the superficial cortex should be grinded, the associated periodontal ligament should be curetted.

5.1.7   Acute necrotizing ulcerative gingivitis

Acute necrotizing ulcerative gingivitis(ANUG) refers to the acute infection and necrosis that occurs on themarginal and papillary gingiva, also named as Vincent gingivitis, fusiform - spirochete gingivitis or trench mouth.

5.1.7.1   Etiology

ANUG is an opportunistic infect of the gingiva caused by varied microorganism including fusiform bacilli and spirochetes with local or systemic immunosuppression. Formerly existed chronic gingivitis or periodontitis may be the important prerequisite for this disease. Furthermore, acute necrotizing ulcerative gingivitis is associated with physical or emotional stress and decreased resistance to infection. Patients under some conditions as varying levels of nutritional deficiency, fatigue caused by chronic sleep deprivation, other unhealthy habits (e. g. , alcohol or drug abuse), psychosocial factors, or systemic disease (e. g. , malignancy, acute infectious disease or blood disease) may be more susceptible.

5.1.7.2   Clinical manifestation

ANUG occurs in the young adults, more common in the male smokers. It is characterized by sudden onset with a short course continuing several days to 1-2 weeks. Characteristic lesions are necroses at the crest of the interdental papillae, subsequently extending to the marginal gingiva and rarely to the attached gingival, more often on the lower anterior teeth. Additional characteristic clinical signs include pronounced bleeding after the slightest stimulation or even spontaneous gingival hemorrhage. The patients usually complain of a constant pain, fetid odor and increased salivation. In mild cases, there are rare systemic signs and symptoms. A slight elevation in temperature and general lassitude are common features of the severe stages of the disease, generally associated with presence of enlarged lymph nodes, especially submaxillary and submental nodes. During the acute stage, failure to treat promptly or suppressed immunity may lead to necrotizing gingivostomatitis. ANUG combined with Achalme's bacillus infection may result in necrotic perforation in the cheek, which is called noma. ANUG can also be changed to chronic necrotic gingivitis if it is treated uncompletely or had a history of repeated remissions and exacerbations. When the lesion leads to a progressive destruction of the periodontium, causing alveolar bone breakdown, it is named necrotizing ulcerative periodontitis.

5.1.7.3 Diagnosis

Diagnosis is based on clinical signs and symptoms of gingival pain, fetid odor, ulceration, and bleeding. Bacteriological smear examination may be helpful in the defferential diagnosis of ANUG and specific infections of the oral cavity.

5.1.7.4 Treatment

The first step of the treatment is alleviation of the acute inflammation by gently removing the necrotic tissue and the superficial calculus. Topical application of oxidants, such as rinsing, irrigating or swabbing with a moistened cotton pellet with 1% – 3% hydrogen peroxide is an adjunctive measure. Patients with severe ANUG and systemic signs or symptoms may take metronidazole, tinidazole or other anaerobic–resistant drugs orally. Supporting therapy as system administration of vitamin C and protein can be adopted when necessary.

The patient should be instructed in plaque control procedures and the systemic predisposing factors should be treated or corrected promptly. After the acute period, initiate therapy like scaling and root planning and reconstructive or esthetic surgery can be adopted. Plaque control procedures are essential to prevent potential recurrences.

5.1.8　Acutepapillary gingivitis

Acutepapillary gingivitis refers to the acute nonspecific inflammation restricted to individual interproximal papilla. It is a common kind of acute lesion on gingiva.

5.1.8.1 Etiology

The direct cause of acutepapillary gingivitis is the mechanical or chemical stimulant on the gingival papilla. Local factors such as food impaction, overhangs, trauma resulted from the misapplication of toothpick may lead to acute inflammation on the interdental papilla.

5.1.8.2 Clinical manifestation

Clinical features include a red and smooth swollen gingival papilla, with tendency of bleeding on tactile stimulation or sucking, spontaneous distending pain and obvious tenderness. Sometimes, the patient complains of a moderate pain that is intensified by caloric stimulation, which should be differentiated with pulpitis. The inflammation and edema of the periodontal ligament below the gingival papilla may cause tooth percussion pain. Local stimulating factors can be found occasionally.

5.1.8.3 Treatment

First of all, the local stimulating factors such as the impacted food, overhang, fishbone or broken toothpick should be removed. Flushing with 3% hydrogen peroxide after removal of the proximal dental plaque and calculus may diminish the acute inflammation of the gingival papilla. When the acute inflammation subsides, the cause of the disease should be removed thoroughly, including eliminating the cause of food impaction, treatment of the proximal cavity and correcting the defective restoration.

5.2   Periodontitis

Periodontitis is a chronic inflammatory disease of the tooth-supporting tissues, not only invaded gingival tissue but also affected the deep periodontal tissue (periodontal membrane, alveolar bone and cementum).

Clinically, the disease has a high prevalence in the adult population and an enormous impact on individuals' health. It is a major cause of tooth loss. And it adversely influences the quality of life via nutrition, speech and oral function.

5.2.1   Dental plaque and periodontal pathogen

In each type of periodontal disease, one or several dominant bacteria can be isolated. Periodontal pathogens, which have significant virulence or pathogenicity, can interfere the host defense ability through a variety of mechanisms, and have the potential to cause periodontal destruction. The evidences of periodontal pathogenic bacteria mainly include actinomycetes, porphyromonas gingivalis and forsythiae.

Dental plaque biofilm is the initial factor of periodontal disease, which is a bacterial plaque in the mouth that can not be washed away. There are three stages: formation of acquired membranes, bacterial adhesion and copolymerization, and maturation of plaque biofilms. Dental plaque biofilms are divided into subgingival plaque biofilms and subgingival plaque biofilms (attached subgingival plaque biofilms and non-attached plaque biofilms). The pathogenic mechanism of periodontal microorganism as follows: ①periodontal colonization, survival and reproduction; ②invade host tissues; ③suppress or evade the host defense system; ④damage the host periodontal tissue; ⑤dental plaque mineralized into calculus.

5.2.2   Promoting factors

The promoting factors of periodontal disease can be divided into local promoting factors and systemic factors. Dental calculus is formed by plaques and sediments that have or are calcifying with the gradual deposit of mineral salts in saliva or gingival crevicular fluid. There is a significant positive correlation between the amount of calculus and the incidence of periodontitis. Other local promoting factors include anatomical factors of tooth, trauma from occlusion, food embedded plug and bad habits such as mouth breathing and tongue spitting. Systemic factors of periodontal disease include genetic factors, sex hormones, smoking, mental stress and related systemic diseases, such as diabetes, AIDS, osteoporosis, decreased number of phagocytes and dysfunction.

5.2.3   Clinical manifestation

The four main symptoms of periodontitis are gingival inflammation, periodontal pocket formation, alveolar bone resorption, loose and displaced teeth.

The main complaint symptom of many periodontal disease patients, mostly occurred when brushing teeth or biting hard objects, occasionally spontaneous bleeding. The initial clinical manifestations were increased gingival crevicular fluid flow and gingival crevicular hemorrhage. Inflammatory congestion in periodontitis patients can affect the attached gingiva. The early manifestation of gingival inflammation is an important marker for further diagnosis and evaluation.

Periodontal pocket is one of the most important pathological changes of periodontitis. The bacteria and its products in gingival groove enter the subgingival connective tissue through the oral epithelium to produce inflammation. The formation of periodontal pocket starts from inflammation in gingival connective tissues, destruction of collagen fibers, and proliferation of binding epithelium. After the formation of periodontal pocket, a good anaerobic environment is formed. The plaque is difficult to remove, and its accumulation further develops the inflammation and forms a vicious circle. According to the changes of tissue formation and the relationship between the bottom of the pocket and adjacent tissues, it can be divided into pseudo periodontal pocket and true periodontal pocket. When suffering from periodontitis, combined with the epithelium to proliferate to the root square, the crown square part of which is separated from the tooth surface to form the periodontal pocket, which is called the true periodontal pocket. The depth of exploration from the bottom of the gingival groove to margin is more than 3 mm.

Inflammation is the most common cause of periodontitis bone destruction. The mechanism of alveolar bone resorption is that plaque bacteria release lipopolysaccharides and other products to gingival crevicular groove, stimulate immune cells and osteoblasts in tissues to release inflammatory mediators, activate macrophages and fibroblasts to secrete cytokines and PGE_2, and induce massive osteoclast formation and alveolar bone resorption. The damage forms of alveolar bone mainly include horizontal vertical and pit-like absorption. X-ray showed that the bony plates on the alveolar ridge were blurred, interrupted and disappeared, and the periodontal space was widened. The height of alveolar bone is decreased, the bone trabeculae arrangement is disordered.

Alveolar ridge absorption, combined trauma, acute inflammation of periodontal membrane, changes in female hormone levels after periodontal surgery can all lead to tooth loosening. The main factors of pathological displacement and enlarged interdentium of teeth are the destruction of periodontal support tissues. In patients with invasive periodontitis, lip displacement of upper and lower anterior teeth occurs, which is called fan-shaped displacement.

The early symptoms of periodontal disease are not easy to be paid attention to, which resulting in long-term chronic periodontal tissue infection and repeated episodes of inflammation. It not only damage the function of oral chewing system, but also affect health. Clinical attention should be paid to the periodontal disease activity. The changes of periodontitis occurred alternately in the stationary phase and the aggravating phase. The resting phase is characterized by a light inflammatory response with little or no loss of bone and connective tissue attachment. The progressive stage starts with the loss of bone and connective tissue adhesion and periodontal pocket deepening.

5.2.4　Chronic periodontitis

Chronic periodontitis(CP) is the most common form of periodontitis in adults, but also in children and adolescents. The morbidity and severity increase with age. There are obvious plaque, tartar and local stimulation factors, which are consistent with the degree of inflammation and destruction of periodontal tissues. The course of the disease progresses slowly or moderately, but there may be a rapid progression period. Patients are generally healthy throughout and may also have certain risk factors, such as smoking, mental stress, osteoporosis, and so on. The main symptoms are bleeding gums, bad breath and weak occlusion. Clinical examination reveals probing bleeding due to gum inflammation. In the early stage of the disease, there are many shallow periodontal pockets, which are generally supraspinal and relatively loose. In the late stage of the disease, deep periodontal pocket often accompanied by periodontal abscess. Alveolar bone is mainly absorbed horizontally, and the degree of alveolar bone resorption is one of the important indexes to judge the severity of lesions. A loose tooth is a sign of decreased dental function. Other complications include gingival recession, root hypersensitivity, root caries, periodontal combined endodonitic lesions, food impaction, secondary occlusion, periodontal abscess.

5.2.5   Aggressive periodontitis

The aggressive periodontitis(AgP) patients are generally below 35 years old, with rapid bone resorption and loss of attachment. The disease has familial aggregation and has been inherited by the maternal line. Patients are generally healthy and have no obvious systemic disease, but some patients have functional defects of neutrophils and/or monocytes. Periodontal tissue destruction in AgP is progressing rapidly, 3－4 times faster than CP. Actinomyces can produce a variety of toxic products and cause destructive effects on periodontal tissues. Periodontal tissue destruction is disproportionate to oral hygiene. Clinically AgP is divided into the localized aggressive periodontitis(LAgP) and generalized aggressive periodontitis(GAgP). LAgP mostly occurs in incisors and first molars, with no more than two other affected teeth(non－first molars and incisors). GAgP shows extensive proximal attachment loss and occurs in incisors and first molars, with more than two other affected teeth(non－first molars and incisors). The teeth are broken loose and displaced at early stage, and fan－shaped separation is frequently seen in anterior teeth. X－ray shows the horizontal absorption in the incisor area, and vertical absorption(arc absorption) in the first molar area.

5.2.6   Other periodontal diseases

Necrotizing ulcerative periodontitis(NUP) is characterized by necrosis of the gingival tissue, periodontal ligament and alveolar bone. The cause of necrotic ulcerative periodontitis is similar to that of necrotic ulcerative gingivitis. This type of periodontitis is the most serious periodontitis caused by bacteria. This disease comes more urgent, ache is apparent. In the early stages of the disease, the gingival papilla between the two teeth is swollen, and the color is bright red or dark red, often seen in the lower anterior teeth. Subsequently, the tip of the interdental papilla is necrotic and the upper end was missing, forming a crater－like change, with a grey－white film on the surface, which is slightly wiped away, and the destruction is visible below. When the disease develops rapidly, the adjacent gums may be affected, and the gum margins are uneven as if bitten by an insect, and the surface is bright red ulcer surface, which will cause severe pain and often spontaneous bleeding. There is a red border between the necrotic area and the unaffected gums. Patients with extremely low body resistance may also be associated with the infection of aeromonas pertussis, resulting in rapid necrosis of the cheek tissue, and even a perforation of the cheek, known as noma chancre, when the patient has systemic poisoning or even death. At present, chancre is basically extinct in China, but it still appears in some poor countries in Africa.

Abscesses of the periodontium can occur in any type of periodontitis. It is localized suppurative inflammation in periodontal pocket wall or deep periodontal tissues, which can cause the destruction of surrounding collagen fibers and bones. It is acute process commonly, also can have chronic periodontal abscess. Periodontitis is a chronic infectious disease of periodontal supporting tissues caused by microorganisms in dental plaque, leading to inflammation and destruction of periodontal supporting tissue, which is the first cause of tooth loss in Chinese adults. Periodontitis develops to middle or late stage, and deep periodontal pockets can accompany periodontal abscess. The gingival abscess is confined to the gingival papilla and the gingival margin and presented localized swelling. No history of periodontitis, no periodontal pocket and loss of attachment, no alveolar bone resorption. There are some obvious stimulation factors, such as foreign body piercing gums, etc., when the foreign body and plaque calculus are removed, no other treatment is needed after discharge and drainage. Periodontal abscess is a local suppurative inflammation in the periodontal supporting tissues, with a deeper periodontal pocket and loss of attachment, and X-ray shows alveolar bone resorption. In chronic periodontal abscess, diffuse bone destruction can also be seen at the root side or around the apices.

Periodontitis with pulp/endodontic lesions is a common complication of periodontitis. The pulp and periodontal tissues are anatomically interconnected, and both periodontal pockets and infected dental pulp contain a mixture of anaerobic bacteria that cause inflammation and immune response. Therefore, the infection and lesion of the pulp and periodontal tissues can affect and diffuse each other, leading to the occurrence of combined lesions. Periodontal disease caused by pulp disease can be seen clinically. The bacterial products of the dead pulp teeth can cause periapical or bifurcation lesions through apical foramen or lateral root canal. The pulp lesions caused by periodontal disease can also be seen clinically. The most common is retrograde pulpitis. Chronic periodontal disease, with chronic, severe and persistent stimulation of the bacteria and toxins in the bag, can also cause inflammation, degeneration, calcification and even necrosis of the pulp of the tooth.

5.2.7　Diagnosis

If the existence of periodontal disease is not detected in time, the optimal treatment time is delayed. In the end, patients can only take the destructive tooth extraction treatment to prevent the deterioration of the disease. Medical record is a comprehensive record of examination, diagnosis and treatment, an important basis and original data for summarizing experience, evaluating medical quality and conducting scientific research. Under certain conditions, it is also a formal basis for legal ruling, so medical records must be written in a serious manner. Medical records are required to be written formally and concisely, accurate in content, complete in items, clear in writing and not to be altered at will. The main contents should be recorded about the evolution and treatment of periodontal disease and the relationship with other oral diseases, and the systemic diseases related to periodontal disease should also be described. To diagnose periodontal disease, we should first know the patient's medical history. It is the basis of the diagnosis of periodontal disease to inquire the patient's history of periodontal disease comprehensively, carry out careful clinical examination and search for risk factors, and analyze the obtained data comprehensively. It should be noted that periodontal disease is closely related to the whole body, including the patient's general condition, periodontal condition and changes in other parts of the mouth during the examination and diagnosis process. Instruments for periodontal tissue examination are routinely performed with oral speculum, dental tweezers and periodontal probes. There should also be a pointed probe, dental floss, occlusion paper and wax tablets. Examination was conducted by means of visual examination, exploratory examination, palpation, percussion, research model and X-ray dental films. With the in-depth understanding of the nature of the disease and the development of diagnostic techniques, some new examination methods have been introduced to assist the diagnosis to improve the accuracy. X-ray is an important and commonly used examination method, which is of great significance in the diagnosis and evaluation of periodontitis. However, it is only an auxiliary diagnosis of periodontitis, which should be combined with clinical examination, comprehensive analysis and judgment, and no diagnosis or treatment plan can be made by X-ray alone. Observation of periodontal bone loss or to compare the effects is given priority to with parallel exposure of root tip. The examination of occlusion is an important content in the diagnosis of periodontal disease. By adjusting the abnormal occlusion relationship and function, the occlusion trauma is eliminated, which is helpful to reduce the degree of tooth looseness, promoting the repair and regeneration of periodontal tissue, and consolidating the curative effect of periodontal disease. The routine examination method of periodontal disease described above is the basis of the diagnosis of periodontal disease. Through these basic clinical examinations, the location, degree of tissue damage and type of disease can be determined. However, the traditional diagnosis can not fully reflect the connotation change of the disease. Because periodontal lesions of different degrees of severity can present the same clinical symptoms, such as exploratory hemorrhage, which can occur in areas without loss of attachment or shallow gingivitis, or in areas with deep periodontal pockets, further examination is needed to determine the nature of the disease. With the rapid development of related disciplines, some new auxiliary diagnostic methods for periodontal disease are of great significance for revealing the nature of the disease, optimizing treatment plan, evaluating curative effect and monitoring during maintenance period. Doctors can choose according to the needs of scientific research and their own working conditions.

5.2.8   Treatment procedures

Overall objectives of periodontal disease treatment: ① Control plaque and eliminate inflammation. ② Restore the function of periodontal tissue. These include restoring or improving the chewing efficiency of natural teeth, repairing missing teeth, adjusting occlusion and correcting bad occlusion habits. ③ Restore the physiological shape of periodontal tissues, including gums and bone tissues, teeth and adjacent relations. ④ Promote the regeneration of periodontal tissue, maintain long-term efficacy and prevent recurrence.

Sequence of periodontal disease treatment is divided into four stages.

Stage 1: basic treatment. The purpose of this stage is to remove all local stimulative pathogenic factors. Periodontal basic treatment includes oral hygiene guidance, supragingival scaling and subgingival scaling. Oral health guidance can be divided into mechanical plaque control (brushing, removing adjacent plaque) and chemical plaque control (0.12% –0.2% chlorhexidine, etc.). The two methods of supragingival scaling include manual scaling and ultrasonic scaling. Subgingival scaling includes ultrasonic subgingival scaling, manual scaling and root surface planning.

At this stage, the physician should explain the treatment plan to the patient and administer the emergency treatment. Besides, temporary fixation of the loose teeth or removal of the teeth that have no hope of retaining. Remove the overhang of the backfill, correct the bad repair, treat food impaction and so on. The drug treatment of periodontal disease, as an auxiliary means of periodontal mechanical treatment, can kill or control pathogenic microorganisms, prevent or reduce the formation of plaque, consolidate curative effect and prevent recurrence. Control the acute infection of periodontal tissue, regulate the host defense function, block the development of the disease, and promote tissue healing. Drug treatment should follow the principle of evidence-based medicine, rational use of drugs. Before the use of drugs to remove dental calculus, plaque destruction of the structure of the biofilm. Local administration should be adopted and the generation of resistant bacteria should be avoided. When choosing antibiotics, try to do bacteriological examination and drug sensitivity test. The most commonly used periodontal drugs are hydrogen peroxide, chlorhexidine, tetracycline and nitroimidazoles.

Stage 2: surgical treatment. The purpose of this stage is to obtain the direct way to clear the pathogenic stimuli and correct the soft and hard tissue configuration. Expose the lesion's root surface and alveolar bone and thoroughly remove plaque, tartar and diseased tissue from the pocket wall and root surface under direct vision. Eliminate periodontal pockets or make periodontal pockets shallow, make it easy to keep clean and reduce the recurrence of inflammation. Repair soft and hard tissue defects and poor appearance, and establish a harmonious tissue form with physiological appearance, which is conducive to plaque control and oral health maintenance. Promote the regeneration of periodontal tissue and establish new periodontal attachment. The restoration of beauty and function is needed to facilitate the restoration of teeth. The timing and indications of periodontal surgery include pocket depth greater than 5 mm after basic treatment, and hemorrhage or abscess after diagnosis; those whose root surface irritation can not be completely cleared by basic treatment; irregular shape of alveolar bone; tooth root bifurcation disease II – III degrees; gingival adhesion is too narrow or gingival recession of individual teeth; dental caries or teeth break under the gingiva. The types of periodontal surgery can be divided into periodontal basic surgery(gingidectomy and gingioplasty, periodontal flap surgery, pocket wall curettage surgery, periodontal resection bone surgery), periodontal regenerative surgery(guided tissue regeneration surgery, bone graft surgery), periodontal surgery(crown lengthening surgery, membranous gingival surgery). Gingivectomy is a surgical procedure to remove periodontal pockets of medium depth in hyperplasia and hypertrophy gingival tissue or parts of the posterior tooth, and to reconstruct the gingival profile and normal gingival groove. Gingivoplasty is similar to gingidectomy but has a single purpose: to repair the shape of the gums and reconstruct the normal physiological appearance of the gums. These two are often used together. The advantages of gingidectomy are simple and easy to operate. However, gingidectomy also has disadvantages, that is, the postoperative wound surface is larger and the healing is slow. When used to eliminate periodontal pocket, the root will be exposed, affecting the appearance, causing sensitive teeth and caries on the root surface, which is not suitable for the removal of periodontal pocket of anterior teeth. Through flap surgery, part of periodontal pocket and inner wall of periodontal pocket are removed by surgical method. The mucosal periosteum flap of the gingiva is rolled up, and the subgingival calculus and granulation tissue are scraped under direct vision, and the alveolar bone could be repaired, and the gingival flap is then reset and sutured to eliminate periodontal pocket or make periodontal pocket shallow. Pocket wall curettage surgery, also known as closed curettage, is a kind of endoscopic curettage, which does not open the mucosal periosteal flap, but penetrates into the bag with an instrument to carry out the bag inner wall curettage and remove the granulation tissue, making the soft and hard tissue stick to each other. Guided tissue regeneration(GTR) technique usually use of membranous materials as a barrier to stop the gingival epithelium and gingival connective tissue to rootward growth in the healing process. GTR provides and guides new adhesive ability of the periodontal ligament cells priority occupation of root surface. Thereafter new fiber embedded with periodontal membrane forms new attachment to heal. Crown – lengthening surgery reduces the gingival margin, removes the corresponding alveolar bone to expose the healthy tooth structure, and lengthens the excessively short clinical crown, so as to facilitate the dental repair or solve aesthetic problems.

Stage 3: prosthodontic and orthodontic treatment. The purpose of this stage is to reconstruct and restore the occlusion function. Normally 3 months after surgery, it suggests to adopt appropriate orthodontic and/or prosthodontic treatment to help establish balanced occlusion state.

Stage 4: maintenance period. Through the oral hygiene instruction, the patient maintains oral hygiene, regular review and rehabilitation to prevent the recurrence of periodontitis. Regularly clinical review should be 3–6 months, and X–ray review once a year. The review included plaque and calculus, gingival inflammation and periodontal pocket depth, occlusion, tooth looseness and other pathological conditions. The first and fourth phases are necessary for each patient, while the second and third phases are arranged as appropriate.

In summary, periodontal disease is a common oral disease. It is one of the main causes of tooth loss in adults, as well as a major oral disease that endangers human teeth and general health. The treatment of periodontal disease is different according to different degrees. Periodontal treatment must have a complete plan and be informed to the patient not to change the plan at will. Supragingival scaling, subgingival scaling and root face leveling should be the first and core treatment. Strengthen the ability of patients to control their own plaque, and pay attention to review and rehabilitation. Regular dental check-up and treatment is necessary to establish good oral hygiene and healthcare.

▶▶ *Summary*

Periodontal diseases comprise gingival diseases and periodontitis. The former are a group of diseases that occur only on the gingival tissues, while the latter are inflammatory destructive periodontal diseases involving all the four kinds of tooth supporting tissues. An understanding of the etiology, clinical manifestation, diagnosis and treatment about different types of gingival diseases and periodontitis is very important for the learners to be qualified clinicians.

▶▶ *Case*

Miss Li was a junior student in Zhengzhou University. She was a beautiful slim girl, 165 cm tall, with long hair. She was diligent, putting her heart and soul into the preparation for the entrance examination for postgraduate school. She had seen the water slobbering from her mouth turn red when she brushed her teeth for years. As the color usually disappeared after she rinsed the mouth with more water, it had not got her attention. That term, she stayed up very late studying every day. She always felt tired. She found most of her teeth loose after she felt uncomfortable when she chewed peanuts a month ago. Her upper right gums began to be swollen and painful last week, and got more and more serious. So she decided to see a doctor.

In Henan Stomatological Hospital, Doctor Zhang in the department of periodontic received Miss Li.

Doctor Zhang: "Good morning, what's wrong with you?"

Miss Li: "I feel most of my teeth loose. "

Doctor Zhang: "How long have you had this condition?"

Miss Li: "About 3 months. "

Doctor Zhang: "Did you have any bleeding from your gums when you brush your teeth or eat hard food, like an apple?"

Miss Li: "Yes, my gums always bled on those occasions you mentioned; sometimes they bled for no apparent reason at all. "

Doctor Zhang: "Have you noticed any bleeding spots on your skin?"

Miss Li: "No, never. "

Doctor Zhang: "Did your gums ever feel uncomfortable?"

Miss Li: "Yes, my upper right gums began to be swollen and painful last week, more and more seriously. That is why I come here. "

Doctor Zhang: "Is there any particular food preference?"

Miss Li: "I prefer to some harder food. "

Doctor Zhang: "Do you have a habit of grinding your teeth at night?"

Miss Li: "No, but when I am nervous I may clench my teeth. "

Doctor Zhang: "Do you notice that you breathe through your mouth?

Miss Li: "No, I don't. "

Doctor Zhang: "Do you have anyone in your family who has serious gums disease?

Miss Li: "Yes. My mother always complains about gums bleeding. She lost her teeth from 40 years old. "

Doctor Zhang: "Have you ever been treated for gingivitis or periodontitis?"

Miss Li: "No. "

Doctor Zhang: "Then, I will ask you about your general health and allergies. How are your health conditions now?"

Miss Li: "Average. In fact, I usually feel tired. Maybe, that is because I am too busy for my study. "

Doctor Zhang: "Have you suffered from any previous disease?

Miss Li: "No. "

Doctor Zhang: "Is your menstrual cycle regular?"

Miss Li: "Yes. "

Doctor Zhang: "When did your last period begin?"

Miss Li: "10 days ago. "

Doctor Zhang: "Are you allergic to anything?"

Miss Li: "No. "

Doctor Zhang: "OK. Now, please sit down in this chair and keep your mouth open. I will give you an oral cavity examination. "

The results of examination:

- Observation of the maxillofacial region was not remarkabale.

- The oral hygiene was very poor. A great deal of calculus and debris could be seen on the lingual surface of lower anterior teeth and the buccal surface of upper posterior teeth.

- The gingivae of most teeth in the mouth were magenta and moderately swollen, bleeding with probing.

The following were the panoramic radiograph(Figure 5-1) and the results of her periodontal examination.

	18	17	16	15	14	13	12	11	21	22	23	24	25	26	27	28	Bu
TM	I	I	III	II	II	I	II		II	II	I	II	I	I			
CI	2 / 1	3 / 2	3 / 1	3 / 1	2 / 1	1 / 1	1 / 1	1 / 2	1 / 2	2 / 1	3 / 2	3 / 2	3 / 2	3 / 2			
R (下)	48	47	46	45	44	43	42	41	31	32	33	34	35	36	37	38	L / Li
TM (下)		I	I	II	II	I	II	III	III	II	I	II	I				Bu

The result of her peridontal examination

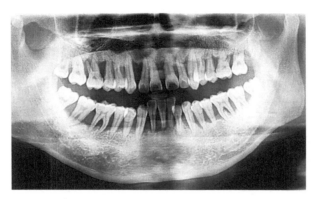

Figure 5-1   The panoramic radiograph

Doctor Zhang gave some advices to Miss Li:

- *Keep good oral hygiene.*

- *Scaling and root planning of all the teeth.*

- *Extraction of heavily loose teeth.*

- *Evaluating the periodontal condition 3 months later.*

- *Periodontal surgery when necessary.*

- *Restoration for the lost teeth when necessary.*

- *Supportive therapy.*

With the consent of Miss Li, doctor Zhang gave her an ultrasonic supragingival scaling for all her teeth and a bottle of mouthwash. He also taught her correct method for tooth brushing and told her to come back for subsequent visit once a week.

One year later, Miss Li came to see doctor Zhang for an examination as usual. She didn't accept the advice of extraction of heavily loose teeth. She said she felt that the tooth mobility reduced significantly. She hadn't seen bleeding when brushed her teeth for a long time. Doctor Zhang checked her periodontal situation and recorded the following table, then let her take an X-ray photograph(Figure 5-2).

Wang Guofang, Guo Zhuling

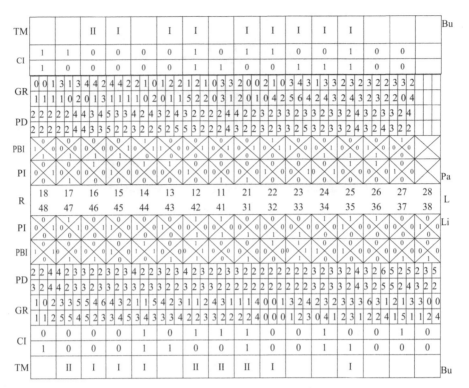

The result of her peridontal examination

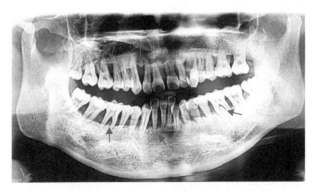

Figure 5-2　The X-ray photograph

▶▶ *Questions*

(1) What is the pathogenesis of periodontal disease?

(2) Why did the patient's gingivae bleed when brushing teeth?

(3) How to differentiate gingivitis and early periodontitis?

(4) What are the classification, diagnosis and treatment of periodontitis?

(5) What is the relationship between system disease and periodontal disease?

(6) What is the reason for tooth mobility?

(7) Is parallel projection periapical radiography or panoramic radiography optical preferential when you want to observe the resorption of alveolar bone? Why?

Chapter 6

Common Diseases of Oral Mucosa

Oral mucosal disease is oral diseases which happen at mucous membrane and soft tissue in oral cavity, including the changes in the normal color, shape, integrity and function of a certain part of the oral cavity. There are many kinds of lesions, which can be combined into complex and diverse damages. Some systemic diseases are also manifested on oral mucosa, and some oral manifestations can be used as clues for the diagnosis of systemic diseases.

6.1　Oral Herpes Simplex

Herpes simplex is a skin mucous membrane disease caused by herpes simplex virus. Clinically, it is characterized by small clustered bullous, self limited and easy to relapse. Epidemiological data show that about 30%–90% of the residents have anti herpes simplex virus antibodies in their sera, indicating that HSV infection has occurred or occurring. About 1%–10% of adults spread the virus periodically in saliva. Herpes simplex virus can survive for hours on body fluids and surfaces. It is generally believed that human beings are the natural hosts of herpes simplex virus, and the oral cavity, skin, eye, perineum and central nervous system are easily involved.

6.1.1　Etiology

Herpes simplex virus(HSV)

Characteristics: clustered small blister, self limited, easy to relapse.

Etiology: type I herpes simplex virus(HSV-I).

Source of infection: oral herpes simplex virus infection and asymptomatic virus carriers.

Transmission routes: droplets, saliva and herpes fluid direct contact, food utensils and clothing indirect infection.

Primary infection: most of them have no clinical symptoms or subclinical infection.

Relapse: some scholars believe that the virus lurks in host epithelial cells, and after division and reproduction, the daughter cells can mutate. Therefore, herpes simplex virus type I may be associated with the occurrence of lip cancer.

6.1.2　Clinical manifestation

6.1.2.1　Primary herpes stomatitis

The most common oral herpes stomatitis caused by herpes simplex virus type Ⅰ may be a more severe gingivitis–acute herpes gingivitis. The clinical symptoms of most of the primary infections are not significant. Most infected children were under 6 years of age, especially 6 months to 2 years old, because most babies have antibodies against herpes simplex virus after birth, a passive immunity from the mother, disappeared at 4–6 months, and no significant antibody titer before the age of 2.

(1) Prodromal stage

Primary herpes simplex infection. The incubation period is 4–7 days, after which fever, headache, fatigue discomfort, whole body muscle pain, and even the sore throat, the submandibular and upper cervical lymph nodes are swollen and sore. Children flow saliva irritable and refuse to eat. After 1–2 days, there was extensive congestion and edema in the oral mucosa, and acute inflammation was also found in the attached gingiva and gingival margin.

(2) Blister stage

A small blisters can be generated at any part of the oral mucosa, similar to the size of the needle, especially the palate and gingival margins of the adjacent molars(adult premolars). Blister wall is thin, transparent, and soon burst, forming superficial ulcers.

(3) Erosion period

Although the blister is small, it can be clustered. After bursting, it can form a large area of erosion, and can cause secondary infection and overlay the yellow false membrane. In addition to the damage in the oral cavity, the skin around the lip and peroral area also has similar lesions.

(4) Healing stage

The erosive surface gradually shrinks, and the healing process takes about 7–10 days. But the recovery is slow without proper treatment. During the illness, antiviral antibodies appear in the blood, the highest level is on 14–21 days. After that, the antibody drops to a lower level, although it can remain for a lifetime, but it can not prevent recurrence.

In a few cases, primary infection can be widely disseminated in the body. In very few cases, HSV can enter the central nervous system, causing encephalitis and meningitis.

6.1.2.2　Recurrent herpetic stomatitis

After primary herpes infection ishealed, no matter what the extent of the disease is, there may be recurrent damage in 30%–50% of cases. Recurrent infection is usually located on the lips or near the lips, so it is also known as recurrent herpes labial herpes.

There are two characteristics of recurrent lip damage.

(1) The damage always starts with blister, often with multiple clusters of blister, and a single blister is rare.

(2) When the lesion recurred, it was always in the place where it had been attacked before. There are many stimulant factors for relapse, including sunshine, local mechanical injury, fever, colds. In many cases, emotional factors also contribute to relapse. In the prodromal stage of recurrence, the patient can feel mild fatigue and discomfort. There are irritation, burning pain, itching and increased tension in the lesion area. About more than 10 hours, there were blisters and mild erythema around them. In general, the blister lasts within 24 hours, then ruptures, followed by erosion and scab. From the beginning to the healing of the contract lasts 10 days, but secondary infection often postpone the healing process, and make small pustules in the lesion, without no scar after healing, but there can be pigmentation.

Although recurrent herpes is the most common recurrence of this disease, a few recurrences may affect the gums and the hard palate, and the recurrent herpes infection in these oral cavity is still self limiting. In general, in the recurrent herpes damage, the body's immunity limits the leision and makes it markedly inhibited.

6.1.3   Diagnosis

In most cases, diagnosis can be made according to clinical manifestations. Primary infection among fants and young children, cause acute attack, heavy systemic reaction, and clusters of small vesicles around any part of the oral mucosa and around the lips. After the blister, the oral mucosa forms superficial ulcers, and the skin around the mouth become scab. The recurrent infection is common in adults. Typical cluster vesicles appear on the, lips and skin.

Laboratory diagnosis of oral herpes simplex virus infection is used only for final diagnosis. The commonly used methods have the following aspects.

(1) The non specific herpes virus examination: including the bullous tissue smear staining to observe the multinucleated giant cells containing the eosinophil inclusion body, and the microscopic examination of the immature virus particles in the damaged cells.

(2) The specific herpes simplex virus examination: including isolation and culture of the virus, direct staining of lesion smears with fluorescein labeled or enzyme labelled monoclonal antibodies, in situ nucleic acid hybridization and polymerase chain reaction (PCR) method.

6.1.4   Treatment

6.1.4.1   Systemic antiviral therapy

(1) Nucleoside antiviral agents: nucleoside drugs are considered to be the most effective anti HSV drugs. There are mainly asilowe, valaciclovir, fanciclovir and ganciclovir.

Primary herpes stomatitis: asilowe 200 mg oral, 5 times a day, 5 days 1 courses; valaciclovir 1,000 mg oral 2 times a day, 10 days 1 courses; valaciclovir 125 mg oral, 2 times a day, 5 days 1 courses.

Patients with severe primary infection: acyclovir 150 mg/(kg · d), divided into 3 intravenous drops, 5 days and 1 courses.

Frequent recurrences (more than 6 recurrences for 1 years): to reduce the number of recurrences, virus inhibition therapy, acyclovir 200 mg, 3 times a day, or valaciclovir 500 mg, 1 times a day for 6-12 months.

(2) Bavirin, a broad-spectrum antiviral drug, mainly by interfering with the synthesis of virus nucleic acid to prevent the replication of the virus and is effective for a variety of DNA viruses or RNA viruses. It can be used for the treatment of herpes virus and so on. Oral 200 mg, 3-4 times a day; intramuscular injection of 5-10 mg/(kg · d), 2 injections every day; the adverse reaction is thirst, leukocyte reduction, etc. , the early pregnancy is forbidden.

The above dosage is for adults. Children's dosage should be calculated according to children's weight and drug instructions.

6.1.4.2   Local treatment

(1) 0.1% -0.2% chlorhexidine gluconate solution, chlorhexidine solution, compound boric acid solution and 0.1% ethacridine solution gargle.

(2) 3% aciclovir ointment or phthalin ointment can be used for local treatment of herpes labial.

(3) Powder, such as tin powder and watermelon frost powder, can be used locally.

(4) Lozenges can be divided into 3-4 times a day with chlorhexidine gluconate tablets 5 mg, lysozyme

tablets 20 mg, cydiodine buccal tablets 1. 5 mg and so on.

(5)Secondary infection of herpes simplex can be treated with warm saline, 0. 1% −0. 2% chlorhexidine chloride or 0. 01% zinc sulfate solution. Zinc can inhibit herpes simplex virus type DNA polymerase, which directly affects the replication of virus. Antibiotic paste, such as 5% chlortetracycline glycerol paste, or 5% tetracycline glycerin paste, topical.

6. 1. 4. 3　Other Treatment

Physical therapy, symptomatic and supportive therapy, and Chinese medicine treatment.

6. 2　Oral Candidiasis

Oral candidiasis is an oral mucosal disease caused by fungal Candida infection. In recent years, due to the widespread application of antibiotics and immunosuppressants in the clinic, the disorder of bacteria and the decrease of immunity have resulted in the increase of the infection of the viscera, skin and mucous membrane, and the incidence of oral mucous candidiasis is also increased.

6.2.1　Etiology

The fungus belong to Cryptococcus, Candida albicans and Candida tropicalis, among which Candida albicans and Candida tropicalis are most pathogenic. Candida albicans is a single cell yeast like fungus with a round or oval shape and gram positive staining. The most suitable pH for growth is 4− 6.

Although healthy people can have Candida, it does not occur. When the host defense function is reduced, this non pathogenic Candida is transformed into pathogenic bacteria, so Candida is a conditional pathogen. Infection caused by Candida albicans is also known as opportunistic infection or conditional infection. Whether pathogens can cause disease after invading the body depends on their virulence, quantity, the adaptability of the invading, the resistance of the body and other related factors. For instance, a variety of reasons lead to the decrease of the skin mucosal barrier, the decrease of primary and secondary immune function, the long−term, misuse of broad−spectrum antibiotics and the disorder of the body and endocrine disorder, which can be the susceptible factors of the host disease.

6.2.2　Clinical manifestation

According to the change of the location of the disease, it can be divided into candidal stomatitis, candidal angular stomatitis and candidal cheilitis.

6.2.2.1　Candidal stomatitis

(1)Acute false membrane candidiasis stomatitis: it can occur at any age of people, more common in the long−term use of hormone, HIV infection, immune deficiency, infant and weak. But the incidence rate is 4%, also known as neonatal thrush or snow mouth disease.

Neonatal thrush usually occurs within 2 − 8 days after birth, and the most frequent locations are buccal, tongue, soft palate and lip. The mucous membrane of the damaged area is hyperemia, with the soft small spots scattered in white as snow, such as the size of the cap needle, which soon fused into white or patches, and can continue to spread to the tonsil, pharynx, and gums. Early mucosal congestion is more obvious, so it is bright red and snow−white contrast. The old lesions were mucosal hyperemia and white patches with yellow color. The patch is not very tight. It can be erased with a little effort, exposing the red mucosal erosion surface and mild bleeding. Children are restless, crying, lactating difficult, sometimes mild fever, general reaction generally lighter; but a few cases, may spread to the esophagus and bronchus, causing candidiasis esophagitis or pulmonary candidiasis. A few patients can also have generalized cutaneous candidiasis and chronic mucocutaneous candidosis. Children with membranous candidal stomatitis may be transient, mild and easily cured.

(2) Acute erythematous Candida stomatitis: it can be primary or secondary to the false membrane type. It's also known as antibiotic stomatitis and antibiotic glossitis. Most commonly seen in long-term use of antibiotics, hormones and HIV infection, and most of the patients suffered from consumptive diseases. The clinical manifestation is the diffuse erythema on the mucousa membrane. The mucous membrane of the tongue is common, and the dorsal mucous membrane of the tongue is bright red and the tongue nipple is atrophied, and the buccal, palate and mouth can also have red plaque. Mucous erythema is due to epithelial atrophy and mucosal hyperemia. Therefore, in recent years, some scholars believe that the type of atrophy which has been replaced by the erythema type is more reasonable. If it is secondary infection, the false membrane is visible. The symptoms are dry mouth, abnormal taste, pain and burning sensation.

(3) Chronic erythematous (atrophic) candidiasis: this type is also known as denture stomatitis. The lesion is often found in the palate and gingival mucosa of the maxillary denture on the side of the palate. Mucous membranes showed brightred edema or yellow white stripe or spotted false membrane, and Candida albicans hyphae and spores could be found.

(4) Chronic proliferative candidiasis is also known as chronic hypertrophic candidal stomatitis and Candida leukoplakia. It is often found in the buccal mucosa, the dorsal tongue and the palate. As the mycelium penetrates into the mucous membrane, it causes keratinization, spinous layer thickening, epitheliosis, micro abscess formation and the infiltration of inflammatory cells in the papilla of the lamina propria, while the membrane of the surface is tightly attached to the epithelium and is not easy to fall off.

6.2.2.2   Recurrent herpetic stomatitis

Candidal cheilitis is a chronic cheilitis caused by Candida infection, mostly in the elderly (over 50 years old). It usually occurs on the lower lip, and can also cause candidal stomatitis or angular stomatitis. The disease is divided into two types: the erosive type in the lower lip the red lip lusts for a long time a fresh red erosive surface, around the phenomenon of hyperkeratosis, surface desquamation; granulated people show the lower lip swelling, lip red skin junction often scattered in the prominent small particles. Candida cheilitis scraped the scaly and small granular tissue on the edge of the erosive site. With microscopic examination of fungi, the spores and mycelium could be found, and it is proved to be Candida albicans by culture.

6.2.2.3   Recurrent herpetic stomatitis

The characteristics of Candida albicans are often bilateral, chapped skin and mucous membrane, adjacent skin and mucous membrane hyperemia, and chapped exudates and exudates, or thin scabs, pain or haemorrhage during mouth opening.

The oral angle of the elderly patients is mostly associated with the shortening of the vertical distance of occlusal. The collapse of the skin in the corner of the mouth is grooved, causing saliva to overflow from the mouth angle, so it is often humid, which is beneficial to the growth and reproduction of fungi.

6.2.3   Diagnosis

It mainly depends on history, clinical features and mycological examination. Laboratory detection methods for Candida include smear, isolation and culture, histopathology, immunology and gene diagnosis.

6.2.4 Treatment

The principle of treatment is to remove the inducing factors, treat the underlying diseases actively, and support therapy if necessary. It was divided into local treatment and general treatment.

6.2.4.1 Local drug therapy

(1)2% – 4% sodium bicarbonate solution: this drug is commonly used in the treatment of infantile thrush. It is used to wash the mouth before and after breast feeding to eliminate the residual curd or sugar that can decompose the acid and make the mouth become an alkaline environment, which can prevent the growth and reproduction of Candida. Mild children do not need other drugs, the lesions can disappear within 2–3 days, but it is still necessary to continue the use of drugs for several days to prevent recurrence. This medicine can also be used to wash the nipples before and after lactation, so as to avoid cross infection or repeated infection.

(2)Chlorhexidine:0.12% or 1% gels can be applied locally, rinsed or gargled, and can also be used as ointment or cream with nystatin to treat oral inflammation, denture stomatitis and so on. Co – washing with chlorhexidine solution and sodium bicarbonate solution can eliminate the synergistic pathogens of Candida albicans.

(3)Western iodine:3–4 times a day,1 tablets each time after swallow. People who allergic to iodine are forbidden to use.

(4)Nystatin:local use of 50 000–100 000 U/mL water suspension coating, once every 2–3 hours, after coating can be swallowed. Gargle can also be used, or tablets, emulsions and so on.

(5)Miconazole:the powder can be used for oral mucosa. The cream is suitable for treating glossitis and stomatitis.

6.2.4.2 Systemic antifungal therapy

(1)Fluconazol:it is the most widely used antifungal drug and has broad antimicrobial spectrum. It is the first choice for the treatment of Candida albicans. The first day is 200 mg, then 100 mg every day for 7–14 consecutive days.

(2)Itraconazole:dose is oral 100 mg daily.

6.2.4.3 Other treatment

(1)Enhance immunity, such as injection of thymosin, transfer factor.

(2) Surgical treatment: for those with abnormal epithelial hyperplasia in Candida leukoplakia, the changes of leukoplakia should be observed regularly. If the treatment effect is not obvious or those with moderate epithelial dysplasia, surgical excision should be considered.

6.3　Recurrent Aphthous Ulcer

Recurrent aphthous ulcers(RAU). The prevalence rate is the first in oral mucosa disease. Epidemiological surveys in various countries show that about 1 people in every 5 people have at least one ulcer, and both men and women, any age, and any species can occur. This disease is characterized by periodicity, recurrence and self limitation.

6.3.1 Etiology

Modern medicine believes that recurrent aphthous ulcers are closely related to immunity. Some patients show immune deficiency and some patients show autoimmune reactions; secondly, it is associated with heredity. In clinical, recurrent aphthous ulcers have a distinct familial genetic tendency. One or more parents have recurrent aphthous ulcers, and their children are more likely to be ill than the average person. In addition, the onset of recurrent aphthous ulcers is associated with some diseases or symptoms such as digestive diseases: gastric ulcers, duodenal ulcers, chronic or migrated ductile hepatitis, colitis, etc., as well as partial food, dyspepsia, fever, sleep deficiency, excessive fatigue, stress, changes of the menstrual cycle, etc. RAV frequently occur as a result of an active or alternation of one or more factors.

6.3.2　Clinical manifestation

There are three main types of clinical manifestations: light aphtha, severe aphtha and herpetiform ulcer.

6.3.2.1　Light aphtha

Light aphtha, also known as mild recurrent aphthous ulcer, accounts for about 80% of RAU patients. The ulcers often occur in the mucosa with no keratinization or keratinization on the lips, tongue, cheek, soft palate, etc. At the beginning of RAU, focal mucosal hyperemia and edema appeared, with miliary red spots, burning pain, and then forming superficial ulcer, round or oval, with a diameter less than 5 mm. About 5 days, the ulcer began to heal. At this time, the ulcer surface had granulation tissue formation, wound narrowing, redness swelling subsided, and pain relieved. About 7−10 days, the ulcer healed without scarring. Mild recurrent aphthous ulcers are usually distributed in 3−5 cases. The interval between ulceration and relapse varies from half a month to a few months. Some patients have a regular onset cycle, such as before and after menstruation, and some patients often suffer from fatigue. General symptoms and signs were not obvious.

6.3.2.2　Severe aphtha

Also known as recurrent necrotizing mucosal periadenitis, the ulcer is large and deep, and it can form scar or tissue defect after healing. It is also known as recurrent scarring aphtha, accounting for about 8%. The ulcer of the periodontic ulcer is large and deep, like a "crater". It can reach the submucosa glands and the tissue of the gland. The diameter of the ulcer is more than 1 cm, the surrounding tissue is red and swollen, and bulge, the basement is slightly hard, the surface has a gray yellow false film or gray white necrotic tissue, which lasted for a long time, up to 1−2 months or longer. Usually 1−2 ulcers, but there are one or several small ulcers during the healing process. The pain is intense and the scar can be left after healing. The initial onset of the mouth, followed by the tendency to move toward the posterior mouth, palate arch, soft and hard palate, which could cause tissue defects and affect talking swallowing. Often accompanied by low fever, fatigue, and other symptoms of systemic discomfort and lymphadenia in the local area of the disease. Ulcers can also recur at the previous healing site, causing greater scarring and tissue defects.

6.3.2.3　Herpetiform ulcer(HU)

About 10% of RAU patients. Oral aphthous ulcers are mostly found in adult women. But the ulcer diameter is smaller, about 2 mm, ulcers can last more than ten or dozens of days, scattered in the distribution, like "full sky star". Adjacent ulcers can be fused into slices, mucosal congestion, redness, the heaviest pain and increased salivary secretion. It can be accompanied by headache, low fever, general discomfort, localized lymphedema and other symptoms.

6.3.3　Diagnosis

The diagnosis can be made according to the medical history and clinical signs. It has periodic recurrent episodes, and the course of disease is limited. If the course of oral ulcer is long or the accompanying symptoms of other diseases, the primary disease should also be checked.

6.3.4 Treatment

The etiology of recurrent aphthous ulcers is not clear, so there are many treatment methods, but there are no special treatment methods, but first, we should keep the mouth clean and give a systemic drug, especially those with abnormal immune function when the condition is serious. Active treatment is necessary for possible factors. Pay attention to the internal mucosa from the friction of hard objects, eat less excellent food, and avoid bites.

6.3.4.1 Local treatment

Local treatment is mainly anti-inflammatory, analgesic, and promote ulcer healing. 0.1% -0.2% chlorhexidine gluconate solution, 0.5% polyvidone iodine solution, 0.1% ethacridine solution, 0.2% cetylpyridnium chloride gargle or compound boric acid solution can be used to gargle. Lysozyme tablets 20 mg and 0.5 mg were added 3-4 times a day. Pain relief can be made by using compound chamomile lidocaine in local ulcer and can be cured by local recombinant human epidermal growth factor for external use. There was no longer healing of the deep sore, with 0.5-1 mL of triamcinolone suspension or prednisolone suspension, and 2% procaine for 0.3-0.5 mL injection in the basal part of the ulcer, once a week.

6.3.4.2 Systemic treatment

Systemic treatment for recurrent, more severe or long-term ulcers may consider systemic treatment to reduce recurrence and promote healing, especially for the cause of treatment, such as immunization with an immune additive in low cellular immune functions, which can often improve the efficacy. In clinic, transfer factor and levamisole are often used to improve the immune function of patients. Transfer factor oral liquid 10 mL, orally, 1-2 times a day, 10 times as a course of treatment. Transfer factor capsules 3 mg, 2 times a day. Adenoid aphtha can be given thalidomide. The adult dose is 100 mg, 2 times a day, orally, 1 week later, 50 mg/d, for 1-2 months. The main adverse reaction is teratogenicity, which is forbidden by pregnant women. Long term application can cause peripheral neuritis, and the total dose should be controlled at 40-50 g.

6.4 Pemphigus

Pemphigus is a group of bullous dermatosis. The clinical manifestation of pemphigus is very easy to break blister appearing on the skin and mucous membrane. There is no obvious inflammation in the basement; it is often difficult to heal without treatment.

6.4.1 Etiology

The cause of pemphigus is still unclear. It is an autoimmune disease, and its autoantigen may be the desmosomes of epidermis (epithelial) cells. Clinically, the following aspects are observed, such as drugs, cancer, and other immune diseases, which are related to pemphigus.

6.4.2 Clinical manifestation

Pemphigus can be classified into four types: vulgaris, proliferative, deciduous and erythematous pemphigus. Common pemphigus type in oral is the vulgaris.

6.4.2.1　Vulgaris pemphigus

(1)Oral cavity:it is the site of early lesions. Before the blister often have a dry mouth, dry throat, or swallowing pain, there are 1-2 or widely different size of the blister, Thin and transparent are, blister easily broken, irregular erosion surface. After breaking the residual blister wall, if the bullous wall is removed or extracted, often together with the adjacent appearance normal sticky. The film is painlessly torn away, leaving behind a bright red wound. This phenomenon is called positive skin lift test. If the probe is gently placed under the mucosa at the edge of the erosive surface, the probe is painless. This is the phenomenon of spinous release. It is meaningful for diagnosis. Damage can occur in the soft palate, hard palate, pharyngeal side and other vulnerable parts. Secondary infection is aggravated and pain is aggravated.

(2)Skin:it often appear in the chest, trunk and scalp, neck, armpit, groin and other vulnerable parts. At the early stage of the disease, systemic symptoms were not obvious. Only 1-2 vesicles were found in the anterior chest or trunk. On normal skin, there is often a sudden appearance of different sizes of blister, the blister does not fuse, the blister wall is thin and slack, the blister is clear or cloudy(it is a light yellow transparent serum). Use hand press blister top, liquid spreads to all round, blister is easy to break, expose the erosive surface that is red wet after breaking. After infection, it can be suppurative and form pus and blood blisters. It has a stench, scabby gradually, and after healing, it leaves a deep pigmentation. If the blister does not break, it can gradually become dry and shrivelled after the turbid.

The bullous bullis can be quickly formed by pushing the normal skin or mucous membrane by the finger laterally;pushing the blister can make it move on the skin;in the mouth, licking and mucous membrane with the tongue can shed or tear the surface of the mucous membrane. These phenomena are called Nissl's sign. The diagnostic value of the examination is compared.

6.4.2.2　Proliferative pemphigus

Oral presentation is the same as pemphigus vulgaris, but there is a significant proliferation in the lip margin. Skin lesions occurred before or after oral mucosa damage, common in the axillary, umbilical and anal and other wrinkles, still the bullous, Nissl's sign positive, after the blisters were broken on the erosive surface mushroom like and papilloma like proliferation, it was covered with yellow thick scab and exudate, smell of odor, surrounded by red halo, conscious pain.

6.4.2.3　Deciduous pemphigus

The primary damage is the erythematous basal surface, which can appear as a blister with, thin wall, and easy to break up, forming a shallow erosive surface, with scab on the erythematous basement. Oral damage is rare.

6.4.2.4　Erythematous pemphigus

Erythematous pemphigus is found in the cheek and other seborrheic areas. No or rare oral damage.

6.4.3　Diagnosis

Oral mucous membrane lesions are most common and usually appear in pemphigus vulgaris. It is important for doctors in department of stomatology to make early diagnosis. According to the clinical manifestation, the blister or bright red erosive surface was found in the oral mucosa, the growth of the edge is positive, the water droplet like blisters of the skin are different, the Nissl's sign is positive, and the diagnosis is easy to be confirmed by the smear of exfoliated cells and the pathological examination of immunology or histopathology.

6.4.4 Treatment

6.4.4.1 Support treatment

Pay attention to supplement protein food, vitamin, appropriate supplement plasma or whole blood. We should pay attention to the nutrition of patients, give high protein and highcalorie diet, and regularly supplement calcium, potassium and various vitamins.

6.4.4.2 Glucocorticoid hormone

The drug is the first choice for the disease. The first dose of light, medium and heavy patients should be 40 mg, 60 mg and 80 mg respectively. If there are still new blisters within 3–7 days, it can be increased by 50% on the first dose until the condition is controlled. After 2 weeks of disappearance, the lesion began to slow down regularly, reduced initially at 2–4 weeks, reduced 1 times in the next 4–8 weeks, and reduced 10%–15% times each time until maintenance.

6.4.4.3 Immunosuppressant

When combined with corticosteroids, such as cyclophosphamide, azathioprine, methotrexate, cyclosporin, and mycophenolate, it may lead to early control of the disease and increase the probability of clinical remission.

6.4.4.4 Local drug use

Mouth erosion and pain, before eating can be 1%–2% lidocaine gel or gargle local wipe or gargle, gargle to help maintain oral hygiene. In addition, topical use of various kinds of ointment, paste and gel suitable for oral cavity helps to promote healing of oral erosion surface.

6.5 Oral Leukoplakia

Oral leukoplakia refers to white patches on oral mucosa, which can not be diagnosed by clinical and histopathological methods. The WHO classified it as a precancerous lesion and defined that oral leukoplakia is a white–based lesion on the oral mucosa and does not have any other definable damage characteristics; a part of oral leukoplakia can be transformed into cancer.

6.5.1 Etiology

The cause of oral leukoplakia is unknown, but it is known to be related to smoking, drinking, chewing areca, Candida infection and toxic substances and carcinogens in the environment. Mechanical stimulation, temperature stimulation, current stimulation or bad repair in the oral cavity can also cause leukoplakia.

6.5.2 Clinical manifestation

According to different clinical manifestations, it can be divided into homogeneous and heterogeneous type. Heterogeneous type can be divided into verrucous, ulcerative and granular type.

6.5.2.1 Homogenization type

White or gray white, homogeneous and hard plaques appear on the oral mucosa. The texture is compact, and the damage is not equal to the area. The surface is crumpled, or there is a small crack. No conscious symptoms, or rough feeling.

6.5.2.2   Particle type

It's also known as granular nodular leukoplakia. Buccal mucosa mouth area is more common. The white lesions are granular like protuberances, resulting in uneven mucosal surface, mucosal hyperemia, and small patches or punctate erosion. Most Candida albicans infection can be found in this type of leukoplakia.

6.5.2.3   Verrucous type

Damage to the uplift, uneven surface, accompanied by papillary or burr shaped, palpation hard. Except for gingiva orpalate, there was no obvious induration on the base, and the rough area was obvious in the lesion area.

6.5.2.4   Ulcerative type

On thickened white plaques, there are erosions or ulcers, with or without local irritation. Patients usually have pain due to the formation of ulcers.

6.5.3   Diagnosis

According to the clinical manifestation, the diagnosis depends on the histopathology. Histopathological examination was simple hyperplasia and abnormal hyperplasia. Leukoplakia is a precancerous lesion with potential malignancy. At present, according to WHO and domestic research data, the incidence of leukoplakia is 3% – 5%.

The following conditions and problems are worth paying attention to the possibility of canceration.

6.5.3.1   Clinical type

The malignant change tendency of leukoplakia is closely related to the clinical type, and the malignant change rate of the granulated and ulcerative type is high, so we should pay special attention to the heterogeneous leukoplakia in clinic to guard against the malignant change.

6.5.3.2   The lesion site

The base of mouth, ventral tongue, buccal mucosa, soft palate complex are the risk factors of malignant transformation.

6.5.3.3   Smoking situation

Long and heavy smoking history.

6.5.3.4   Histopathology

Pathological examination showed atypical hyperplasia of epithelium.

6.5.3.5   Candida albicans infection

Leukoplakia combined with Candida albicans infection has a more malignant tendency.

6.5.3.6   Leukoplakia without obvious causes

Clinically, it is found that female patients with unknown cause should be prevented from malignant transformation.

6.5.3.7   Pathological changes

For patients with longer pathological changes, heavier symptoms, irritation or spontaneous pain.

6.5.4   Treatment

(1) Removal of possible pathogenic factors, such as smoking cessation and removing the bad denture. For small area lesions, surgical removal, laser and cryopreservation can be used. But it must be reviewed

regularly.

(2) Conservative treatment: the 0.2% dimensional A acid solution is suitable for topical application, but it does not apply to the damage associated with congestion and erosion. Close follow-up should be made during conservative treatment.

(3) The disease with Candida albicans infection can be combined with antifungal therapy.

(4) In the leukoplakia area, it is necessary to remove the ulcer as early as possible when it is found that the ulcer or the base is hard and the surface is thickened.

6.6 Oral Lichen Planus

Oral lichen planus(OLP) is a chronic inflammatory disease of skin and mucous membrane, which can occur alonein the oral cavity or skin, and can also occur at the same time. Damage can be seen in the oral cavity, but also in the genitals, nails and/or toenails, but relatively rare. There are more women pawents in middle age. WHO is included in precancerous condition because of its malignant degeneration.

6.6.1 Etiology

The etiology of lichen planus is unknown. It is generally believed that the pathogenesis of lichen planus may be related to psychological factors, endocrine factors, viral infection, autoimmunity and heredity.

6.6.1.1 Psychological factors

In clinic, it is common to cause dysfunction of the body due to psychological abnormality, which causes the onset of OLP, aggravates the condition, or recurs and delays.

6.6.1.2 Endocrine factors

Epidemiological survey showed that the incidence of OLP was higher in middle-aged women. Studies have shown that some female OLP patients are relieved during pregnancy and relapse after menstrual recovery after lactation.

6.6.1.3 Immune factors

The pathological examination shows that a largenumber of lymphocytes in the lamina propria of OLP are one of the typical pathological manifestations, so OLP is considered to be related to the immune factors. Clinically, the use of corticosteroids and chloroquine and other immunosuppressive agents is effective, and it is also proved that the disease is related to immune factors.

6.6.1.4 Factors of infection

Virus infection may be one of the pathogenic factors.

6.6.1.5 Systemic disease

Many patients with lichen planus are associated with the existence of some systemic diseases, such as diabetes, chronic hepatitis, hypertension, and thyroid diseases.

6.6.1.6 Factors of microcirculation disorder

The microvascular morphology of OLP patients was significantly changed, and their expansion and congestion were significantly higher than those of the normal group.

6.6.1.7 Genetic factors

The disease has a familial hereditary tendency.

6.6.2   Clinical manifestation

6.6.2.1   Oral mucosa damage

The main feature is pearlite white papules or stripes. White stripes can be woven into mesh orden-drites. They can also be single lines or circular. Damage often has obvious left and right symmetry, soft mu-cous membrane, normal elasticity, but rough feeling, mild irritation pain.

Oral cavity is more common in buccal mucosa and vestibular groove, followed by tongue, lip and gingi-va. The lesion is often symmetrical. The incidence of mucosal damage is about 25%, which can be seen in mucous membrane and concurrent with skin. The most common damage is white stripes. It is divided into the following types.

(1) Papular type

Gray papules strewn on mucous membranes, sometimes aggregated to form small plaques. There were no clinical symptoms.

(2) Mesh type

White reticulate stripe is found on the oral mucosa. Asymptomatic in clinical, occasionally rough feel-ing.

(3) Plaque type

This type is commonly seen in smokers and occurs on the back of the tongue and cheek. Atrophy of the dorsal lingual papilla results in a white, glossy patch.

(4) Atrophic type

It is commonly seen in the gums, often in the attached gingiva, and also in the buccal mucosa. Lesions tend to form erosive surfaces and are sensitive to irritating food.

(5) Erosive type (ulcerative type)

The lesion is ulcerated to form erosive surface and is easy to merge secondary infection. The patient has a sense of pain.

(6) Blister type

It is rare. It often occurs on the back of the tongue or gingiva, and is prone to erosion.

6.6.2.2   Skin damage

The skin lesion of lichen planus is characterized by shallow and glossy light purple red polygonal pap-ules. The papules are like the size of the mung bean. The edge is clear, the texture is hard and dry, and the fusion is the moss. The lesion area is rough, and the skin is wrinkled between papules. There are many scratches due to itching. Paraffin oil is applied to the papule surface. Under the magnifying glass, we can see fine white stripes, called Wickham's lines.

6.6.2.3   Damage to nails and (or) toenails

It is usually symmetrical. The body is thinner and without gloss. There are sunken in press. The surface of the armor body can be shown as the longitudinal furrow, point gap and cutting surface of the fine scale. Serious injuries to the fingers and toenails can cause abscission of the nail body and ulcers.

6.6.3   Diagnosis

The diagnosis can be made according to the clinical manifestation. Oral lichen planus has been consid-ered as a precancerous state, such as lesions that occur in dangerous areas, plaque type, atrophic type and recurrent erosion are recommended for pathological examination.

6.6.4 Treatment

(1)Patients without symptoms also need to be treated and observed regularly.

(2)Limited erosive lesions can be injected with steroids at the erosive base(prednisolone 0.5 mL plus lidocaine 0.3-0.5 mL).1 times a week.0.1%-0.2% chlorhexidine solution,0.5% povidone iodine solution,0.1% ethacridine solution,0.2% cetylpyridnium chloride gargle or compound boric acid solution can be used. Lysozyme tablets 20 mg and 0.5 mg are added 3-4 times a day.

(3)Patients with extensive erosive lichen planus may consider local and systemic treatment.

1)Glucocorticoid:careful consideration should be given to a small dose and short course of treatment. Adults can choose prednisone 15-30 mg/d for 1-4 weeks.

2)Hydroxychloroquine:the initial dose of 0.125 mg/d,can be added to 0.25 mg for 3 months to half a year after 1 weeks of medication.

3)Tripterygium glycosides:10-20 mg,orally,3 times a day.1 months for a course of treatment.

(4)Long term ulcers or histologic manifestations of atypical epithelial hyperplasia can be surgically removed.

(5)Treatment of traditional Chinese medicine.

6.7　Oral Manifestations of Sexually Transmitted Diseases

6.7.1　Syphilis

Syphilis is a common sexually transmitted disease,which is infected by the pallid spirals. It has been published for hundreds of years. It is now distributed worldwide and is a very important sexually transmitted disease. It can be divided into congenital syphilis,acquired syphilis,etc.

6.7.1.1　Etiology

The pathogen of syphilis is Treponema pallidum,an anaerobic microorganism,which is not easy to survive after leaving the human body. Boiling,drying,daylight,soapy water and ordinary disinfectants can kill it quickly. The cold tolerance is strong,and it can survive for 3 days at 4 ℃,and it is still contagious for several years at -78 ℃.

The only source of contagion for syphilis is syphilis. Helicoid was found in skin lesions,blood, semen,milk and saliva. Treponema pallidum can only pass through the mucosa but can not pass through the normal skin. It is easy to survive in the humid parts of the pudendum. Therefore,syphilis is mainly transmitted by sexual behavior.

6.7.1.2　Clinical manifestation

Syphilis is divided into corgential syphilis and acquired syphilis. The latter is divided into 3 stages,1st stage 2nd stage syphilis and late syphilis. The first stage and the second stage of the disease in 2 years are called early syphilis. Over 2 years,it is called late syphilis.

(1)Acquired syphilis

1)1st stage syphilis:treponema pallidum enters the skin or mucosa. It begins to propagate and cause local inflammation. After 2-4 weeks,the ulcer and erosion occur at the entry site of helicoid,called chancre. Chancre is most common in males,such as coronal sulcus,glans and penis. Chancre is more than 1,sometimes also more hair,a single diameter is 1-2 cm,a circular or oval painless ulcer,the edge of a bulge,a clean surface without pus,the touch of cartilage-like hardness,it is also called hard chancre. A few days after the chancre,the regional lymph node enlargement,the perineum infection is the inguinal lymph node inflammation,its characteristic is the lymph node enlargement,the activity,but does not ache nor break. The chancre usually subsidise in 1 month. Lips,palate,pharynx and other parts of the oral mucosal syphilis lesion site,showing a single diameter 1-2 cm round or oval painless ulcers.

2)2nd stage syphilis:after the chancre subsided,the helicoid still continued to propagate in the body. After a period of syphilis,it could invade the skin mucous membrane and the whole body within 1-2 months. Most of the two syphilis symptoms occur successively or simultaneously within 2 years after infection.

Syphilis plague rash is the most important symptom. It is characterized by wide symmetrical distribution of the whole body,and the most frequently invaded parts of the palms,metatarsus,anus,and genitals. After a few weeks or months,the rash naturally subsided. The rash in the two stage of syphilis is mainly macular and papules. The most common form of rash is the symmetrical distribution of the whole body,which occurs in the palm and feet with copper red scales. Papules can be either large or small,and small group of patients with integrated or mossy syphilis. A small number of patients,especially those with HIV infection,have obvious prodromal symptoms and appear diffuse papules,pustules and ulcers,known as malignant syphilis.

Mucous patches on the lips,cheeks and tongue can be seen as round or oval gray mucous patches. The patches with gray,white,light,and micro roots are usually round,oval or annular,and the central part is prone to congestion and erosion. These lesions may have a large number of spirals on the surface and are highly contagious.

3)3rd stage syphilis:untreated syphilis patients still have 40% late onset symptoms after 2-3 or 10 years of infection. Late syphilis can invade all organs of the body,and syphilis is the most common skin and mucous membrane. The number of Borrelia in the lesion is very low,and the infection gradually decreases,but the severity of the damage is increased. The damage of skin,mucous membrane and bone marrow began to be limited to some parts,in which the limbs,head,face and back are good locations. Although without pain,it often causes great damage,and the scar is often left behind. 10 years later,it gradually invades important organs such as cardiovascular system and central nervous system.

The gum swelling can occur at any part of the mouth,the tongue,the hard palate and the soft palate are often infringed. The syphilis or the gum swelling is the granulation tissue produced by the third stage syphilis,showing an elastic mass,the central necrosis,the wave motion,and then break,so the palate syphilis can lead to the perforation of the soft and hard tissue. Most of the syphilis of the tongue are diffuse interstitial glossitis,so it is lobulated,with cleft and atrophy of the tongue,and often accompanied by white keratosis of the tongue and leukoplakia on the edge of atrophy.

(2)Congenital syphilis

Pregnant women with early syphilis are prone to stillbirth or preterm birth; the infants of late syphilis may have congenital syphilis at the age of 4 or at the age of 10-16,known as early and late congenital syphilis,and the latter has no infection. The Hutchinson teeth and mulberry teeth are the characteristics of advanced congenital syphilis.

6.7.1.3 Diagnosis

The diagnosis of syphilis should be based on the history and clinical manifestations,and reliable laboratory examinations. For example,spiral body examination,Syphilis serological test,etc.

6.7.1.4 Treatment

Principles of treatment:early,adequate,regular medication,regular follow-up after treatment. There should be no sexual life during the treatment. Sexual partners should be treated at the same time.

(1) Early syphilis (including first, second stage, early late syphilis): penicillin 800 thousand units, 1 times a day for 10–15 days, the total amount of 8 million U to 12 million U. Benzyl penicillin 2 400 000 U, on both sides of the hip muscle intramuscular injection, 1 times a week, a total of 2–3 times. For penicillin allergy, erythromycin or doxycycline was used, erythromycin 500 mg daily, 4 times a day, orally for 30 days, and 2 times a day.

(2) Late syphilis (including third stage, second stage relapse and late latent syphilis): penicillin 800 thousand U, once a day, muscle injection, 15 consecutive days, the total amount of 12 million U, 2 weeks interval for second courses, the total amount of 24 million U. Benzyl penicillin 2 million 400 thousand U, on both sides of the hip muscle intramuscular injection, once a week, a total of 3 times. Erythromycin or doxycycline can be used for penicillin allergy with early syphilis.

After the treatment of syphilis, it should be regularly followed up for 2–3 years.

6.7.2 Acquired immuno deficiency syndrome (AIDS)

AIDS is the abbreviation of acquired immunodeficiency syndrome. It is caused by the sexual transmission with by the human immunodeficiency virus (HIV) and the infectious disease that can be transmitted through the blood. Its characteristic is that CD4 cell immune function is seriously damaged by HIV, which leads to various opportunistic infections. Finally, many malignant tumors occur and cause death.

6.7.2.1 Etiology

AIDS is caused by HIV. HIV is a retroviral RNA virus, and the cell membrane is sprout. The size of the virus particles is 100–140 nm and has a special tendency to T lymphocytes. For the heat sensitive, 56 ℃ and 30 minutes inactivation, many chemicals can inactivate HIV quickly, such as ether, acetone, 2% hypochlorite, 50% ethanol, 10% bleaching powder, 2% amyl glycol with 4% Formaldehyde Solution and so on. But it is not sensitive to ultraviolet light.

AIDS patients and asymptomatic HIV carriers are the source of infection. Especially the latter is more dangerous because of their latent illness. Viruses can exist in patients' blood, semen, uterus and vaginal secretions, saliva, tears, milk, urine, cerebrospinal fluid and amniotic fluid.

6.7.2.2 Clinical manifestation

(1) General manifestation

1) Acute HIV infection: fever, fatigue, myalgia, joint pain, pharynx, diarrhea, and general discomfort like influenza symptoms, it can be scattered in the rash, mainly in the torso spot papules, rose rash or urticaria; a few patients have headache, meningoencephalitis, peripheral phlogistic or acute multiple neuritis; there are enlarged lymph nodes in the neck, armpit and occipital region, similar to infectious mononucleosis.

2) Asymptomatic HIV infection: often without any symptoms and signs, some patients with infection may develop persistent systemic lymphadenopathy. This period is the incubation period of AIDS, usually 2 – 15 years, with an average of 8–10 years, but it can also be short to several months or prolonged to 20 years.

3) AIDS period: unexplained immune function; persistent irregular low fever for more than 1 months; persistent generalized lymphadenopathy (lymph node diameter greater than 1 cm); chronic diarrhea more than 4–5 times/d, weight loss more than 10% in 3 months; combined oral Candida infection, Pneumocystis carinii pneumonia infection of cytomegalovirus (CMV), herpes virus infection, toxoplasmosis, Cryptococcus neoformans meningitis, rapid active tuberculosis, Kaposi sarcoma of skin mucosa, lymphoma and so on. Dementia is found in young patients.

(2) Oral manifestation

The oral presentation of AIDS is one of the important diagnostic indicators of the disease. Most HIV infected patients have oral manifestations. Many patients developed oral lesions at the initial stage and first visited the Department of Stomatology. The most common oral manifestations are Candida albicans infection, hairy leukoplakia and Kaposi sarcoma.

1) Oral candidal infection: oral candidiasis is the most common oral lesion in HIV infection. More than 90% of the HIV infected patients can have false membrane, atrophic Candida infection or candidal stomatitis at different stages of the disease.

2) Oral hairy leukoplakia: about 30% HIV of the infected person developed oral hairy leukoplakia during the course of the disease. The damage is most common in the bilateral lingual border mucosa, which extends to the back of the tongue mucosa and abdomen. The damage is white wrinkles and can not be erased. More common in men. Hairy leukoplakia is now widely recognized as a special oral damage of AIDS infected people, highly suggestive of AIDS, and other diseases rarely appear hairy leukoplakia.

3) Kaposi sarcoma: a common tumor of HIV infection. The tumor can occur in the skin and in the oral mucosa. In the oral cavity, the palate is the best part and the second is the gum. The tumor has deep red or purplish red nodules or patches. The finger pressure does not fade, and there are yellow brown ecchymosis around it.

4) AIDS related periodontitis: a series of periodontal diseases can occur in AIDS patients.

Linear gingival erythema: the gingival margin is characterized by obvious red andred congestion, with clear boundaries, spontaneous gingival bleeding or bleeding after brushing. Oral local treatment is not effective.

Acute necrotizing gingivitis periodontitis: gingival ulcer, necrosis, alveolar bone destruction and obvious pain in the short term.

6.7.2.3 Diagnosis

The diagnosis must be based on comprehensive analysis of epidemiological contact history, clinical manifestations and laboratory findings, and careful diagnosis. In any stage of HIV infection, laboratory tests for anti HIV antibodies or HIV antigens are necessary.

HIV laboratory examination methods include virus isolation and culture, antibody detection, antigen detection, viral nucleic acid detection and viral load detection.

6.7.2.4 Treatment

Treatment principle: for asymptomatic HIV infection, in general, only pay attention to rest, strengthen nutrition, avoid infecting others. For symptomatic patients, the anti HIV treatment should be adopted according to the HIV infection in different periods of the disease, the treatment of pathogens and various complications, including support, immunoregulation and psychotherapy.

(1) Antiretroviral therapy has three broad categories of chemotherapeutic agents. These include nucleoside reverse transcriptase inhibitors, non nucleoside reverse transcriptase inhibitors and protease inhibitors, which should be combined.

(2) Immunoregulatory therapy is used mainly for immunomodulating drugs such as interferon alpha, interleukin 2(IL-2), and gamma globulin, such as letinous edodespolysaccharide, Salvia miltiorrhiza, Astragalus and glycyrrhizin.

(3) The treatment of comorbidities is aimed at the treatment of various infections and tumors.

1) Oral candidiasis: local and systemic use of antifungal drugs, such as oral fluconazole 100 mg/d(the highest dose to 800 mg/d) or itraconazole 200 mg/d. In patients with tolerance to fluconazole or other azolic drugs, the suspension of amphotericin B was 1-5 mL, 4 times a day, swallowed after gargling, and itraconazole 200 mg/d. Local use of clotrimazole lozenge 10 mg, 4 times a day, alkaline mouthwash gargle, angular

stomatitis can be used miconazole ointment erasure. The lesions disappeared after 10-14 days of treatment. Effective antiviral therapy should be carried out at the same time to rebuild immune function, otherwise it will relapse easily. In order to prevent recurrence, maintenance treatment is often used, local use of the same, the whole body use of fluconazole 100 mg/d or itraconazole 200 mg/d, the treatment of the patient's liver function should be monitored.

2) Hairy leukoplakia: severe cases can be treated with acyclic guanosine 2-3 g/d for 2-3 weeks. It is easy to relapse after withdrawal. High dose acyclic guanosine (A Silowe) can be used for maintenance treatment. Ganciclovir is the same effective drug as acyclic guanosine. Hairy leukoplakia can also disappear after highly active antiretroviral therapy.

3) Kaposi sarcoma: surgical excision, cauterization, curettage or cryotherapy. Attention should be paid to preventing secondary infection, which can be combined with radiotherapy and local chemotherapy. Chemotherapeutic drugs often include vincristine, doxorubicin, anthracycline antibiotics and etoposide. In addition, it can also be combined with biologic therapy.

6.7.2.5 Prevention

AIDS is not yet cured, and its vaccine research has not yet been successful. Prevention is particularly important.

(1) Carry out health education, popularize basic knowledge of AIDS prevention and control, and understand its transmission routes and main protective measures. We should strengthen moral education, ban commercial sex workers and prohibit sexual promiscuity, especially avoid sexual contact with HIV infected persons, AIDS patients and high-risk groups. Promote safe sex and use condoms. Carry out consultation on HIV infection and AIDS.

(2) The use of blood, blood components and blood products, must be tested by HIV, encouraging and implementing the voluntary blood donation system, donation of blood, organ, tissue and semen should betested by HIV.

(3) To prevent iatrogenic infection, sterilized syringes, needles and surgical instruments must be sterilized. Disposable syringes and needles should be used where conditions permit.

(4) Women who are infected with HIV or HIV should avoid pregnancy. They should be given abortion if they are pregnant, and direct breastfeeding should be avoided for babies who have been born.

(5) Oral doctors and nurses should have a high degree of responsibility and good professional habits, pay attention to self protection, avoid direct contact with HIV blood or body fluids, wear latex gloves, eye mask, mask, isolation clothes, and totally sterilize. The protocol disinfection and sterilization should be carried out.

Zhao Hongyu

Chapter 7

Local Dental Anesthesia

Local anesthesia is the use of local anesthetics to temporarily block the sensory conduction of nerve terminals and fibers in a certain area and make the part lose the sense of pain. The exact meaning is local painless, but other feelings, such as touch pressure and sense of temperature, still remain, and the patient remains conscious.

7.1 Characteristics of Local Anesthesia

Dentists can operate independently, without anesthesiologists participation, also do not need special equipment, no special preoperative preparation, postoperative patients awake, without special care. It's much safer. The combined use of local anesthetic and vasoconstrictor can obviously prolong the time of anesthesia, and make the operation area clear and easy to operate. But local anesthesia is not suitable for patient who can not cooperation(such as disorientation and pediatric patients) and local to the site of inflammation.

7.2 Selection of Local Anesthetics

The local anesthetic has the nerve impulse conduction block, and should have the following properties: pharmacological anesthetic effect completely, to the injection site organization without stimulation, does not cause the unreversible neural structures trauma; fast, lasting for a long time; safe, no obvious toxic reaction after absorbed; soluble in a proper solvent, particularly soluble in water; stable, resistant to high temperature high pressure disinfection, and other ingredients such as vasoconstriction medicines and not easy decomposition. There are many kinds of local anesthetics, which can be divided into esters and amides according to their chemical structure. The common local drugs in China are procaine and tetracaine, and lidocaine, bupivacaine and articaine.

7.2.1 Procaine(or novocaine)

The water solution of procaine is unstable when it is alkaline, and it is easily decomposed and failed.

The anesthetic effect is true, the toxicity and side effect is small, the price is low, so it is a kind of local anesthesia medicine which is widely used in clinical practice. The quality of this product is poor in penetration and dispersion, so it is not suitable for surface anesthesia. Because of its obvious vasodilating effect, a small amount of adrenaline is often applied to slow down the absorption of procaine and prolong the time of anesthesia. The commonly used solution with a concentration of 1% –2% is not more than 1 g per time. Procaine and other esters of local anesthetics are used together because they sometimes produce anaphylaxis, and an allergy test is needed before it is used, so it is not used for local anesthesia at present.

7.2.2　Lidocaine(or xylocaine)

Lidocaine is much more stable than procaine in hydrochloride solution. The local anesthetic effect is stronger than procaine, and the maintenance time is longer, and has strong tissue penetrability and diffusivity, so it can also be used as surface anesthesia. However, the clinical application is mainly based on 1% –2% lidocaine containing 1 : 100,000−1 : 200,000 adrenaline. It is the most widely used local anesthetic in Department of Stomatology. Lidocaine also has a rapid and safe effect on ventricular arrhythmias and is often the preferred local anesthetic for patients with arrhythmia. The toxicity of this product is larger than procaine. When used as local anesthetic, the dosage should be smaller than procaine, and not more than 0. 4 g per time.

7.2.3　Bupivacaine(or marcaine)

The duration of anesthesia of lidocaine, usually up to more than 5 h, which is 4 times the strength of lidocaine anesthesia. Usually 0. 5% solution is shared with 1 : 200,000 epinephrine. The drug has low concentration in blood and little accumulation in body. It is a safe and long−acting local anesthetic, especially suitable for time −consuming operation. Postoperative analgesia time is longer. The maximum amount is not more than 200 mg per time.

7.2.4　Tetracaine(or pantocaine)

Tetracaine is soluble in water, strong penetration. It is mainly used as a surface anaesthesia. The anesthetic effect was 10−15 times stronger than procaine, and the toxicity was 10−20 times larger than procaine. As a result of large toxicity, no infiltration anesthesia is usually done. That is, the use of surface anesthesia also should pay attention to the dose, usually 1% –2% solution, each 3 mL added 0. 1% adrenaline solution 1 drops, the total amount is not more than 20 mg. Sustainable 20−40 minutes. It is not used in clinical anesthesia and block anesthesia.

7.2.5　Articaine(or primacaine)

The onset time is 2−3 minutes. It is tissue permeability, anesthesia high efficiency, little side effects, and now it has been widely used in clinical.

7.2.6　The function and use of vasoconstrictor

The clinical application of local anesthesia often adds vasoconstrictor in the anesthetic solution, which is due to the rich blood flow in the oral and maxillofacial region and the rapid absorption of local anesthetics. In order to postpone the absorption, enhance the analgesic effect, prolong the time of local anesthesia, reduce the toxic reaction and reduce the bleeding in the operative area, it is necessary to add the vasoconstrictor in the local anesthetic solution.

The common adrenaline is added to the local anesthetic solution at the concentration of 1 : 100,000. The trace adrenaline(1 : 200,000 – 1 : 400,000) does not cause significant change in blood pressure. It will not cause adverse reactions to cardiovascular disease or diabetes. It has good analgesic effect, and therefore is an important measure to eliminate the fear and unease of the sick and avoid the sharp fluctuation of blood pressure caused by the pain.

7.3 Method of Local Anesthesia

The common local anesthesia methods in oral and maxillofacial surgery include surface anesthesia, infiltration anaesthesia and block(conduction) anesthesia.

7.3.1 Surface anesthesia

Surface anesthesia is also known as coating anesthesia, which is to coat or spray anesthetic drugs on the surface of the operative area, and anesthetic drugs are absorbed to make peripheral nerve palsy, so as to achieve the effect of pain relief. This method is adapted to the superficial submucosal abscess incision and drainage, the removal of loose teeth or permanent teeth, and the mucosal surface anaesthesia before endotracheal intubation. The commonly used drug is 2% tetracaine hydrochloride, which has a strong anesthetic effect. However, because of the large toxicity and vasodilator effect, it should increase the speed of drug absorption. For topical anesthesia, we should pay special attention to dosage(not more than 20 mg) or add a small amount of epinephrine to slow down the absorption of tissue into tetracaine.

7.3.2 Infiltration anesthesia

Infiltration anesthesia is injected into the tissue of the local anesthetic, which is mainly used in the nerve endings to lose the ability to transmit the pain and to produce the anesthetic effect. When the dosage of liquid is large, the concentration is low. The commonly used local anesthetic solution is 0.5% – 1% of procaine or 0.25% – 0.75% of lidocaine. The surgery of the soft tissue in the oral and maxillofacial region is often used for the nerve endings. The commonly used methods of infiltration anesthesia are as below.

7.3.2.1 Wheal injection

Wheal injection: the method for injecting a small amount of local anesthetic solution to the skin and mucosa to form a small wheal, then the incision along the line, from shallow to deep layer is injected into the area of the operation send organization, local anesthetics and diffuse to nerve endings, with a good anesthetic effect. At the same time because of local anesthetic solution produced in the tissue tension, it can make blood capillary infiltration operation area significantly reduced, the operative field is clear, to facilitate the separation operation organization.

7.3.2.2 Infiltration of the periosteum

The infiltration of the periosteum, also known as the local infiltration, is used to inject the anesthetic into the superficial periosteum of the root tip of the tooth. From the labial and buccal or lingual palatal gingival marginof about 1 cm, equivalent to the root tip into the needle, the needle and the mucosal surface at an angle of 45 degrees, into the mucous membrane, periosteum, bone needles after the withdrawal of about 2 mm, and then injected anesthetics 0.5–2 mL, 2–4 minutes markedly. Be careful not to enter the periosteum so as not to cause postoperative pain and local response. This method of infiltration is mainly used for maxillary teeth, mandibular anterior teeth and alveolar bone surgery.

7.3.2.3 Periodontal ligament injection

It uses short and relatively fine syringe needle to pierce the periodontal ligament from the proximal and distal side of the tooth to a depth of about 0.5 cm, and then inject the local anesthetic 0.2 mL into the periodontal ligament. The disadvantage of this method is anesthesia injection pain. Because of the damage caused by the injection is small, it is suitable for hemophilia and similar bleeding tendency of patients; it can also avoid other deep tissue hematoma caused by other infiltration anesthesia or nerve block anesthesia. In addition, the simple use of submucosal infiltration or block anesthesia with incomplete analgesic effect, combined with periodontal membrane injection, can often achieve better analgesic effect.

7.3.3 Block anesthesia

Block anesthesia is injecting local anesthetics into the vicinity of the main nerve stem or its main branches, so as to block the stimulation of nerve terminals and make the anesthetic effect of the blocked nerve areas. Because the branches of trigeminal nerve that govern jaws and teeth are mostly penetrated by deep bone or bone canals, the infiltration of local infiltration anesthesia is poor. If block anesthesia is applied, it can not only reduce the dosage and injection times of anesthetics, but also achieve good anesthetic effect, as well as reduce pain and avoid infection and spread.

When blocking anesthesia, we must grasp the oral and maxillofacial anatomy and the trigerminal nerve's behavior and distribution, and introduce the injection mark with the related anatomical structure. In operation, the principle of sterility should be strictly observed in order to prevent concurrent infection. When the needle reaches near the nerve trunk, before the injection of local anesthetics, we must pull back the plunger, check whether the return of blood; if the blood return, it should be a little needle back, change direction after the assassination, until withdrawing without blood before the injection of narcotic drugs.

7.3.3.1 Block anaesthesia of posterior alveolar nerve

Posterior alveolar nerve block anesthesia is injection of local anesthetic fluid in the maxillary nodule to anaesthetized the upper alveolar nerve, so it is also called the maxillary nodule injection.

Indications: operation of maxillary molar extraction, buccal gingival, mucous membrane and maxillary nodule.

(1) Method

1) Intra-oral injection: the general method of the maxillary second molar buccal root oral vestibule at the entry point; as in maxillary second molars of children not yet adorable in the vestibule, distobuccal root of the first molar as the entry point; as in the maxillary molar missing patients is in the vestibule of zygomatic ridge for the ently point. Injection when patients take seat, head slightly back, half open mouth, teeth of maxillary and plane ground plane at an angle of 45 degrees, the needle and maxillary long axis 45 degrees upward after the side piercing tip; sliding along the leading nodules surface, needle depth of about 2 cm, catheter when no blood can be injected anesthetic medicine from 1.5−2 mL. Note that needles should not be too deep in order to avoid deep hematoma caused by the wing plexus behind the maxillary nodule.

2) Extra-oral injection method (tuberosity injection): fingers in the cheek a palpable zygomatic ridge, indicating the angle with the maxillary zygomatic margin formed under the selection of 5 or 7 injection needle, piercing the skin to the bone surface, then upward direction within about 2 cm, can give the injection of 2−3 mL.

(2) The scope of anesthesia

The periosteum, and gingival mucosa of the same lateral molar (except the middle root of the first molar), the alveolar process and the buccal side, and the periosteum, and the gingival mucosa can be anesthetized.

7.3.3.2 Block anaesthesia of the anterior palatine nerve

Injecting anesthetic into the palatine orifice or near its anterior palatine nerve, so it is also called the injection of the palatine foramen.

Indication: palatine anaesthesia, palatine protuberance resection and cleft palate restoration of maxillary premolar and molar extraction.

(1) Method

The anatomic location of the palatine foramen is seen by the injection of the pterygopalatine tube. Injection method: patients with head back, mouth maxillary plane and the ground plane form an angle of 60 degrees. The needle was injected into the palatine mucosa at the front of the palatine hole and pushed up to the palatine foramen, and the anesthetic was injected 0.3–0.5 mL.

(2) The scope of anesthesia

The tissue of the ipsilateral molar, the mucous periosteum of the palatine side of the premolar, the gingival and the alveolar bone.

The anesthetic should not be overdose, and the injection point must not be partial, so as not to simultaneously anesthese the palatine and posterior palatine nerves, causing nausea or vomiting due to palsy and palatal paralysis.

7.3.3.3 Nasalpalatal nerve block anesthesia

Injection of anesthetic into the anterior palatal hole (incisor hole) to narcotic nasalpalatal nerve, so it is also called the injection of the palatine foramen. The anatomical position of the anterior palatine foramen is on the intersection of the left and right canine lines with the middle palatine line. The anterior teeth laced with labial frenulum, 0.5 cm behind the alveolar ridge, which was the palatine papilla.

Indication: extraction of maxillary anterior teeth and local operation of maxillary anterior teeth area.

(1) Method

Patients head backward, open big mouth, needle injection from the edge of the gingival papilla to the mucosa, then put the needle to the middle line, making it parallel to the long axis of the central incisor, pushing about 0.5 cm above the back, and then enter the anterior palatal foramen. It is dense and requires greater pressure when injecting anesthetic, and the general injection amount is 0.2–0.5 mL.

(2) The scope of anesthesia

The gingival, palatine mucous periosteum and alveolar bone in front of the palatine of both sides of the canine. The distal palatine tissue is intersecting with the anterior palatine nerve, so it can not be completely anesthetized. It is necessary to be assisted with the anesthesia of the anterior palatine nerve block or the local infiltration anesthesia.

7.3.3.4 Block anaesthesia of infraorbital nerve

Inject the anesthetic into the orbital foramen or the infraorbital canal to anaesthetized the suborbital nerve and its branches, also known as the orbital foramen or the orbital infraorbital injection. Injection of anesthetic into the infraorbital canal can anesthetized the upper alveolar, middle nerve, and even the posterior alveolar nerve, so the whole upper alveolar nerve plexus can be anaesthetized.

(1) Method

1) Extra-oral injection: the orbital foramen is located 0.5–1 cm below the middle point of the orbital margin. With the left index finger when the injection of infraorbital margin, right hand holding the syringe needle from the same side of the nose by about 1 cm to penetrate the skin; the injection needle and the skin

was 45 degrees upward the needle depth is about 1.5 cm, can be directly into the infraorbital foramen, sometimes tip bone surface can not enter the conflict tube holes which make the injection of a small amount of local anesthetic, painless, and then move the needle for probing the infraorbital foramen, until you feel resistance that has disappeared into the hole. Then the anesthetics are injected 1–1.5 mL. The injection needle should not be too deep into the supraorbital tube to prevent the eyeball damage.

2) Intra-oral injection: pulling the upper lip forward and upward, the injection needle and the midline of the maxilla are 45 degree angle, and entered the oral vestibular groove at the corresponding part of the root tip, then reached the upper and posterior needles, and the infraorbital foramen, but it was not easy to enter the infraorbital canal.

(2) The scope of anesthesia

It is the same side, lower eyelids, nose, infraorbital area, upper lip, maxillary anterior teeth, premolars, and alveolar bone, periosteum, gingiva and mucosa of these teeth.

7.3.3.5　Block anesthesia of inferior alveolar nerve

The anesthetic is injected into the mandibular foramen near the pterygoid space, and the anesthetic alveolar nerve can be anesthetized after the diffusion of narcotic drugs, so it is also called the pterygoid mandibular injection. The inferior alveolar nerve block anesthesia has two kinds of injection methods in the mouth and outside the mouth. Intraoral injection is commonly used in clinical practice.

(1) Intra-oral injection

1) Injection marks: patients with opening big mouth, visible molar palatopharyngeal arch in front of the rear, with a mucosal folds, as pterygomandibular plica, the deep surface pterygomandibular ligament. In addition, the cheek has a triangular buccal fat pad formed by the protuberance of the adipose tissue, and its tip is located at the midpoint of the pterygoid ligament and slightly lateral. At the large opening, the intersection of the middle point line between the upper and lower mandibular alveolar ridge and the 3–4 mm outside the pterygommandibular fold is the injection point.

2) Injection method: big mouth in patients with mandibular and parallel to the ground plane. The syringe is placed in the anterior molar area of the opposite side of the mouth, and the angle is 45 degrees to the middle line. The injection should be higher than the mandibular tooth surface 1 cm parallel needle 2.5 cm, up to the mandibular bone surface of the mandible and the nerve groove, back to the blood injection of 1–2 mL after injection of anesthetic.

3) The scope of anesthesia: the ipsilateral mandible and related teeth, periodontal membrane, premolar to the middle incisor lip(cheek) side gingival, mucous periosteum and lower lip.

4) Notes the greater the width of the mandibular branch, the greater the distance between the mandibular and the anterior edge of the mandibular branch, and the depth of the needle also be increased. The wider the mandibular arch, the injection syringe should try mare to move towards the opposite side of the molar area, that is to increase the angle between the central line and the medial line, avoiding the obstruction of the oblique ridge in the mandible, and making it get near the mandibular foramen. The greater the angle of the mandibular angle, the position of the mandibular hole is higher, and the needle point should be moved up properly when the injection is injected. After injection of anesthetic 10 minutes, there is still no anesthetic sign, which may be inaccurate and need to be reinjected.

7.3.3.6　Lingual nerve block anesthesia

The lingual nerve is parallel to the inferior alveolar nerve from the mandibular nerve, and between the pterygoid muscles and the lateral pterygoid muscles, at the level equivalent to the mandibular sulcus, the lingual nerve is located at the anterior 1 cm of the inferior alveolar nerve.

（1）Injection method

After the injection of the inferior alveolar nerve block in the mouth, the injection needle is withdrawn from 1 cm. At this time, the anesthetic is 0.5-1 mL, and the tongue nerve could be anaesthetized.

（2）The scope of anesthesia

The gingival, mucous periosteum, mucous membrane of the mouth of the mouth and the 2/3 area anterior of the tongue in the same side of the mandibular tongue.

7.3.3.7   Buccal(cheek)nerve block anesthesia

The buccal nerve is separated from the mandibular nerve, and is parallel to the temporomandibular tendon in the medial front of the mandibular branch. About the equivalent of mandibular molar, left buccal nerve sheath, buccal mucosa, muscle, distributed in buccal and mandibular first premolar after skin.

（1）Injection marks and methods

The area of the buccal nerve distribution around the insertion point of the lower alveolar nerve is close to the buccal nerve trunk. During the anesthesia of the inferior alveolar nerve block, the buccal nerve can be anaesthetized when the tip of the needle falls back to the submucosa and injections of 0.5-1 mL of the anesthetic.

（2）The scope of anesthesia

The buccal gums, mucous membrane, buccal mucosa, muscle and skin of the mandibular molar.

7.3.3.8   Block anesthesia of maxillary nerve

The opening of the maxillary nerve is carried out in the pterygopalatine fossa, and the local anesthetic is injected into the area of the maxillary nerve block anesthesia. So it is also known as round hole injection or pterygopalatine fossa injection. This is a deep injection of anesthesia, it is difficult and generally less use now, unless necessary.

▶▶ *Method*

（1）Intra-oral injection of pterygopalatine tube: the surface of the palatine is a large palatine hole. At the junction of sphenopalatine foramen in the maxillary third molars or second molars in the palatal gingival and palatal midline foreign 1/3, the junction of soft and hard before about 0.5 cm; the overlying mucosa showed small sag, is symbol of the needle. If the third molar has not yet erupted, it should be on the palatine side of the second molar. When the injection of length 7 needle, since the surface markers of contralateral oblique projection into the sphenopalatine foramen mucosa depression. The injection of a small amount of local anesthetic, to be effective after the syringe to the same side, and then carefully explore the thorn enters the pterygopalatine canal; the angle between the maxillary plate and earth is 45 degrees, slowly upward and backward needle is about 3 mm, withdrawing without blood, and inject drug 2-3 mL. Sometimes it is difficult to push the injection into the proper depth, and the osmosis can be used to make the anesthetic ooze the pterygopalatine and anesthetized the maxillary nerve. If it is difficult to push forward, do not push strongly in order to prevent the needle from breaking. Before the injection, the patient should be explained in detail: when the local anesthesia is carried out, the head position should be kept stable to prevent the needle from breaking.

（2）Extra-oral injection: away from coronoid process, in the front or rear, from below the zygomatic arch into the needle through the pterygopalatine fossa in anesthesia of the maxillary nerve. Commonly used for posterior coronoid process injection. The 7-8 cm length 7 needle is selected and a sterilized rubber sheet is placed at 5 cm from the tip of the needle as the limiting depth of the needle. The middle point between the zygomatic arch and the sigmoid notch of the mandibular branch is first marked as the needle entry point. The injection of a small amount of anesthetic in the skin, then the skin vertically into the needle to the lateral pterygoid plate. At this time, the position of the rubber sheet is adjusted to the skin about 1 cm, that is, the depth of the needle to the pterygopalatine fossa, the general total depth is no more than 5 cm. Then the needle tip to the subcutaneous, reupward 10–15 degrees forward into the needle, until the rubber sign reached pterygopalatine fossa. Before the injection of anesthetic, it is necessary to withdraw without blood, so that the drug can be injected.

7.3.3.9　Block anaesthesia of the mandibular nerve

Injecting the anesthetic into the foramen ovale, so it is also called the oval hole injection.

Indications: the diagnosis, differential diagnosis and radiofrequency treatment of facial pain, such as trigeminal neuralgia and atypical facial pain.

▶▶ *Method*

(1) Length 7 needle sleeve disinfection rubber, to the zygomatic arch and the lower edge of the sigmoid notch for piercing the skin, and vertically into the needle, leading to the pterygoid plate. Fix the rubber sheet at 1 cm from the skin and mark the depth. Then the needle to the subcutaneous injection needle, back to back on the inner deflection angle of 15 degrees to mark the depth of needle is near the foramen ovale. After withdrawal of blood, 3–4 mL of anesthetics are injected.

(2) The scope of anesthesia is the same lateral mandibular teeth, tongue, bottom of mouth, mandible and periodontal tissue, maxillary muscle group and temporal skin.

7.4　Complications of Local Anesthesia

7.4.1　Syncope

Syncope is a sudden and temporary loss of consciousness. It is due to a temporary central ischemia.

7.4.1.1　Diagnostic points

(1) There are factors such as fear, hunger, fatigue, pain, poor body position and poor body health.

(2) When the local anesthetics injected, there are dizziness, chest tightness, pale complexion, sweating all over the body, cold limbs, cold, nausea, dyspnea and so on.

(3) A serious person may have a slow heart rate decline, a sharp drop in blood pressure, and a transient loss of consciousness.

7.4.1.2　The prevention and treatment principle

Do a good job of examination and ideological work, to eliminate tension, to avoid operation on an empty stomach.

7.4.1.3　Key points of treatment

(1) Stop the injection immediately, flat out the seat quickly, and put the patient at the head low.

(2) Loosening the collar and keeping the breath open.

(3) Aromatic ammonia alcohol or ammonia water stimulates respiration.

(4) Acupuncture at the middle point.

(5) Oxygen inhalation and intravenous injection of hypertonic glucose solution.

7.4.2　Anaphylaxis

Anaphylaxis mainly occurs in ester anesthetics, but is rare. There are two kinds of delayed reaction and immediate reaction.

7.4.2.1　Delayed response

The common resaon is vascular neuroedema, and it is seldom caused by urticaria, drug rash, asthma and anaphylactoid purpura.

7.4.2.2　Immediately response

After the use of a very small number of drugs can immediately have very serious similar toxic reactions, such as sudden convulsions, coma, sudden cardiac arrest and death.

The same kind of anesthetics have a cross phenomenon, such as those allergic to procaine, and tetracaine can not be used.

7.4.2.3　The principle of prevention and treatment

Before surgery, ask for details about whether there are any local anesthetics such as procaine hydrochloride allergy, patients who are allergic to ester local anesthetics and allergic constitution. They can use amide drugs, such as lidocaine, and do allergy test ahead of time.

7.4.2.4　Key points of treatment

(1) The mild allergic reaction, to desensitization drugs such as chlorpheniramine or oral calcium, promethazine, cortisone like bowel intramuscular injection or intravenous injection and oxygen inhalation.

(2) Acute anaphylaxis should be immediately injected with adrenaline to give oxygen.

(3) If the respiratory heartbeat stops, it should be according to the method of cardiopulmonary resuscitation.

7.4.3　Poisoning

When the local anesthetic enters the blood circulation faster than the decomposition rate per unit time, the blood concentration increases, and the toxic symptoms or anaphylaxis caused by a certain concentration.

7.4.3.1　Diagnostic points

(1) Excessive injection of drug or local anesthetic is injected into the blood vessel quickly.

(2) Excitatory manifested as irritability, words, tremor, nausea and vomiting, shortness of breath, sweating, increased blood pressure, severe cases, convulsions, hypoxia, cyanosis.

(3) Suppressed the rapid emergence of weak pulse, blood pressure drops, unconsciousness, then breathing and heart beating.

7.4.3.2　Key points for prevention and treatment

(1) Before using the drug, we should know the size of the drug toxicity and the maximum dosage of the drug.

(2) To adhere without blood, and then slow injection of anesthetics to avoid direct and rapid injection of blood vessels.

(3) Elderly patients, children, physical weakness, heart disease, kidney disease, diabetes, severe anemia, vitamin deficiency and other diseases have low tolerance to narcotics. Appropriate dosage of anesthetics should be controlled.

(4) Once the toxic reaction occurs, the injection of anesthetics should be stopped immediately.

(5) A slight poisoning patients in the supine position, loosening the neck up, keep the airway open.

(6) The heavy people need to give oxygen, rehydration, anticonvulsant, the use of hormone and boost drugs and other measures.

7.4.4 Local complication

7.4.4.1 Hematoma

The hematoma caused by injection needle puncture is more common in the posterior alveolar nerve and infraorbital nerve block anesthesia. Especially after puncturing the venous plexus, there may be bleeding within the tissue, and there are purple or red congestion spots or masses on the submucosa or subcutaneous. After a few days, the color of the hematoma began to fade into yellow green, and slowly absorbed and disappeared.

The principle of prevention and control:

(1) Injections do not repeat punctureing, injection needles can not have inverted hook, so as not to increase the opportunity to puncture blood vessels.

(2) If the hematoma has appeared in the local area, the hemostasis can be oppressed immediately and the cold compress should be given. After the bleeding is stopped within 24 hours, the hematomas are used to make the hematoma absorbed and dissipated.

(3) The antibiotics and hemostatic drugs can be properly given.

7.4.4.2 Infection

Injection needle contaminated, local or anesthetic disinfection not strict, or infection in the injection can cause infection into deep tissue, causing infection of infratemporal fossa, pterygoid space, parapharyngeal space or floor space. The serious person may also cause systemic infection through the circulation of blood. In general, 1 – 5 days after the injection, the local red, swelling, heat and pain are obvious, even there are restricted or dysphagia due to difficult and systemic symptoms.

The principle of prevention and control:

(1) The injection equipment and the injection area must be sterilized strictly.

(2) Prevent injecting needle pollution and avoid through or direct injection in the area of inflammation.

(3) Those who have been infected should be treated according to the principles of the treatment of inflammation.

7.4.4.3 Temporary facial paralysis

It is usually seen in block anesthesia of inferior alveolar nerve. When the syringe needle is biased, it can not touch the bone surface or exceed the sigmoid notch, resulting in temporary paralysis of the anesthetic facial nerve injected into the parotid gland, and occasionally seen in the nerve block of masticatory muscles. After the effect of the anesthetic effect, the function of the nerve can be recovered without special treatment.

7.4.4.4 Broken of needle

The needles are poor in quality, lack of elasticity and so on. The broken part is common in the junction of needle and needle body. Due to the improper operation of the injection, the needle is overturned and broken; or the patient is restless and uncoordinated.

The principle of prevention and control:

(1) Routine examination of the quality of the injection needle before injection.

(2) The appropriate length and model of the syringe, at least 1 cm length should be retained outside the organization.

(3) Attention to the operation method, change the direction of injection should not be over bending injection needle, when there is resistance, it should not be forced to push.

(4) If the needle is broken, the patient is asked to maintain the static state of the mouth immediately; if the needle is exposed, it can be carried by a toothed tweezers.

(5) If the needle has completely entered the tissue, the other needle can be inserted into the same part into a mark, and X-ray location is taken. After determining the location of the broken needle, the operation is removed again.

7.4.4.5　Pain and edema in the injection area

(1) Reasons

1) Anaesthetized liquid is metamorphosed or mixed with impurities or unmatched isosotic solutions.

2) The injecting needle is blunt and bent, or the barb can easily damage the tissue or nerve.

3) No strict aseptic operation is carried out to bring the source of infection into the tissue and cause infection.

(2) Principle of prevention and control

1) Careful examination of anesthetics and instruments.

2) Pay attention to disinfection and isolation in the injection and avoid repeating injections in the same part.

3) If there has been pain, edema, and inflammation, the local hot compress can be used for physical therapy, closure, or to give antiphlogistic and analgesic drugs.

7.4.4.6　Nerve injury

Injection needle puncture, or injection of mixed alcohol solution, can cause nerve damage, sensory abnormalities or numbness, neuralgia and other symptoms.

▶▶ *Treatment points*:

(1) Most of the nerve injuries are temporary and reversible.

(2) The light will recover after a few days, without treatment.

(3) Some of the severe nerve injuries recover slowly and are completely unable to recover.

(4) It is difficult to judge the degree of nerve injury. Therefore, all the symptoms of postoperative numbness should be treated actively to promote the complete recovery of nerve function. Acupuncture, physiotherapy, hormone(early injury), vitamin B_1 or B_{12} can be used.

7.4.4.7　Temporary trismus

It is rare that it can occur during the anesthesia of the inferior alveolar nerve. Because the injection is not accurate, anesthetic the masseter muscle, lose the function of contraction and relaxation and stagnation in contraction, resulting in trismus. Generally, it is temporary. Most recover within 2-3 hours (caused by infection of trismus is except).

7.4.4.8　Temporary diplopia or blindness

In the mouth inferior alveolar nerve block anesthesia, the injection needle into the inferior alveolar artery without confirmation, the local anesthetic is injected into the blood vessels, the middle meningeal artery, ophthalmic artery or its main branches into orbit, causing ophthalmoplegia and optic nerve paralysis and temporary diplopia or blindness. After the general anesthetic effect disappear, eye movement and visual acuity can be recovered.

7.4.5　Complications of cervical plexus block anesthesia

7.4.5.1　Cervical sympathetic nerve syndrome

It is also known as Horner syndrome. The anesthetic infiltration of the sympathetic nerve is caused by the anesthesia of the deep cervical nerve block.

Diagnostic points: Ipsilateral mydriasis, ptosis, conjunctival congestion, small fission, flushing of face, dry facial skin, no sweat, auricular redness, congestion of nasal mucosa and nasal congestion. In general, symptoms disappear with the disappearance of anaesthesia, and no special treatment is required.

7.4.5.2　The hoarseness of the voice

It is caused by the obstruction of the vagus nerve due to the infiltration of the vagus nerve, which causes the obstruction of the recurrent laryngeal nerve conduction. Generally do not have to deal with, after the anaesthesia effect disappeared, that is self recovery.

▶▶ *Note*

Bilateral deep nerve plexus anesthesia can not be performed at the same time in order to prevent the vagus nerve from being infiltrated by anesthetics and the vocal cords are completely paralyzed, which can lead to acute upper respiratory obstruction.

7.4.5.3　Total spinal anaesthesia

It is a serious complication caused by anaesthesia in the subarachnoid cavity of the cervical spinal canal.

(1) Key points of diagnosis

The rare symptoms of decreased blood pressure, skin cold, cyanosis, dyspnea, loss of consciousness, etc. A serious person can lead to death.

(2) Key points for prevention and control

1) Assure the master mark and injection method, not the anesthetic into the spinal canal.

2) If the blood pressure has been reduced, or the blood pressure has a downward trend, the rapid intravenous infusion and the adjustment of the body position can be corrected.

3) Intravenous injection of 10-15 mg of ephedrine, a vasoconstrictor, can be used to correct hypotension.

4) Patients with bradycardia are given atropine by intravenous injection of 0.3-0.5 mg.

He Wei

Chapter 8

Tooth Extraction

Tooth extraction is one of the most important clinical treatments for oral diseases. The tooth, which can not be retained after treatment or have a negative impact on the local or systemic health condition, should be removed as soon as possible.

8.1 Instruments for Tooth Extraction

8.1.1 Dental forceps

An assortment of forceps has been designed for specific teeth in the dental arch, to enable the surgeon to achieve the most appropriate adaptation and to facilitate control of the forces applied to the tooth. The basic components of dental extraction forceps are the handle, hinge and beaks. The concave shape of the blades allows the surgeon to apply the maximum surface area of the blades on the tooth, distributing the forces evenly and thus giving a greater degree of control. Usually the beaks of maxillary forceps are parallel to the handles and the mandibular forceps are perpendicular to the handles. The hinge of the forceps connects the handle to the beak, transferring the force from the handle to the beak. The handles are mainly straight but may be curved, which provides the operator with a sense of "better fit". So sufficient pressure and leverage can be delivered to remove the required tooth.

8.1.2 Dental elevators

Many different types of elevators are available for the extraction of teeth, tooth roots and root tips. Three major components of the elevator are the handle, shank and blade. The biggest variation in the type of elevator is in the shape and size of the blade. Three basic types of elevators are the straight type, the Cryer and the pick type. The straight elevator is the most common type. It is a single-bladed instrument that is placed between the tooth and the alveolar bone, to luxate tooth from the surrounding bone. The Cryer elevator is particularly useful when a single retained root from an extraction of a mandibular molar remains in the alveolar bone. A Cryer elevator is placed apically into the empty root socket, and the point of the blade is rotated toward the residual root which forces the remaining root vertically out of the socket.

The instrument is held in the palm of the hand with the index finger extended along the shaft of the elevator to control the forces applied to the tooth. Without using this technique, the elevator may slip and damage adjacent tissues. Because the elevator acts as a lever, the fulcrum must be against bone so as not to dislodge an adjacent tooth.

8.1.3 Other instruments

The dental extraction instruments also include the instruments for incising tissue, elevating mucoperiosteum, retracting soft tissue, controlling hemorrhage, grasping tissue, removing bone and suture mucosa.

8.2 Tooth Extraction Indications and Contraindications

8.2.1 Indications

In the past many of the teeth belonging to tooth extraction indications, can now be retained. Tooth extraction indications are relative, and the decision to extract should be made individually according to different cases.

8.2.1.1 Caries

The tooth is subjected to severe caries with extensive loss of surface that may not permit restorative procedures.

8.2.1.2 Severe periodontal disease

Periodontal disease is accompanied with severe attachment and bone loss, irreversible tooth hypermobility, and its prognosis is poor for periodontal treatment.

8.2.1.3 Pulp disease

Irreversible pulpitis, pulp necrosis, the internal resorption of root canal or the obliterated root canal where endodontic procedures are not possible or has failed.

8.2.1.4 Impacted teeth

The impacted teeth do not always reach the functional occlusion, and they should be considered for extraction if the potential for the development of root resorption or bone loss of the adjacent teeth, or other pathologies such as cysts.

8.2.1.5 Pathological lesions in relation to teeth

The tooth extraction may be considered during the treatment of other related pathological lesions, for example in the treatment of osteomyelitis, or tumor of jaw.

8.2.1.6 Crown and root fracture

Sometimes successful restorative therapy can not be achieved for the tooth with crown, crown and root or the root fracture, and tooth extraction is the only alternative.

8.2.1.7 Malpositon teeth and supernumerary teeth

Malposition of teeth with conditions such as trauma to soft tissue or teeth crowding and supernumerary teeth with potential for future pathology are indications for extraction.

8.2.1.8 Before other treatments

Sometimes teeth have to be removed prior to orthodontic treatments, prosthetic procedures, other surgical procedures or radiation therapy due to tumors in the head and neck region.

8.2.1.9   Other reasons for extraction

Extraction can sometimes be performed due to economic or esthetic reasons. The patient might choose to extract the teeth rather than the more expensive endodontic treatment or restorative procedure. In these situations it is especially important to tell other choices and inform preoperatively so the surgeon and the patient agree on the same choice.

8.2.2   Contraindications

Contraindications for tooth extractiom are often relative. Patient's local conditions and general health should be taken into consideration before tooth extraction. Some disease used to be contraindications can be changed after proper treatment.

8.2.2.1   Systemic contraindications

These constitute all health factors and mental factors which affect the patient's ability to withstand the surgical procedure. In general, patients with hemophilia or other coagulopathies should first have their disorder controlled before extraction. The uncontrolled metabolic diseases, such as diabetes, constitute a relative contraindication until they brought under control. Similarly, patients with severe hypertension and cardiac diseases should be ideally treated. The chemo and (or) radiotherapy is also a relative contraindication. In all cases, one should be aware of the medication that affect the immune system, delaying the healing process or interrupting the medications. Severe dental anxiety can be a relative contradiction to extraction in local anesthesia and in some cases can be treated in general anesthesia.

8.2.2.2   Local contraindications

The most common local contraindications is the acute infection which should be treated first before the proceeding of extraction. The extraction of the lower third molar during on-going pericoronitis could lead to life-threatening infection after surgery. However, there are situations where the acute abscess is best drained by tooth extraction even during the acute phase. So the acute infection should not be considered the absolute contraindication for extraction. One of the most important contraindication to extraction is the radiation, past or present, involving the jaws. Delayed healing, dehiscence, necrosis are the complications due to the extraction in irradiated bone. The tooth in the area of the malignant tumor should not be removed before the planned tumor treatment.

After a complete history and review of systems, the surgeon may ask the patient about certain medical conditions that may make the patient unsuitable for a routine dental extraction under local anesthesia. Some examples are bleeding dyscrasias, liver disease, immunocompromised conditions, cardiac disease, and coronary artery disease. A thorough history of radiation and bisphosphonate therapy should be determined and appropriate measures taken.

8.3   Preparation Before Tooth Extraction

It is important to consider the patient's overall health during the initial consult appointment. No aspect of simple tooth extraction is more important than the careful preoperative examination of the patient. This includes an updated medical history, any indicated laboratory tests, physical exam, oral exam, and dental radiographs.

During the clinical and radiographic assessments, a routine dental extraction may need to be converted to a surgical approach based on certain key findings, such as teeth with gross amounts of decay through the furcation or below the level of the alveolus, root dilacerations, and a previous history of endodontic therapy. Certain anatomic barriers may require additional skill and expertise, such barriers include extraction of a maxillary molar in the presence of a pneumatized maxillary sinus or extraction of a mandibular molar with roots that approximate the inferior alveolar nerve canal.

8.3.1 Patient position

For optimal control of the procedure, the surgeon and patient must be in a proper chair position. This allows for ideal visibility, lighting, and access. When extractions are being performed in the upper arch, the patient should be reclined so the maxillary occlusal plane is 45–60 degrees to the plane of the floor. When extracting a mandibular tooth, the patient is positioned so the mandible is parallel to the floor. In both cases, the height of the chair should be adjusted so the surgeon's elbows remain comfortably relaxed, without tensing the shoulders to reach into the mouth with extraction instruments. The surgeon's position relative to the patient also varies, depending on which tooth is being extracted and on the surgeon's dominant hand.

8.3.2 Preparation for the surgical area

For oral procedures, even a relatively clean field is difficult to maintain because of oral and upper respiratory tract contamination, but the sterile procedure should not be neglected. 1% or 2% iodine can be used for the sterilization of the mucosa area with the diameter no more than 2 cm, because of the iodine irritation to the oral mucosa. For the open surgical approach, 75% ethanol is used to disinfect the perioral skin and the lower 1/3 part of the face.

8.4　Principle of Simple Tooth Extraction

Simple tooth extraction is accomplished by applying controlled and focused force to the tooth.

After a local anesthetic has been administered and allowed to take effect, the surgeon usually begins by relieving the superior portion of the attached gingiva from the tooth. This maneuver also serves to verify soft tissue anesthesia at the site.

A straight dental elevator is used to begin moving the tooth. This instrument may be inserted into the mesial interproximal space, perpendicular to the tooth being removed, and then rotated. Alternatively, the instrument may be inserted vertically along the mesiobuccal line angle of the root and direct it apically, facilitating the coronal movement of the tooth or tooth root.

Choosing the right forceps is to securely grasp the cervical portion of the tooth. The beaks of the forceps are adapted to the buccal and lingual surfaces of the tooth with the beaks pointed apically, parallel to the long axis of the tooth. This allows the most effective alveolar bone expansion and reduces the risk of fracture at the root apex. Careful buccal–palatal movement is repeated, allowing time for the bone to expand under firm pressure. Rotational force can be applied when extracting maxillary incisors. Once the tooth is mobile, it is generally delivered from the socket by gentle traction toward the path of least resistance. In most cases, this is toward the buccal, but lower second and third molars may be delivered lingually.

Once the tooth has been removed, the calculus, amalgam, or tooth fragment remaining in the socket should be gently removed with a curette. If a periapical lesion is visible on the preoperative radiograph, the periapical region should be carefully curetted to remove the granuloma or cyst. It is important to carefully palpate the bony margins of the socket and the loose bone fragments or sharp, splayed bone margins must be removed or smoothed to prevent lingering pain and impaired healing.

After the tooth extraction, the initial maneuver starts with the placement of a small piece of gauze directly over the socket to control bleeding. The patient should be instructed to bite firmly on this gauze for at least 30 minutes. Food in the first 12 hours should be soft and cool. To avoid hard spitting or sucking on straws. Patients should keep their teeth and the whole mouth reasonably clean which will result in a more rapid healing of surgical wounds. A minimal amount of postsurgical bleeding is normal and expected following dental extractions. However, bleeding that persists or recurs beyond the first 24−48 hours are indications for a return visit. Simple extractions generally result in mild pain for 1 or 2 days, which is well managed by pain medications. Pain lasting more than a few days often indicates a healing complication, so a new assessment of the patient is necessary.

8.5 Specific Techniques for the Removal of Each Tooth

8.5.1 Maxillary incisors and canine

Usually maxillary incisors and canine have conic roots and alveolar bone is thin on the labial side compared to the palatal side. The initial movement should be labial with slow, steady, and firm froce and a less vigorous palatal force, followed by a slow, firm, rotation. The tooth is delivered from the socket in a labial incisal direction with labial tractional forces.

8.5.2 Maxillary premolars

The maxillary first premolar is a single−rooted tooth in its first two thirds, with a bifurcation into a buccolingual root usually occurring in the apical. Initial movements is buccal direction. Palatal movements are made with small amounts of force to prevent fracture of the palatal root tip, which is harder to retrieve. No rotational force. Final delivery of the tooth from the tooth socket is with tractional force in the buccal−occlusal direction.

The maxillary second premolar has a single thick root with blunt end. The extraction requires relatively strong movements to the buccal back to the palate, and then in the bucco−occlusal direction with a rotational, tractional force.

8.5.3 Maxillary molars

The maxillary first molar has three large and strong roots. Buccal roots are close, and the palatal root diverges widely toward the palate. The buccal plate is thin and the palatal is thick and heavy. Slow, strong, steady buccal pressure expands the buccocortical plate and only a minimum palatal forces should be used. Rotational forces are not useful for extraction of this tooth.

Compared with the first molar, the anatomy of the maxillary second molar is similar except that the roots tend to be shorter and less divergent, with the buccal roots more commonly fused into a single root. So the tooth is more easily extracted by the same technique described for the first molar.

The erupted maxillary third molar is usually easily removed because buccal bone is thin and the roots are usually fused and conic. However the root anatomy of this tooth is variable and often small, dilacerated, hooked. Retrieval of fractured roots in this area is difficult due to more limited access.

8.5.4   Mandibular anterior teeth

The extraction movements are equal pressures in the labial and lingual directions. Once the tooth has become luxated and mobile, rotational movement may be used to expand alveolar bone further for canines. The tooth is removed from the socket with tractional forces in a labial-incisal direction.

8.5.5   Mandibular premolars

The roots of mandibular premolars tend to be straight and conic, albeit sometimes slender. The overlying alveolar bone is thin on the buccal side. The forceps are apically forced as far as possible, with the basic movements directed toward the buccal aspect, returning to the lingual aspect. Rotational movement is used when extracting these teeth except that root curvature exists in the apical third of the tooth. The tooth is then delivered in the occluso–buccal direction.

8.5.6   Mandibular molars

Mandibular molars usually have two roots. The roots of the first molar are more widely divergent than those of the second molar. Additionally, the roots may converge at the apical one. Strong buccolingual motion is then used to expand the tooth socket and allow the tooth to be delivered in the bucco–occlusal direction. The second molar can be removed more easily with stronger lingual pressure, because the linguoalveolar bone around the second molar is thinner than the buccal bone.

Erupted mandibular third molars usually have fused conic roots. The lingual plate of bone is definitely thinner than the buccocortical plate, so most of the extraction forces should be delivered to the lingual aspect.

8.5.7   Primary teeth

The roots of the primary teeth are long and delicate. The roots are subject to fracture, especially when there is resorption of coronal portions of the root structure caused by the succedaneous tooth. The initial movements are slow, steady pressures toward the buccal aspect and return movements toward the lingual aspect. The dentist should pay careful attention to the direction of least resistance and deliver the tooth into that path.

8.6   Procedures for Impacted Tooth Extraction

Any tooth in the mouth may be impacted, but third molars are the most commonly impacted teeth, followed by maxillary canines and mandibular premolars.

8.6.1   Indications for impaction removal

Prevention of periodontal diseases, dental caries, pericoronitis; prevention of root resorption; prevention of odontogenic cysts and tumors; treatment of pain of unexplained origin; prevention of jaw fracture and facilitation of orthodontic or prosthesis treatment.

8.6.2   Contraindications for impaction removal

Like all surgical procedures, elective removal of impacted teeth should not be performed if the risks outweigh the expected benefits. Clearly patients with significantly compromised or unstable medical conditions are not candidate for elective removal of impacted teeth showing no evidence of active pathology.

8.6.3   Classification of impacted mandibular third molar

8.6.3.1   Angulation

The most commonly used classification system uses a determination of the angulation between the long axis of the impacted third molar and the adjacent second molar. The impacted third molar can be classified into the mesioangular impaction, horizontal impaction, vertical impaction, distoangular impaction. In addition, teeth can also be angled in buccal or lingual directions. Rarely, a transverse impaction or inversion impaction occurs.

8.6.3.2   Relationship to anterior border of ramus

This method is based on the amount of impacted tooth covered by the bone of the mandibular ramus. If the mesiodistal diameter of the crown is completely anterior to the anterior border of the mandibular ramus, it is in a class Ⅰ relationship. If the tooth is positioned posteriorly so that approximately one half is covered by the ramus, it is in a class Ⅱ relationship. A class Ⅲ relationship between the tooth and ramus occurs when the tooth is located completely within the mandibular ramus.

8.6.3.3   Relationship to the occlusal plane

In this classification, the degree of difficulty is measured by the depth of the impacted tooth compared with the height of the adjacent second molar. The class a impaction is one in which the occlusal surface of the impacted tooth is level or nearly level with the occlusal plane of the second molar. The class B impaction involves an impacted tooth with an occlusal surface between the occlusal plane and the cervical line of the second molar. Finally, the class C impaction is one in which the occlusal surface of the impacted tooth is below the cervical line of the second molar.

8.6.4   Surgical technique

8.6.4.1   Reflecting adequate flaps for accessibility

The preferred incision for the removal of an impacted mandibular third molar is an envelope incision that extends from the mesial papilla of the mandibular first molar, around the necks of the teeth to the distobuccal line angle of the second molar, and then posteriorly to and laterally up the anterior border of the mandibular ramus. The incision on the retromolar pad should keep angled buccally in order to avoid the lingual nerve. A mesial release incision can be made from the distobuccal of the second molar and drops inferiorly into the buccal vestibule.

The recommended incision for the maxillary third molar is also an envelope incision. The incision extends posteriorly over the tuberosity from the distal of the second molar and anteriorly to the mesial aspect of the first molar. In situations in which greater access is required, a release incision extending from the mesial aspect of the second molar can be used.

8.6.4.2   Removal of overlying bone

Bone is removed with a bur under copious saline irrigation until most of the occlusal surface and the buccal surface are exposed to the level of the cervical height of contour or the cemento-enamel junction. The amount of bone that needs to be removed varies with the angulation of the tooth, the depth of the impaction and the morphology of the roots. No bone is removed from the lingual aspect so as to avoid the lingual nerve injury.

8.6.4.3　Sectioning the tooth

After bone removal, the surgeon should assess the need to section the tooth, which depends primarily on the angulation of the impacted tooth and any root curvature. In all cases, care is taken not to cut too deeply either toward the lingual or inferiorly, where the lingual or inferior alveolar nerves may be at risk of injury. A straight elevator is inserted into the slot made by the bur and rotated to split the tooth. More complicated impactions may require a series of sometimes delicate divisions, followed by careful separation and elevation of small segments.

8.7　Complications of Tooth Removal

As in the case of tooth extraction, the best and easiest way to manage a surgical complication is to prevent it from ever happening. Prevention of surgical complications is best accomplished by a thorough preoperative assessment and comprehensive treatment plan, followed by careful execution of the surgical procedure.

8.7.1　Intraoperative complications

8.7.1.1　Soft tissue injuries

Injuries of the oral soft tissue are always the result of the surgeon's lack of adequate attention or the use of excessive and uncontrolled force.

The most common one is the tearing of the mucosal flap as the surgeon tries to gain needed access during surgical extraction of a tooth. Instruments may slip from the surgical field and damage adjacent soft tissues, due to the improper technique. Abrasions or burns to lips, corners of the mouth usually result from the rotating shank of the bur rubbing on soft tissue. Prevention of this complication: ①adequate attention during operation; ②adequately sized flaps to prevent excess tension on the flap; ③controlled amounts of force. If a tear does occur in the flap, the flap should be carefully repositioned once the surgery is completed. The treatment of puncture wound is aimed at preventing infection and allowing healing to occur. If an area of oral mucosa is abraded or burned, little treatment is possible other than keeping the area clean with regular oral rinsing.

8.7.1.2　Root fracture

Root fracture is one of the most frequent problems encountered in tooth extraction. Long, curved, divergent roots that lie in dense bone are the most likely to be fractured. The main methods of preventing fracture of roots is to perform surgery in the manner described in previous chapters or to use an open extraction technique and remove bone to decrease the amount of force necessary to remove the tooth. Sometimes small root tip left has been shown to remain in place without postoperative complications if it is not grossly infected. Radiographic follow-up may be all that is required.

8.7.1.3　Fracture of the alveolar process

In some situations, the alveolar bone fractures is removed with the tooth, because of the use of excessive force with the forceps. The most likely places for bone fractures are the buccal cortical plate over the maxillary canine and molars, the portions of the floor of the maxillary sinus that are associated with maxillary molars, the maxillary tuberosity, and labial bone over mandibular incisors.

Preoperative radiographic and clinical assessments, proper use of controlled force and the early decision to perform an open extraction are needed to prevent the fractures of large portions of the cortical plate. If the bone has been completely removed from the tooth socket along with the tooth, it should not be replaced. When the bone remains attached to the periosteum, the bone and the attached soft tissue dissected away from the tooth are repositoned and secured with sutures.

8.7.1.4 Fracture of the mandible

Fracture of the mandible is a rare occurrence. The typical situation is a deeply impacted third molar, most commonly in an older individual with dense bone. It often occurs during the forceful use of dental elevators. When such a fracture occurs, the surgeon should perform an immediate reduction and fixation of the fracture.

8.7.1.5 Oroantral communications

If the maxillary sinus is greatly pneumatized with little or no bone existing between the roots of the teeth and the maxillary sinus, and if the roots of the tooth are widely divergent, it is common for a communication to be created between the oral cavity and the maxillary sinus.

The tooth-sinus relationship must be carefully evaluated by preoperative radiographs whenever maxillary molars are to be extracted. If the sinus floor appears close to the tooth roots and the tooth roots are widely divergent, the surgeon should perform a surgical removal with sectioning of tooth roots and excessive force should be avoided.

The nose-blowing test could be used to confirm the presence of a communication. If a communication exists, there will be bubbling of blood in the socket area. The treatment depends on the approximate size of the communication. If the communication is small(2 mm in diameter or less), no additional surgical treatment is necessary. Measures should be taken to ensure the formation of a high-quality blood clot in the socket. Patients also should be advised to avoid blowing the nose, sneezing violently, sucking on straws, and smoking. If the communication is of moderate size(2-6 mm), a figure-of-eight suture should be placed over the tooth socket. Patients should be followed up carefully for several weeks to ensure that healing has occurred. If the sinus opening is large(7 mm or larger), repair with a flap procedure should be considered.

8.7.1.6 Nerve disturbance

The regional nerves which are most likely to be injured during tooth extraction are the lingual nerve and the inferior alveolar nerve. The lingual nerve is often injured during soft tissue flap reflection, so the incisions made for surgical exposure of impacted third molars should be made well to the buccal aspect of the mandible. The inferior alveolar nerve is injured when the roots of the teeth are manipulated and elevated from the socket. This complication is common enough during extraction of third molars that it is important routinely to inform patients preoperatively.

8.7.1.7 Injury of adjacent tooth or tooth in the opposite arch

Inappropriate use of the extraction instruments may luxate an adjacent tooth. The treatment goal is to reposition the tooth into its appropriate position and stabilize it so that adequate healing occurs. Teeth in the opposite arch may also be injured as a result of uncontrolled forces. If such an injury occurs, the tooth should be smoothed or restored, as necessary.

8.7.1.8 Others

The displacement of tooth or tooth tip into the related anatomy should be also considered. Three-dimensional localization of the displaced tooth or root should be used for appropriate planning. Sometimes tooth might be lost into the pharynx and swallowed. The chest and abdominal radiographs should be taken to determine the specific location of the tooth and it is highly probable that it will pass through the gastrointestinal tract within 2-4 days. Sometimes wrong tooth could be extracted. Careful preoperative planning, clear communication with referring dentists, and attentive clinical assessment of the tooth to be removed before the elevator and forceps are applied are the main methods of preventing this complication.

8.7.2 Postoperative complications

8.7.2.1 Bleeding

Before tooth extraction, a thorough patient history should be taken with regard to any existing problems with coagulation. The patient ought to be questioned about any history of bleeding, particularly after injury or surgery, and any medications currently being taken that might interfere with coagulation.

The treatment of bleeding begins with local measurements, pressure with gauze, and packing. In the case of prolonged postoperative bleeding, the patient should be instructed to remove loose clots and bite firmly and continuously on amoist gauze pack for 30 minutes. If this is unsuccessful, exploration and debridement of the wound should be completed under local anesthesia without vasoconstrictor to allow for diagnosis of the cause of bleeding. Soft tissues can usually be controlled with cautery, and bone tissue should be checked for small nutrient artery bleeding or general oozing. Granulation tissue should be debrided, irregular sharp bony edges smoothed or removed, and hemostatic agents used within the alveolus to assist in bleeding control.

If hemostasis is not achieved by any of the local measures above discussed, additional laboratory screening tests should be performed to determine whether the patient has a profound hemostatic defect.

8.7.2.2 Infection

Infections are a rare complication after routine dental extraction. The risk of infection increases with degree of impaction, need for bone removal or sectioning of the tooth, the presence of gingivitis, periodontal disease, surgeon experience and increasing age.

(1) Acute infection

Acute infection usually arises the sencond day after surgery. Clinical signs can vary from localized swelling to fluctuance and trismus or systemic manifestations with fevers, etc. The treatment involves surgical drainage in addition to the administration of systemic antibiotics. Careful asepsis and thorough wound debridement after surgery can best prevent infection. Some patients who are predisposed to postoperative wound infections should be given prophylactic antibiotics.

(2) Dry socket

Almost all dry sockets occur after the removal of lower molars. Dry socket typically arises on the third or fourth day after surgery, leaving a painful, slow–healing defect with exposed alveolar bone. The pain is moderate to severe, and frequently radiates to the patient's ear. On examination, the tooth socket appears to be empty with a bad odor, a partially or completely lost blood clot. And some bony surfaces of the socket are exposed.

Atraumatic surgery with clean incisions and soft tissue reflection should be performed to prevent dry socket syndrome. After the surgical procedure, thorough irrigation with saline delivered under pressure is needed. Small amounts of antibiotic placed in the socket alone or on a gelatin sponge have been shown to substantially decrease the incidence of dry socket in mandibular third molars and other lower molar sockets.

The single therapeutic goal of dry socket is to relieve the patient's pain during the period of healing. Treatment consists of irrigation and insertion of a medicated dressing. The tooth socket is gently irrigated with sterile saline and then a small strip of iodoform gauze soaked in or coated with the medication (eugenol, benzocaine, peru, etc.) is inserted into the socket with a small tag of gauze left trailing out of the wound. The initial healing may take 2 weeks or more.

Fu Kun

Chapter 9

Implant Dentistry

Implant dentistry concerns the use of artificial tooth roots and crowns made of biological materials to replace or restore missing teeth so as to achieve long-term stable and comfortable chewing function and aesthetic appearance. Oral implantology is an interdisciplinary subject, which involves oral prosthodontics, maxillofacial surgery and periodontal disease, biomaterials, bioengineering mechanics and oral prosthodontics. Oral implantology is regarded as the most breakthrough subject in the history of stomatology in the 20th century and one of the fastest developing clinical subjects in the world stomatology in the past decades.

9.1   Oral Implant

In ancient times, people in Europe, the Middle East and Central America tried to use all kinds of homologous or different materials, including human and animal teeth, carved bones and shells, etc. , to implant jaw bone instead of missing teeth. In modern times, people have tried to use artificial materials to make implants of various shapes, and to repair the missing teeth or provide support for dental prostheses through the implantation of internal or external bone. However, these implants fail to meet the requirements of the complex oral environment, resulting in a large number of shedding failures. In the middle of the 20th century, the Swede Branemark (father of modern oral implantology) observed that the animal's bone tissue can bind tightly to an implanted titanium device. He laterly defined the phenomenon as osseointegration. In 1965, he successfully repaired a cleft palate defect in the first clinical case using an osteo-bound titanium implant. In 1982, at the Toronto conference, Branemark has reported a great deal of research on bone bonding over 15 years, which is considered a breakthrough in oral medicine. It laid the foundation of oral implantology, a new branch of oral medicine. In the following decades, dental implantology has developed rapidly and become mature. Dental implantology, as a repair method that is very similar to the function, structure and aesthetic effect of natural teeth, has become the best choice for oral medicine and patients with tooth loss at present.

Implant restoration can also be called "implant teeth": a method of restoration of the missing teeth, which is based on the underlying structure of the implanted bone tissue to support and retain the upper dental prosthesis. It includes the dental implant on the lower part and the dental prosthesis on the upper part. It adopts artificial materials (such as metal, ceramics) to make implants (generally similar to the root morphology of teeth), which are implanted into the tissue (usually maxilla and mandible) by surgical method and obtain solid retention support of bone tissue. The upper dental prosthesis is connected to support by special devices and methods. The implant repair system is usually classified with the implant material, shape structure, surface structure and connection mode. According to site of the implant, dental implants can be divided into bone eal implant, and soft tissue level implant. According to planting materials, dental implants can be divided into ceramic implant, carbon implant, polymer implant and composite implant. According to the number of operations, dental implants can be divided into one-stage implant and two-stage implant. According to the shape of the implant, dental implants can be divided into spiral implant, columnar implant, leaf-shaped implant, anchor implant and implant base frame. Currently, there is no standard classification for dental implants. The clinical practice of oral implantology makes the present oral implant materials and implant morphology tend to be single. The implant is mainly made of grade four commercial pure titanium. The threaded column and root implant have become widely accepted in the world. Studies have shown that moderately rough surface structure can increase the surface area of the implant and bone bonding. Therefore, the current clinical planting system is generally a rough surface with different roughness obtained through various surface treatments. The implant and the upper prosthesis are connected by a certain structure, which is mainly divided into external connection and internal connection.

Implant denture has great function of support, retention and stability. Dental implants do not pose a risk of clogging the airways or esophagus as normal removable dentures may fall off during eating or speaking. The artificial tooth root is deeply implanted in the alveolar bone, which has functional stimulation to the alveolar bone. It can protect the alveolar bone structure and avoid its atrophy. Through the retention device on the foundation pile, the upper denture is fixed. Good retention and stability can increase comfort and chewing strength. Just like natural teeth, speaking with dental implants when facial expression is as natural as before, increase self-confidence. Dental implants are relatively expensive due to high material and process. The whole treatment time of dental implantation is relatively long, and the implantation technology is more demanding to doctors. In the past 30 years, the technology of dental implantation has developed rapidly, and the success rate of dental implantation has increased greatly. However, dental implants are not suitable for everyone. The adult with good general condition, healthy body and mind, and fixed bone and tooth development is suitable for dental implants. If there are any system diseases such as hemorrhagic disease, hypertension, heart disease, diabetes, etc. , dental implants can be accepted after the treatment is stable.

9.2　The Biological Basis of Oral Implant

9.2.1　Implant-bone interface

The bone-binding theory proposed by Branemark is a milestone in the development of implant denture. It provides a reliable basis for the development and clinical application of dental implants, and the condition of osseointegration has also become a prerequisite for predicting the success of implant dentures. Initially, "bone osseointegration" was described as "the interface between an inactive metal surface and active bone tissue, without the insertion of other tissues, it was a direct bond between the two interfaces", this concept just relied on optical microscopy by which histological phenomena were observed, so the interface status of the implant under functional loading was not considered, nor was there a chemical binding at the molecular level between the implant and the surrounding bone tissue. Thus, Zarb et al. suggested that "bone binding" be defined as "rigid binding to bone tissue without obvious clinical symptoms of heterologous material and can remain in bone during functional load". The process of osseointegration should include mechanical locking between the early implant and the alveolar bone(initial stability), and the subsequent generation and alteration of new bone around the implant(later stability). Recent studies have found that the interface between the implant and bone tissue is very complex. It includes various components of the implant surface, bone tissue, and various cells and proteins between these two interfaces. The diversity of interfaces depends on the mutual recognition and interaction between the implant and bone tissue. A variety of interface−binding theories have been proposed, involving a range of related disciplines, which have greatly promoted the basic research and development of implantology.

9.2.1.1   The formation of the bone−implant interface

The osseointegration of implants has a similar physiological process to the healing of fractures, which can be roughly divided into the initial stage of implants inserted at the beginning of new bone formation, the reconstruction of bone−implant interface and the period of new bone maturation around implants. Implants are implanted in the host sites during surgery and the primary implant stability is achieved through mechanical locking and then bone tissue begins to metabolise. Several hours after implantation, platelets chemotized and adhered to the implants and released a variety of bone growth factors, such as platelet derived growth factor(PDGF) and transforming growth factor beta 1 (TGF−β_1). Several days after implantation, mastocyte began to secrete growth factors (PDGF, TGF−β_1, MDAF, bFGF, IGF and OAF, etc.), and various growth factors jointly regulate the formation of new bone. New born bone cells are abundant and the contents of collagens are high. It has bundle structures called woven bone. After 2 weeks, the bone tissue around the implants was gradually densified, and the gap between the implant surface and bone tissue was filled by woven bone and the stability of the implant was enhanced. At the beginning of the third week, the vascularization of the woven bone was evident and the amount of new bone increased rapidly. After 4 weeks, the new woven bone around the implant and the loose trabecular bone formed the primary bone unit, and the layers were arranged in lamellar bone structure. As the blood circulation is affected by surgical trauma or aseptic inflammatory reaction, necrosis occurs in the cortical bone with a thickness of 0. 5 − 1. 0 mm around the post−surgical implant holes and they can provide adequate primary stability, at the same time, they closed the implant interface in order to separate connective tissue. During the process of new bone formation, they can also be used as a scaffold for osteoblast adhesion, growth, and proliferation At the same time, new capillaries can grow into the area of bone necrosis and then provided adequate nutrient metabolism, and regenerated the active implant−bone interface, finally formd the lamellar bone. The lamellar bone was further mineralized and the bone density around the implant was increased. At 6 weeks the implant has been able to withstand non−functional loads. After 8 weeks, the bone tissue in direct contact with the implant was completely replaced by the mature lamellar bone. After wearing the superstructure, healing process got into the functional weight − bearing stage and with the generation and change of the mechanical stress, the new bone had a series of changes such as increased bone density, rearrangement of bone trabecula, and bone structure adjustment. Sub−mineralization occured and the thickness and strength continued to increase. Bone remodeling is the result of continued bone resorption near the surface of the implant(≤1 mm), reflecting the spread of mechanical stress to the implant−bone interface. Similar to the normal physiological activity of bone tissue, bone remodeling will be carried out for life, and it is a necessary physiological reaction to maintain the osseointegration and long−term stability of implants.

9.2.1.2　Confirmation of osseointegration

(1) There is no loosening in the clinical examination and a crisp sound is produced when slamming with a metal rod.

(2) X-rays show that the implant and bone tissue are in close contact and no transmissive gap.

The histology of animal experiments showed that the protrusions of osteoblasts were attached to the surface of the implant, the bone cells matured, and the interface was free of connective tissue.

9.2.2　Implant-gingival soft tissue interface

Keeping the stability of the marginal bones and soft tissue of the implants neck is an important guarantee for the long-term, stable functioning of implants and the maintenance of their aesthetic effects. Clinical studies have found that bone resorption occurs in the first year after implantation for two-stage implants, and the resorption of alveolar crest usually reaches 1.5-2.0 mm and generally up to the first or second thread of the implant, after that 0.2 mm of bone resorption will occur annually. Because implants were implanted in the first year and the abutments were installed, the interface between the implants and the abutments, soft tissues, and bone tissues was remodeled to affect the bone absorption around the implants.

The interface formed by the contact between the gingival soft tissue and the implant is the gingival interface. Epithelial cells adhere to the surface of the implant and form a biological seal, known as the cuff. The success of implants is directly related to the quality of the closure of the gums. The gingival soft tissue cells adhere to each other through the special proteoglycans and serum protein on the implant surface. The epithelial cells secrete the extracellular matrix, and then form hemidesmosomes between the cell membrane and the titanium oxide film, then adhesion occurred through hemidesmosomes. However, the specific mechanism is still inconclusive. Biological width (BW) studies have shown that the soft tissue healing stage after implant restorations is similar to that of natural teeth. The BW form by the junctional epithelium and connective tissue also exists on the implant surface. Among them, the width of junctional epithelium is approximately 2 mm, and the connective tissue is approximately 1 mm, so the average BW of the implant is approximately 3 mm. Epithelial connective tissue around the implant forms a biologic seal, which blocks oral bacteria and their metabolites from entering the bone tissue. However, the attachment of the epithelium in the implant cuffs is weaker than that of natural teeth: On the one hand, unlike natural teeth, the implant lacks cementum, and there is no perpendicular fiber bundle to its surface. The gingival fibers are aligned parallelly to the surface of the implant and the alveolar dome. The upper soft tissue is oriented parallelly to the implant and does not penetrate the surface of the implant. On the other hand, a few fibroblasts and blood vessels in the inner tissue surround the implant. When the bacteria invade, there is weak inflammatory reaction and low defense capacity, which makes the sites become vulnerable parts of peri-implantitis.

Soft tissue thickness establishes a good implant-soft tissue interface that requires a certain thickness of soft tissue to ensure proper epithelial connective tissue attachment. When the vertical thickness of the local soft tissue is insufficient, the soft tissue attachment space is provided through the bone absorption at the neck and finally a suitable BW is formed. Linkevicius et al. found that if the thickness of soft tissue is less than 2 mm, the bone of the implant neck can be absorbed by 1.45 mm after 1 year. If the soft tissue thickness is above 2.5 mm, the bone resorption is only 0.2 mm. In a subsequent study, Linkevicius et al. found that even when the initial soft tissue is thin, even platform switching implants can not be more conducive to bone preservation than flush-bottomed implants. Therefore, in the BW formation process, thin soft tissue is more likely to cause alveolar bone resorption. Cochran et al. suggested that in order to maintain the stability of the bone around the implant at least 3 mm thick soft tissue is needed around the implant to form a stable epithelial and connective tissue attachment. Linkevicius suggested that soft tissue thickness should be routinely measured prior to implant placement to assess the effect of soft tissue thickness on bone resorption at the margin of the implant.

9.2.3 Factors affecting osseointegration

9.2.3.1 Biocompatibility of planting materials

The essence of osseointegration is to form a stable direct contact between implant and bone, so the biocompatibility of the material is very important for osseointegration Titanium and titanium alloys have excellent biocompatibility, good galvanic corrosion resistance, high strength, and low elastic modulus, and have been commonly used as dental implant materials. Currently, the latest generation of ITI implants (SLActive surface), with its unique surface treatment method, greatly improve the biocompatibility and bone-binding ability, and can achieve perfect osseointegration within 4 weeks after implantation, shortening the treatment procedure.

9.2.3.2 The surface structure and performance of the implant

The surface structure of the implant includes macrostructure and microstructure. In the aspect of the macrostructure of the implant, the shape is irregular, and the implants with holes, grooves, and sockets are easy to mechanically interlock with the bone tissue to increase the binding force. The microstructure of the implant surface also affects the function of the cells and the binding force between the implant and the bone. Roughness of the implant surface can be divided into four categories: smooth surface ($Sa < 0.5$ μm), low-rough surface($0.5\ \mu m < Sa < 1.0\ \mu m$), moderately rough surface($1.0\ \mu m < Sa < 2.0\ \mu m$) and the rough surface($Sa \geq 2.0\ \mu m$). The roughness of the implant surface is determined by the geometry of the implant and the micromorphology of the surface after treatment. Experiments have shown that moderate rough surfaces can provide good mechanical locking shortly after placement, allowing implants to gain more bone contact and greater binding force, as well as good initial stability. Materials with different surface energy implanted in the body will have different protein layers adsorbed on surfaces. This will determine the attachment of cells and the interaction between cells and protein layers. Implants with low surface energy often form a low-binding fiber layer in the interface region, while high surface energy substances form a tight bond with the tissue on the surface. The increase in surface energy of implants is manifested as enhanced hydrophilicity, which will more effectively promote the attachment of osteogenic related factors such as adhesion proteins, growth factors, finally promote osteoblast adhesion, extension, and proliferation.

9.2.3.3 Implant trauma

During the process of preparation implant holes, the mechanical cutting of the drill bit and the resulting heat will damage the bone tissue, resulting in a necrotic bone with a thickness of about 1 mm on the inner surface of the planting nest. When the temperature exceeds 47 ℃, the layer organization increases by 1 time. Since healing involves the removal of necrotic bone and hyperplasia of new bone, the greater the trauma was made, the greater the inflammatory response, the longer the healing process and the less likely to form osseointegration would have. Therefore, during the operation, the drilling rate should be controlled below 2,000 r/min and continued to be cooled with 4 ℃ saline. In addition, the accuracy of preparing the implant bed is also closely related to the formation of osseointegration. If the gap between the surface of the implant and the bone tissue is > 0.5 mm, the bone callus tissue will not be able to connect bone, resulting in a fibro-bone junctional interface Therefore, the diameter of the implant hole should be slightly smaller (spiral implant) or consistent(non-spiral implant)than the diameter of the selected implant in order to obtain good early stabilization of the implant.

9.2.3.4　The healing ability of the planting bed

Bone mineral density in the planting area is one of the factors affecting the interface formation. The higher the bone density is, the higher the binding rate of the implant and bone will be. Patients with systemic diseases such as osteoporosis and diabetes, as well as patients undergoing radiochemotherapy and immunosuppressive drugs, suffer from bone and mineral metabolism abnormalities, which reduce bone formation rate, change bone remodeling and increase bone density. The healing of the window in the area is affected, so care should be taken to assess the patient's status and determine the appropriate repair plan. In recent years, many reports have confirmed that low intensity pulsed ultrasound(LIPUS) can accelerate the healing of fractures and enhance the mechanical properties of the healing tissue. Liu et al. reported that the punctuated cavitation and microcaloric effects produced by LIPUS can accelerate bone repair in implanted areas, shorten healing time after implant placement, and enhance bone mass around the implant.

9.2.3.5　The loading status of the implant

Load is an important factor in determining the interface of implant bone tissue. Pilliar et al. believe that osteoblasts and fibroblasts are differentiated from mesenchymal cells. If the implant is loaded at an early stage, there will be some degree of motion. In the interfacial region, the cells are mechanically stimulated by the loosening of the implant, which promotes the formation of fibroblasts and eventually forms a fibro−osteoporotic interface. With the further study of histology and biomechanics, it was found that implants can also form osseointegration under certain physiological loads. The osseointegrated implant will have a 30 μm fretting under normal conditions. If the load exceeds the physiological range and the fretting exceeds 150 μm, the osseointegration conditions may be converted to fibrous osseointegration. Therefore, when the implant is implanted, special attention should be paid to the direction of implantation, minimizing the level or torsion force, so that the newly formed osseointegration can be maintained for a long time.

9.3　Dental Implant Surgery

With the continuous improvement of implantation system and the development of imaging technology and digital technology, implantation repair technology can be accepted in theory for patients with single tooth loss, multiple tooth loss and edentulous jaw. If there is an adverse reaction to implantation repair, it may lead to poor general health, serious endocrine and metabolic disorders, such as uncontrolled diabetes. Dental implant surgery is contraindicated in patients with poor systemic conditions or who cannot afford surgery due to serious systemic diseases: diseases of the blood system, such as erythrocyte or leukocyte hematopathy, coagulation disorders. Cardiovascular disease, which can not tolerate surgery. Long−term use of special drugs affecting clotting or tissue healing, severe systemic immune disease, pregnancy, excessive addiction to alcohol, tobacco, nerve and mental disorders. Dental implant surgery is also contraindicated in patients with local restrictions on oral and maxillofacial conditions: acute and chronic inflammation in the mouth, such as gingival, mucosa and maxillary sinus. Benign and malignant tumors in oral or maxilla, and some bone diseases, such as osteoporosis and osteomalacia. Serious habitual bruxism and inadequate distance between the jaw. Poor oral hygiene.

The procedures of implantation repair: clinical examination and imaging examination, diagnosis and treatment design, surgery, denture making and repair, and implant and prosthesis maintenance. According to the time relationship between implant placement and tooth extraction, implantation can be divided into immediate implantation, and delayed implantation(3 months after tooth extraction and longer). According to the relationship between the load on the prosthesis and the implantation time, the implant restoration can be divided into immediate load, early load and delayed load. With the development of prosthodontics, the treatment cycle is being significantly shortened, and it is possible for implants to be implanted and even tooth extraction to be implanted.

Dental implantation should follow the basic principles. It is in line with the most basic principles of surgical bacteria concept and aseptic operation to ensure that the implant and the implanted bed are free of contamination. The operation is delicate and gentle. The trauma is minimized and the implanted tissue is retained to ensure the initial stability of the implant and to achieve bone healing. Prevention of secondary injury, such as nerve vascular bundle, maxillary sinus, nasal cavity and lateral bone perforation should be avoided. Reduction of thermal damage. When drilling in full planting bed, a large amount of normal saline should be used to cool down. Pay attention to the relationship with the superstructure. The placement of dental implants should take into account the uniform stress distribution of the implant denture. The placement of the terminal implant should not be too close to the middle. Dental implants should not be located near the buccal or lingual side of the alveolar ridge. The direction of the dental implant is related to the fabrication and repair effect of the superstructure. During the operation, the directional bar is put into the unfinished implant socket, and the relationship with other foundation piles or natural tooth direction is measured visually. If it is not ideal, it should be adjusted.

Before the implant surgery, the surgeon will perform a pre-implant surgery, including soft tissue surgery, alveoloplasty, alveolar bone augmentation, and maxillary sinus elevation, which can not be performed at the same time as the implant. It is recommended to use dental implant guide plate for implantation. The method of making implantable implant guide for non-total tooth loss is divided into CT data collection, bone 3D model reconstruction, the patient's bone conditions, and the simulated cylinder of the implant socket according to the implant position design the implant scheme. Preoperative routine cleaning, oral disinfection should be applied with 2% iodine tincture or 0.2% iodov, but 75% ethanol must be used to remove iodine, because iodine is harmful to metal implants. Local incision should also be used for infiltration anesthesia to stop bleeding. Anesthetic drugs are generally available with 2% procaine, 2% lidocaine or 0.5% bupivacaine. The patient is usually in a supine position with the surgeon on the side of the head. The assistant is on the right and the instrument nurse is on the left. After incision of the mucosa, the incision of the periosteum was cut roughly 0.5 cm along the submucosa toward the top of the alveolar ridge. Then all alveolar processes were exposed and separated along the bone surface. According to the predesigned template, prepare planting nest. According to the bone quantity of alveolar bone, the suitable length of implant and corresponding series of drill are selected. The rapid drill of dental implant machine is used to rinse with a large amount of normal saline. First, the drilling is positioned with a circular drill, followed by the gradual reaming with a crack drill and navigation drill, and then the upper opening is expanded and the wound is rinsed. A slow drill was used instead, a large amount of saline was also used to rinse and cool down, and a tap was used to prepare the threads on the implant socket wall. The implant is gently inserted into the prepared implant socket and carefully tightened with special tools to make the top edge of the implant level with the bone surface. The implant fixation screw is required to be in place, and the fixation is tightened and fixed, but the bone socket thread can not be damaged. The upper end of the implant can be struck with a metal rod, and the sound of crisp metal percussion indicates that the implant is in place and fixed satisfactorily. Finally screw in the cover nut. In order to achieve good healing of the gingival mucosa, the mucosa should be tightly encircled by the reposition of the mucosa flap with strict suture, especially around the base. Finally, the wound surface was covered with gauze, and the mandible was padded with gauze to make it bite pressure for 1 hour. After 7 days, remove the thread and continue to wear the original removable denture, but a part should be rubbed off at the implantation site of the implant on its base tissue surface, as a buffer to avoid crushing the mucosa. 3 – 6 months after the operation, along with the implant and the alveolar bone close tightly, the whole process of dental implantation was completed after the installation of the porcelain crown.

The reduction of postoperative infection and the improvement of patient satisfaction are related to the implementation of quality care in perioperative period. Warm yarn ball is used for compression and hemostasis, and ice compress is used to relieve swelling and pain. If obvious swelling appears the next day, remove 1–2 lines to make the discharge drainage unobstructed, then clean the wound. The patients were treated with antibiotics 5–7 days after surgery. If the secretions were large or accompanied by other systemic symptoms, the patients should immediately increase the dosage of antibiotics or switch to other antibiotics. After setting porcelain teeth, should gradually adapt to increase the hardness of chewing food. To prevent the impact of external forces, do not immediately chew hard things. Once the impact of the root of the tooth may be injured, immediately to the hospital for examination and treatment. Postoperative follow-up is of great significance to improve the success rate of implant. Medical workers should also do regular follow-up work to understand the postoperative situation and patients' inner thoughts, and actively respond to post operative emergencies. Patients should be reviewed every 3 months in the first year after surgery, and the follow-up interval should be adjusted according to the patient's own situation. Patients with periodontitis with poor oral health control should be reviewed once every 3 – 6 months, and the interval of follow – up for patients with good oral health can be prolonged.

Currently, the well-accepted standards for successful dental implants include the following: Implant stability and tightness index < 0. No bone density reduction around the implant. Vertical bone resorption <3 mm. No nerve, maxillary sinus and nasal injuries. Periodontal pocket depth in all directions <5 mm. 5–year success rate is over 85% of maxilla and 95% of mandible; and 10–year success rate is over 80%. Complications caused by planting generally fall into two categories: biological and mechanical. Biological complications include surgical bleeding, nerve damage, maxillary sinus perforation, adjacent tooth injury, postoperative infection, periimplant inflammation and abscission. Mechanical complications mainly include implant and prosthesis related screws, abutment, implant fracture, restoration damage, etc. Suture too tight or loose, especially in the case of an infection should debridement in time and suture again. Hemorrhage is mostly caused by large injury or extensive submucosal dissection and insufficient postoperative compression. Early cold compress and late hot compress are advocated. Lower lip numbness is mainly caused by intraoperative damage to the mental nerve or the alveolar nerve. The former is mostly recoverable. The latter should remove the implant and avoid nerve reimplantation. Progressive marginal bone resorption mostly occurs in the bone tissue of the neck of the implant, and is associated with gingivitis, periimplant inflammation, overconcentration of implant stress, and prolonged uncorrected mechanical fracture of the implant.

9.4 Bone Augmentation Procedure

9.4.1 Guided bone regeneration technology

9.4.1.1 Introduction

Guided bone regeneration (GBR) technology, which uses the principle of barrier membrane for guided tissue regeneration (GTR) to establish an isolation space through the membrane to allow angiogenic cells and osteogenic cells migrate to the defect area and prevents fibroblasts from forming new bone. It provides an effective treatment for the bone defect caused by peri-implantitis or some other disease in implantology.

The materials used for GBR include both the barrier membrane materials and bone substitutes. Restoration of bone tissue, especially completed bone regeneration requires basal bone to provide adequate blood supplement, mechanical stability, requires abundant osteogenic cells, angiogenic cells and tension-free soft tissue to coverage and exist a critical value for bone defects (1 mm defect is the critical value for direct bridging of woven bone).

GBR, by increasing the growth of bone progenitors and vascular progenitor cells, which provides space for its growth, promotes the differentiation and proliferation of osteogenic cells, activates osteoblasts, promotes bone matrix secretion, and activates undifferentiated mesenchymal cells to increase the bone.

The barrier membrane is placed between the bone defect and the mucoperiosteal flap to prevent the growth of fibroblasts and connective tissue, providing an isolated environment for bone repairing and reconstruction. The barrier membrane needs to be biocompatible, with no cytotoxicity, immunological rejection, and its degradation does not affect the formation of new bone; it makes cell isolated, which isolates the connective tissue cells that affect bone regeneration, maintains space, and ensures new bone bone mass and profile tissue integration; the barrier membrane, surface-covered soft tissue and underlying blood clot can be quickly integrated into a whole.

The bone substitute material can support the barrier membrane to avoid its collapse, guide cell migration, provide its growth scaffold, and at the same time stabilize blood clots. It is absorbed slowly and promotes bone formation and osseointegration.

Bone substitutes are divided into autologous bone substitutes (bulk bone, granular bone, bone chips, bone mud), allogeneic bone substitutes (fresh frozen bone, allogeneic freeze-dried bone, allogeneic demineralized freeze-dried bone), xenogeneic bone substitutes (animal-derived bone matrix, such as deproteinized bovine bone matrix; animal-derived bone-like matrix, extracted from corals, algae), heterogeneous bone substitute materials (calcium phosphate, bioactive glass, polymer).

9.4.1.2   Inical procedure

(1) Complete debridement in the area of the operation.

(2) Bone substitute is wetted by 0.9% normal saline or mixed with growth factors prepared from autologous blood, and is strictly implanted into the bone graft area. (Figure 9-1-Figure 9-3).

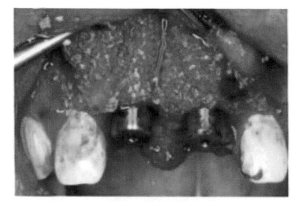
Figure 9-1   Overlying bamier membrane materials

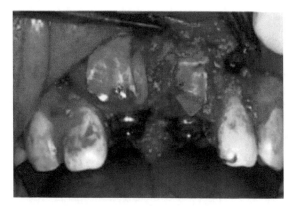
Figure 9-2   Covering membrane

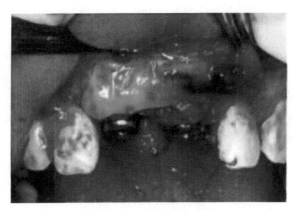

Figure 9-3 Covering A-PRF

9.4.1.3 Alveolar ridge preservation

(1) Introduction

After removal of the residual root and residual crown of the implant site, the healing of the tooth extraction fossa and the reconstruction of the bone and soft tissue will appear. After 3 months of healing, the horizontal resorption of the alveolar bone was 2.2 mm at the crest, and 1.3, 0.59, and 0.3 mm at 3, 6, and 9 mm apical to the crest, respectively; after 6 months of healing, the vertical resorption of the alveolar bone was 11% –22%, whereas the horizontal resorption of the alveolar bone was 29% – 63%.

It is difficult to avoid the absorption of the lip bone and the change of the soft tissue, and affect the final effect of the implant. In this case, the preservation of the tooth extraction site can reduce the alveolar ridge absorption, increase the bone support for the soft tissue, and avoid or reduce the atrophy of the soft tissue during the healing process of the tooth socket. Improving the quality of new bone and mucosa will create conditions for aesthetic restoration.

(2) Clinical procedure

1) Minimally invasive extraction of teeth: using Minimally invasive extraction instruments to separate periodontal ligament and extract teeth in order to avoid the injury of bone wall. Debridement of the tooth pit (Figure 9-4).

2) Clear tooth extraction: scratch the extraction socket and thoroughly remove the residual lesion tissue. Implant bone substitutes (Figure 9-5).

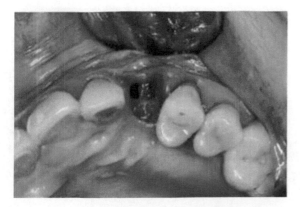

Figure 9-4 Debridement of the tooth pit

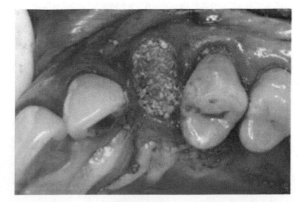

Figure 9-5 Implant bone substitutes

Bone substitutes were filled in the tooth extraction fossa. Seal extraction socket (Figure 9-6, Figure 9-7).

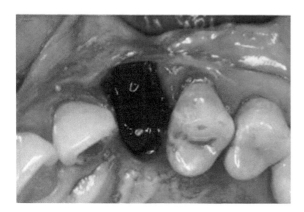

Figure 9-6　**Covering A-PRF**

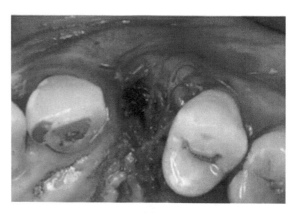

Figure 9-7　**Sealed extraction socket**

Transplant soft tissues, such as palatal mucosal flap, collagen membrane. And CBCT shown at before the surgery (Figure 9-8), after the surgery (Figure 9-9), after surgery for 7 months (Figure 9-10).

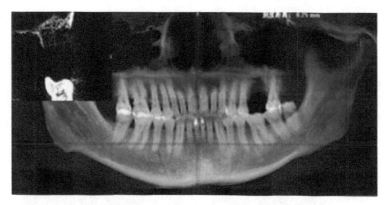

Figure 9-8　**CBCT before surgery**

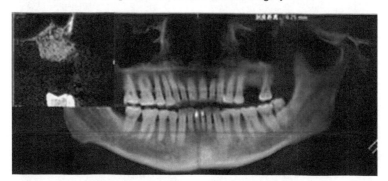

Figure 9-9　**CBCT before surgery**

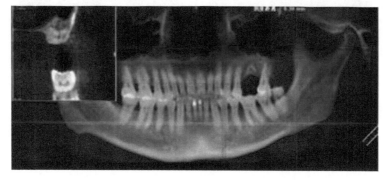

Figure 9-10　**CBCT after surgery for 7 months**

9.4.1.4 Autogenous bone augumentation

(1) Introduction

Autogenous bone has been the gold standard for bone graft. Autologous bone substitute is the use of autologous bone for bone grafting without or rarely using bone substitutes. The advantage of autogenous bone is better bone induction and bone guidance ability, but the disadvantage lies in opening up the second operative area and easily producing complications.

(2) Clinical procedure

1) Donor bone: the parts of the bone can be divided into the mouth (the joint of the mandible, the maxillary tuberosity, the posterior molar area and the ramus mandible) and the outside of the mouth (ilium, rib, outer plate of the skull, frontal bone), but the former can be more accepted by the patients because of the bone marrow in the mouth.

2) Onlay bone grafting: massive bone embedded in the bone surface of the recipient area can effectively increase the width and height of the severely absorbed alveolar ridge. In addition, an important factor in the survival of massive bone is the stabilization of bone fragments.

Autogenous bone augumentation(Figure 9–11–Figure 9–16).

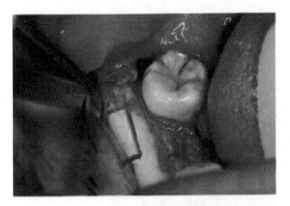

Figure 9–11　**Bone taking**

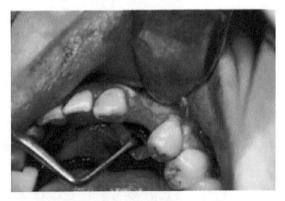

Figure 9–12　**Full-thickness flap**

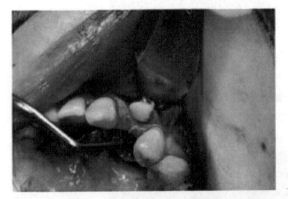

Figure 9–13　**Onlay bone graft**

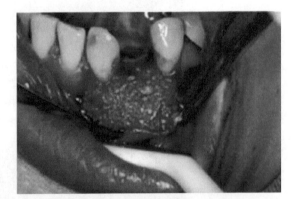

Figure 9–14　**Input bone substitutes**

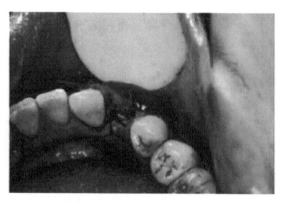

Figure 9-15 **Stitch**

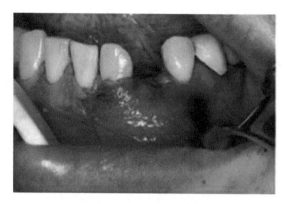

Figure 9-16 **Sealed**

9.4.1.5 Maxillary sinus floor elevation

Maxillary sinus floor elevation or maxillary sinus augmentation refers to a case in which the maxillary sinus floor is too low due to maxillary sinus gasification and the height of the alveolar ridge does not meet the implant length requirement. The mucous membrane of the sinus floor is lifted and the bone augmentation material is employed into the space and the implant will be implanted simultaneously or in stages. At present, the maxillary sinus floor elevation operation mainly includes elevation of maxillary sinus floor with alveolar crest approach and elevation of maxillary sinus floor by opening of the lateral wall of maxillary sinus.

(1) Elevation of maxillary sinus floor with alveolar crest approach

Summers proposed a maxillary sinus floor elevation technique to lift maxillary sinus. The technology uses a Summers-designed top-end sharp, concave-shaped osteotomer (Summers osteotomers) to break the maxillary sinus floor plate with a hammer and lifts the maxillary sinus floor and the bone plate simultaneously in order to obtain more space. Although many scholars have controversial about the elevation of the maxillary sinus, the type of technique is still favored by physicians and patients, which is considered to be a conventional technique in implant therapy. In the Chinese literature, it is known as maxillary sinus lift or cap lift.

Instruments of elevation of maxillary sinus floor with alveolar crest approach (Figure 9 – 17 – Figure 9–19).

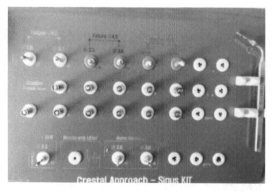

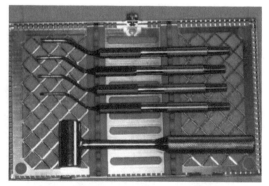

Figure 9-17 **Maxillary sinus lifting tool box**

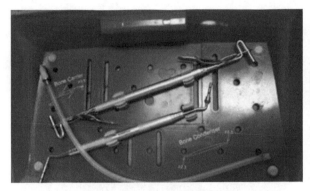

Figure 9-18   Bone carrier bone condenser hydraulic lifter hydraulic lifting tube

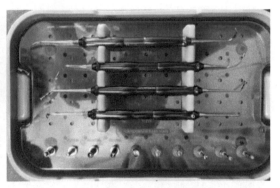

Figure 9-19   Maxillary sinus lift kit

(2) Clinical procedure

1) Routinely disinfectant paving, under the local anesthesia, cutting along the side of the alveolar crest to the bone surface and bluntly separating the mucoperiosteum to expose the alveolar crest at the odontic area.

2) Identify the site of implantation for maxillary sinus elevation. The traditional method used the Summers bone chisel hammer method to break the maxillary sinus floor plate, carefully separating the maxillary sinus floor mucosa, lifting the maxillary sinus floor and the fractured bone plate simultaneously, and employing the bone substitute material in the lifting space. The current advanced method uses a CAS-KIT or DASK drill with different diameters in the maxillary sinus lifting kit to fracture the sinus floor plate, raising the maxillary sinus mucosa, and carefully implant the bone substitute material to the desired height.

3) The maxillary sinus mucosal integrity must be ensured during surgery, and the balloon method is usually to judge the integrity of maxillary sinus mucosa. The method inject a proper amount of physiological saline into the implantation cavity, and when the resistance of the mucous membrane is felt, multiple repeated injections and withdrawal are required until physiological saline can be injected into the gap between the bottom of implantation cavity and the maxillary sinus mucosa without resistance, so that the maxillary sinus mucosa is gradually separated from the maxillary sinus floor. After saline injection, it can be withdrawn back to the syringe to assist in judging that the mucosa is not damaged. Confirming that the nasal ventilation experiment is negative, the bone substitute material is employed in the lifting space.

4) Case report (Figure 9-20-Figure 9-22).

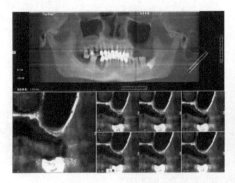
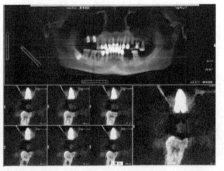

Figure 9-20   Preoperative and postoperative CBCT of left maxillary first molar

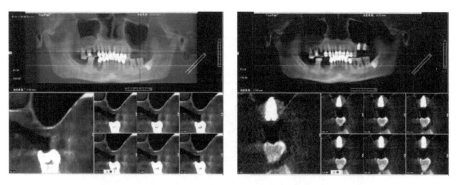

Figure 9-21　Preoperative and postoperative CBCT of left maxillary second molar

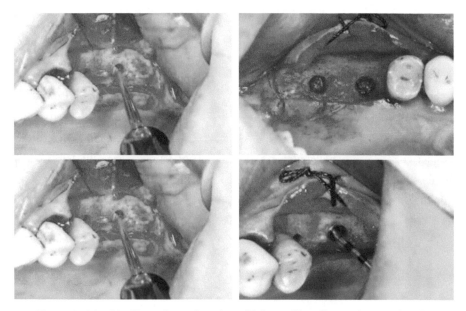

Figure 9-22　Maxillary sinus elevation of left maxillary first and second molar

(3) Elevation of maxillary sinus floor by opening of the lateral wall of maxillary sinus

1) Introduction: In 1980, Boyne applied Caldwell-Lucopening to remove maxillary sinus mucosa filed with autologous cancellous granules and lifted the maxillary sinus floor and three months later implanted bladed implants. Subsequently, Taum et al. performed a maxillary sinus floor elevation using the same method, but did not peel the fenestrational lateral bone plate and retained it as the maxillary sinus sinus floor. Prior to this, the maxillary sinus site was a restricted area for implant therapy. In 1996, the Society of Osseointegration held a consensus seminar on maxillary sinus floor elevation, which included bone graft materials, implant types, timing of implant placement, analysis of implant failure, radiation analysis, indications, contraindications, and implant restorations. At present, the maxillary sinus lateral wall opening technique has become a routine surgical procedure for implant surgery. It is known as a maxillary sinus floor elevation technique in the Chinese literature.

2) Instruments of elevation of maxillary sinus floor by opening of the lateral wall of maxillary sinus (Figure 9-23).

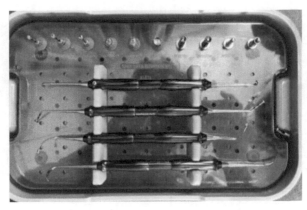

Figure 9-23　Maxillary sinus lift kit

3) Clinical procedure

● Routinely disinfectant paving, under the local anesthesia, the incision was made by horizontal incision of the alveolar ridge at the humeral side and vertical incision at the middle and distal sides.

● DASK drill was used to open the window in the wall of maxillary sinus. The position of the bone wall was the position which the lower edge of the bone window was located 3 – 5 mm above the maxillary sinus floor, and the upper edge of the bone window was located about 10 mm above the lower edge.

● Peeling the sinus floor mucosa along the perimeter of the manufacturing side window with a curved sinus spoon (the thickness of maxillary sinus mucosa is only 1 mm).

● Implantation of bone substitutes in the lifted maxillary sinus space.

4) Case report: see Figure 9-24.

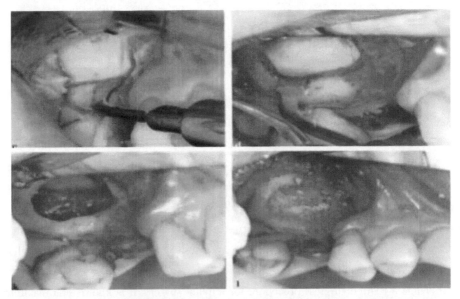

Figure 9-24　Side wall window maxillary sinus floor elevation of right first molar

(4) Osteotomy

1) Introduction: Split-ridge technique uses a bone chisel to gradually open a narrow alveolar ridge and increases the width of the alveolar ridge. The bucco-lingual gap is obtained after splitting of the alveolar bone and satisfies the implantation of the implant and the employs the GBR at the same time in order to ensures the initial stability of the implant and reduces the amount of bone graft.

2) Instruments of osteotomy (Figure 9-25).

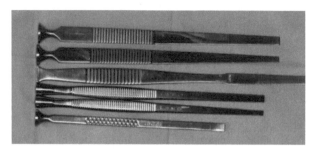

Figure 9-25   **Osteotomy instruments**

3) Clinical procedure

● Routinely disinfectant paving, under the local anesthesia, cutting along the side of the alveolar crest to the bone surface and bluntly separate the mucoperiosteum to expose the alveolar crest at the edentulous region and root ossification in the edentulous region.

● Designation of the bone opening path: It uses an ultrasonic bone knife to cut the root of the alveolar ridge, controls the direction of the bone opening path, and places the bone opening path on the thickened temporal bone wall of the bone plate.

● Osteotomy: The alveolar ridge is splited along a bone splitting path using a single-sided osteotome, with the osteotomy plane facing the temporal side and the oblique side facing the buccal side. The tip of the instrument indicates the depth.

● Bone substitute material was implanted in the space around the implant and on the surface of the buccal bone plate.

4) Case Report: see Figure 9-26.

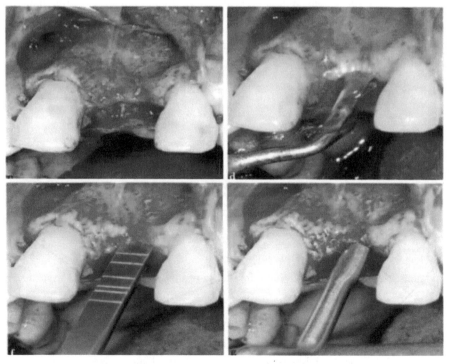

Figure 9-26   **Bony splitting bilateral bone grafting and guided bone regeneration**

9.5　Implant Maintenance

There is a relationship between the implant and periodontology tissues which are similar to the natural tooth. It is necessary to perform special implant cleaning around the implant tooth and conventional cleaning of the surrounding natural tooth to maintain the long-term stability of the implant. The dental implant should be coordinated with the natural teeth to maintain the normal function of oral and maxillofacial system, and the dental implant should be coordinated regularly to adapt to the changing relationship. Dental implants, like natural teeth, are composed of multiple parts, but each part of the natural teeth is organically combined together. Ddental implants are connected by screws or adhesives, so it should be regularly checked in the hospital to see if the various parts of the dental implants have lesions, so as to timely treatment. Patients who have received dental implants should pay close attention to their own cleaning and maintenance, and visit professional dental hospitals regularly for the re-examination of dental calculus and plaque removal. If patient has a large number of different kinds of bacteria in the gingival crevicular and surrounding tissues, the bacteria can easily adhere to the surface of the implant and multiply a lot, causing infection, which may complicate the bone integration process and cause the implant failure. The length of life of each implant is not only related to the treatment quality, but also closely related to the patient's physical condition, use and self-maintenance in the future, which is one of the important factors to determine the implant life. Records show that one of the earliest modern dental implants has been perfectly serviced for tooth loss for over 40 years.

Implant surrounding gingival sulcus for microorganisms colonize provides a unique ecological environment, compared with non-smokers, smokers in gingival sulcus around implants healthy microbial diversity is reduced, and microorganisms related to disease, such as lactic acid bacteria, treponema, propionic acid bacillus, pseudomonas, carbon fiber autophagy bacteria, cilia bacteria present significant enrichment phenomenon. Smoking increases the reproduction of bacteria, which invades the implant and interferes with the immune system, causing inflammation around the implant. Changes in the level of inflammatory factors may affect the good formation of the implant-bone interface, and even damage the existing implant-bone interface, causing the implant to loosen and fall off. Smoking can inhibit the proliferation and function of B and T cells, and enhance the survival ability of polymorphonuclear white blood cells, thereby interfering with humoral and cellular immunity. High expression of the protease inhibitors, tumor necrosis factor alpha, bone protection element can reduce periodontal tissue anti-infection ability, interfere with wound healing. Some scholars reported that the annual absorbance rate of alveolar bone in patients with smoking was significantly higher than that in the non-smoking group 5-10 years post implantation. The success rate of using surface modified implants by smokers and non-smokers is not much different from that of bone loss. A moderately rough implant surface can accelerate bone formation at the implant interface, promote implant stability and shorten treatment. Reducing smoking and even quitting smoking are still seen as key factors to improve the success rate of implant repair in patients. Implanting patients, especially those with periodontal disease, should strictly control tobacco, correct bad oral habits, and improve oral hygiene environment. After the periodontal tissue is in a stable period, the implant denture repair stage can be started. Postoperative care-giving, regular follow-up, control of periodontal disease and systemic disease, and improve the implant function repair effect.

▶▶ *Summary*

Dental implant can achieve a repair effect very similar to natural tooth function, structure and aesthetic effect, and has become the preferred repair method for more and more patients with tooth loss. The success of implantation therapy is closely related to the healthy status of the surrounding tissues, good oral hygiene and regular maintenance of professional implants. Patients should pay attention to oral hygiene, control inflammation and adopt positive postoperative care, which is crucial to the stability of periodontal tissue and the success of implantation.

Yin Lihua, Guo Zhuling

Chapter 10

Orofacial and Neck Infection

10.1 Introduction

Infections of orofacial and neck region, particularly those of odontogenic origin, have been one of the most common diseases in human beings. Despite great advances in health care, these infections remain a major problem; quite often faced by oral and maxillofacial surgeons. These infections range from periapical abscess to superficial and deep neck infections. The infections generally spread by following the path of least resistance through connective tissue and along fascial planes. The infections spread to such an extent, distant from the site of origin, causing considerable morbidity and occasional death.

Early recognition of orofacial infection and prompt, appropriate therapy are absolutely essential. A thorough knowledge of anatomy of the face and neck is necessary to predict pathways of spread of these infections and to drain these spaces adequately.

This chapter deals with various types of orofacial and neck infections, with necessary description of numerous fascial spaces; with special reference to their involvement, surgical anatomy, clinical features, principles of their management with the surgical techniques used for drainage or decompression of the infections by intraoral orextra oral routes, and finally modes of their spread and the complications that would be encountered if these cases are left untreated, are also discussed.

10.2 Etiology

Infections in the orofacial and neck region usually originate from following sources.

10.2.1 General classification: it is based on the origin of the infection

(1) Odontogenic: the majority of infections in orofacial and neck region belong to this group. Odontogenic infections arise within jaw bones, and can be classified as those arising from: ①pulp disease. ②periodontal disease. ③secondarily infected cysts or odontomes. ④remaining root fragment. ⑤residual infection. ⑥pericoronal infection.

These manifest in the following forms：① periapical abscess. ② periodontal abscess. ③ infected cyst. ④ residual abscess. ⑤ pericoronal abscess.

（2）Traumatic：occasionally，trauma from penetrating wounds of soft and hard tissues of the face can lead to orofacial infection.

（3）Implant surgery.

（4）Reconstructive surgery.

（5）Infections arising from contaminated needle punctures.

（6）Others：this group includes instances of orofacial infections arising from other factors such as infected antrum，salivary gland afflictions.

（7）Secondary to oral malignancies.

10.2.2　On the basis of causative organisms：orofacial infections can be classified

（1）Bacterial infections

①The odontogenic infections encountered in orofacial region are mostly bacterial infections. ② Non-odontogenic infections：tonsillar，nasal infections which are more common in children，and furuncle of overlying skin.

（2）Fungal infections

These infections have a slow rate of spread. These are difficult to diagnose in early stages.

（3）Viral infections

The literature does not show sufficient reports about these conditions of odontogenic origin.

Irrespective of the original source of infection，once it has been established within the soft tissues，its further spread tends to occur in uniform fashion.

10.3　Odontogenic Infection

10.3.1　Pathways of odontogenic infection

Serious dental infection，spreading beyond the tooth socket，is more common due to the pulpal infection than the periodontal infection.

10.3.2　Anatomic location

The anatomic spaces of the head and neck can be graded in severity by the level to which they threaten the airway or vital structures，such as the heart and mediastinum or the cranial contents. The buccal，infraorbital vestibular，and subperiosteal spaces can be categorized as having low severity because infections in these spaces do not threaten the airway or vital structures. Infections of anatomic spaces that can hinder access to the airway due to swelling or trismus can be classified as having moderate severity. Such anatomic spaces include the masticatory space，whose components may be considered separately as the submasseteric，pterygomandibular，and superficial and deep temporal spaces，and the perimandibular spaces （submandibular，submental，and sublingual）. Infections that have high severity are those in which swelling can directly obstruct or deviate the airway or threaten vital structures. These anatomic spaces are the lateral pharyngeal and retropharyngeal，the danger space，and the mediastinum. Cavernous sinus thrombosis and other intracranial infection also have high severity.

The clinical presentation and relevant surgical anatomy of infections of the various deep fascial spaces of the head and neck have been well described in other texts. The borders, contents, and relations of the various anatomic deep spaces that are likely to be invaded by odontogenic infections are described in Table 10-1 and Table 10-2.

Table 10-1 Borders of the deep spaces of the head and neck

Space	Borders					
	Anterior	Posterior	Superior	Inferior	Superficial or medial	Deep or lateral
Buccal	Corner of mouth	Masseter m. pterygomandibular space	Maxilla, infraorbital space	Mandible tissue and skin	Subcutaneous	Buccinator m.
Infraorbital	Nasal cartilages	Buccal space	Quadratus labii superioris m.	Oral mucosa	Quadratus labii superioris m.	Levator anguli oris m. , maxilla
Submandibular	Ant. belly digastric m.	Post. belly digastric, stylohyoid, stylopharyngeus mm.	Inf. and med. surfaces of mandible	Digastric tendon	Platysma m. , investing fascia	Mylohyoid, hyoglossus, sup. constrictor mm.
Submental	Inf. border of mandible	Hyoid bone	Mylohyoid m.	Investing fascia	Investing fascia	Ant. bellies digastric m.
Sublingual	Lingual surface of mandible	Submandibular space	Oral mucosa	Mylohyoid m.	Muscles of tongue	Lingual surface of mandible
Pterygomandibular	Buccal space	Parotid gland	Lateral pterygoid m.	Inf. border of mandible	Med. pterygoid muscle	Ascending ramus of mandible
Lateral pharyngeal	Sup. and mid. pharyngeal constrictor mm.	Carotid sheath and scalene fascia	Skull base	Hyoid bone	Pharyngeal constrictors and retropharyngeal space	Medial pterygoid m.
Retropharyngeal	Sup. and mid. constrictor mm.	Alar fascia	Skull base	Fusion of alar and prevertebral fasciae at C_6-T_4 space	None	Carotid sheath and lateral pharyngeal space
Pretracheal	Sternothyroid-thyrohyoid fascia	Retropharyngeal space	Thyroid cartilage	Superior mediastinum	Sternothyroid-thyrohyoid fascia	Visceral fascia over trachea and thyroid gland

Adapted from Flynn TR.[1] ant. = anterior; inf. = inferior; lat. = lateral; m. = muscle; mm. = muscles; med. = medial; mid. = middle; post. = posterior; sup. = superior.

Table 10-2   **Relations of deep spaces in infections**

Space	Likely cause	Contents	Neighboring spaces	Approach for incision and drainage
Buccal	Upper bicuspids, upper molars, lower bicuspids	Parotid duct Ant. facial a. and v. , transverse facial a. and v. , buccal fat pad	Infraorbital, pterygomandibular, infratemporal	Intraoral (small) Extraoral (large)
Infraorbital	Upper cuspid	Angular a. and v. , infraorbital n.	Buccal	Intraoral
Submandibular	Lower molars	Submandibular gland, facial a. and v. , lymph nodes	Sublingual submental Lateral pharyngeal Buccal	Extraoral
Submental	Loweranteriors, fracture of symphysis	Ant. jugular v. , lymph nodes	Submandibular (on either side)	Extraoral
Sublingual	Lower bicuspids, lower molars, direct trauma	Sublingual glands, Wharton's ducts, lingual n. , sublingual a. and v.	Submandibular, lateral pharyngeal, visceral (trachea and esophagus)	Intraoral Intraoral–extraoral
Pterygomandibular	Lower third molars, fracture of angle of mandible	Mandibular div. of trigeminal n. Inf. alveolar a. and v.	Buccal, lateral pharyngeal, submasseteric, deep temporal, parotid Peritonsillar	Intraoral Intraoral–extraoral
Submasseteric	Lower third molars, fracture of angle of mandible	Masseteric a. and v.	Buccal, pterygomandibular, Superf, temporal, parotid	Intraoral Intraoral–extraoral
Infratemporal and deep temporal	Upper molars	Pterygoid plexus, internal maxillary a. and v. , mandibular div. of trigeminal n. , skull base foramina	Buccal Superf. temporal Inf. petrosal sinus	Intraoral Extraoral Intraoral–extraoral
Superficial temporal	Upper molars, lower molars	Temporal fatpad, temporal branch of facial n.	Buccal Deep temporal	Intraoral Extraoral Intraoral–extraoral
Lateral pharyngeal	Lower third molars, tonsillar infection in neighboring spaces	Carotid a. , internal jugular v. , vagus n. , cervical sympathetic chain	Pterygomandibular intraoral Submandibular Sublingual Peritonsillar Retropharyngeal	Intraoral–extraoral

Adapted from Flynn TR. [2] a. =artery; div. =division; inf. =inferior; n. =nerve; superf. =superficial; v. =vein; ant. =anterior.

Table 10-3 lists the severity score for each of the various deep fascial spaces. Thus, a patient with cellulitis or abscess of the right buccal (SS=1), right pterygomandibular (SS=2), and right lateral pharyngeal (SS=3) spaces would have a total severity score of 6, which is the sum of the values assigned to each of the three anatomic spaces. Flynn and colleagues were able to explain by correlation analysis 66% of the length of hospital stay with a model that used the initial SS and the white blood cell count on admission.

Table 10-3 Severity scores of fascial space infections

Severity score	Anatomic space
Severity score=1 (low risk to airway or vital structures)	Vestibular
	Subperiosteal
	Space of the body of the mandible
	Infraorbital
	Buccal
Severity score=2 (moderate risk to airway or vital structures)	Submandibular
	Submental
	Sublingual
	Pterygomandibular
	Submasseteric
	Superficial temporal
	Deep temporal (or infratemporal)
Severity score=3 (high risk to airway or vital structures)	Lateral pharyngeal
	Retropharyngeal
	Pretracheal
Severity score=4 (extreme risk to airway or vital structures)	Danger space (space 4)
	Mediastinum
	Intracranial infection

The severity score for a given patient is the sum of the severity scores for all of the spaces involved by cellulitis or abscess, based on clinical and radiographic examination.

10.4 Types of Odontogenic Infections

Types of infection: acute and chronic.

10.4.1 Acute stage

In the acute stage, the infection spreading in the soft tissues can take the following forms in the clinical situations.

(1) Abscess

It is a circumscribed collection of pus in a pathological tissue space. A true abscess is a thick-walled cavity containing pus. The suppurative infections are characteristic of staphylococci, often with anaerobes, such as bacteroides, and are usually associated with large accumulation of pus, which require immediate drainage. These microorganisms. produce coagulase, an enzyme, that may cause fibrin deposition in citrated or oxalated blood.

(2) Cellulitis

It is spreading infection of loose connective tissues. It is a diffuse, erythematous, mucosal or cutaneous infection. It is characteristically the result of streptococci infection; and does not normally result in large accumulation of pus (Table 10-4). Streptococci produce enzymes such as streptokinase (fibrinolysin), hyaluronidase, and streptodornase. These enzymes break down fibrin and connective tissue ground substance and lyse cellular debris, thus facilitate rapid spread of bacteria along the tissue planes. Antibiotics may arrest the spread of infection; and may bring about complete resolution of the condition. However, in cases refractory to antibiotic coverage, pus pockets should be suspected; and in such cases, exploration and drainage should be done.

(3) Fulminating infections

Fulminating infections of the various spaces in the orofacial region. Here, the infection involves the secondary spaces involving vital structures, along the pathway of least resistance.

Table 10-4　Differences between cellulitis and abscess

Characteristics	Cellulitis	Abscess
Duration	Acute phase	Chronic phase
Pain	Severe and generalized	Localized
Size	Large	Small
Localization	Diffuse borders	Well-circumscribed
Palpation	Doughy to indurated	Fluctuant
Presence of pus	No	Yes
Degree of seriousness	Greater	Less
Bacteria	Aerobic	Anaerobic / mixed

10.4.2　Chronic stage

In the chronic stage, the odontogenic infection can present itself in the following forms.

(1) Chronic fistulous tract or sinus formation: abscesses neglected for a long time discharge intraorally or extra orally. When the abscess discharges through the skin; the sinus may appear in a location unfavorable for drainage; and the resulting scar is always thickened, puckered, and depressed and more obvious esthetically prominent.

(2) Chronic osteomyelitis.

(3) Cervicofacial actinomycosis.

10.5　Evaluation of the Patient with Orofacial Infection

Patients with an orofacial infection may present themselves with various signs and symptoms ranging from unimportant to the extremely serious. A quick assessment of the situation is a must.

If the patient:

(1) Toxic.

(2) Exhibits central nervous system changes and:

(3) Airway compromise.

Then:

(1) Immediate hospitalization.

(2) Aggressive medical treatment.

(3) Aggressive surgical intervention (including intubation and tracheostomy) should be done. The basic principles of patient evaluation must be followed: complete history, physical examination, clinical features, appropriate laboratory investigations, radiological investigations, and proper interpretation of findings. Adherence to the basic principles helps in arriving at an accurate diagnosis and instituting appropriate treatment.

10.5.1 History taking

It helps in obtaining information regarding the origin, extent, location and potential seriousness of the problem. The following information may be stressed: ①history of present illness, especially, onset. ②History of toothache; or headache, or chills; their nature, location, and duration. ③Previous hospitalization with infection; the treatment instituted and its response. ④Previous trauma to soft and hard tissues in the region. ⑤History of recurrent infections, ⑥History of recent rate of increase in extent of swelling, or airway difficulty.

10.5.2 Physical examination

10.5.2.1 General examination

①examination of thorax. ②abdomen. ③extremities. ④heart and its murmurs. ⑤recording the vital signs: this serves as a useful baseline for noting progression or regression of disease process. Pulse rate is increased, 10 beats/minute for each degree F of rise in temperature.

10.5.2.2 Regional examination

It comprises of a comprehensive physical examination and includes the following: ①skin of face, head and neck. ②swellings, injuries and areas of tenderness over maxillary and frontal sinuses. ③sinus tracts and fistula formation. ④enlargement of underlying bone. ⑤enlargement of salivary glands. ⑥enlargement of lymph nodes.

(1) Extraoral examination

A comprehensive regional examination would include as follows:

1) Inspection: ① skin of face (redness), head and neck. ② swelling, injuries. ③ fixation of skin, or mucosa to underlying bone. ④sinus or fistula formation.

2) Palpation: ①size of swelling. ②tenderness. ③local temperature. ④fluctuation. ⑤enlargement of underlying bone. ⑥salivary glands. ⑦regional lymph nodes (enlargement, tenderness).

(2) Intraoral examination

The examiner should have a good light for the examination of the oropharynx, while slightly depressing the tongue, in order to visualize swelling of tonsillar pillar and deviation of uvula away from the affected side.

① Trismus: The interincisal opening should be measured. ② Teeth: their number, presence of caries, and large restorations, and mobility. ③Localized swelling and fistulae. ④Sites of tooth extraction. ⑤Percussion: It is useful in determining hypersensitivity. It is performed with a metallic instrument or a tongue blade. ⑥Heat and cold testing. ⑦Electric pulp testing. ⑧Visualization of Stenson's and Wharton's ducts: The flow of saliva from the two ducts on both the sides should be examined. ⑨Soft palate, tonsillar fossa, uvula and oropharynx. ⑩ Displacement of tissues, presence of swelling, and drainage of pus.

(3) Ophthalmologic examination

It includes, assessment of extraocular muscle function, proptosis, or swelling of eyelids, and dorsum of root of the nose.

10.5.3   Clinical features

(1) Signs of infections

The cardinal signs of inflammation, are usually present to some extent.

1) Rubor or redness: this is usually present, when the infection is close to the tissue surface; especially in individuals with light complexion. It is due to vasodilation.

2) Tumor or swelling: it is due to the accumulation of inflammatory exudate or pus.

3) Calor or heat: it is due to pouring of warm blood from deeper tissues at the site of infection, increased velocity of blood flow, and increased rate of metabolism.

4) Dolor or pain: ① The pressure on sensory nerve endings, caused by distension of tissues (edema or spreading of infection). ② Increased tissue tension: the action of liberated or activated factors; such as kinins, histamin, or bradykinin like substances. ③ Loss of tonicity of injured tissues. ④ Functio laesa: or loss of function of the affected part. It is caused by mechanical factors and reflex inhibition of muscle movements associated with pain. This is reflected in difficulty in chewing and swallowing and respiratory embarrassment.

(2) Fever/Pyrexia

It is one of the most consistent signs of infection. Other conditions, which may manifest pyrexia include the following:

1) Noninfectious inflammatory disorders; such as rheumatoid arthritis.

2) Excess catabolism as in thyrotoxicosis.

3) Neoplastic disease such as lymphoma.

4) Postoperative: release of endogenous pyrogens, which stimulate the hypothalamic thermoregulation centers.

(3) Repeated chills

It is common in bacteremia and pyogenic abscesses.

(4) Headache

It is usually associated with fever, and is thought to be due to stretching of sensitive structures surrounding dilated intracranial arteries.

(5) Lymphadenopathy

The condition of lymph nodes depends upon whether the condition is acute or chronic. In acute infections, the lymph nodes are soft, tender and enlarged. The surrounding tissues are edematous and overlying skin is erythematous/reddish. In chronic infection, the lymph nodes are firm nontender and enlarged. The edema of surrounding tissues may not be present. The location of enlarged lymph nodes often indicates the site of infection.

Suppuration of lymph nodes occurs, when the causative organism has overcome the local defence mechanism in the node; resulting in excessive cellular reaction and collection of pus.

(6) Others

① Presence of draining sinuses or fistulae. ② Difficulty in opening mouth. ③ Difficulty in swallowing. ④ Increased salivation. ⑤ Changes in phonation. ⑥ Difficulty in breathing. ⑦ Bad breath.

Clinical symptoms of possible life threatening infections:

- Respiratory impairment.
- Difficulty in swallowing.
- Impaired vision or eye movement or both.
- Change in voice quality.
- Lethargy.
- Decreased level of consciousness.
- Agitation, restlessness due to hypoxia.

Toxicity—signs and symptoms:

- Pallor.
- Rapid respiration, throbbing pulse.
- Fever, shivering.
- Appearance of illness.
- Lethargy.
- Diaphoresis.

Central nervous system changes associated with infection:

- Decreased level of consciousness.
- Evidence of meningeal irritation—severe headache, stiff neck, vomiting.
- Edema of eyelids and abnormal eye signs.

10.5.4　Radiological examination

10.5.4.1　Conventional radiography

The radiological examination: the radiological examination is helpful in locating the offending teeth or other underlying causes. The various radiographs are useful: ① Intraoral periapical radiographs. ② Orthopantomography (OPG). ③ Lateral oblique view of the mandible. ④ AP, and lateral view of the neck for soft tissues can be helpful in detecting retropharyngeal space infections.

10.5.4.2　Other diagnostic aids

The other diagnostic imaging aids play a vital role in the management of infection of fascial spaces of face and neck. It helps the surgeon to know the anatomic extent of the fascial space infections, which aids in surgical drainage of the abscess and inflammatory exudate. CT guided needle aspiration of fluid collections can be used to obtain material for microbial analysis.

The imaging techniques can be broadly classified into following: ① Computed tomography (CT scan). ② Magnetic resonance imaging (MRI). ③ Nuclear medicine. ④ Xeroradiography.

These help in diagnosing extension of infection beyond maxillofacial region. CT scan: It is the "gold-standard", in head and neck imaging. CT and other X-ray images are based on a single factor, i. e. , the X-ray beam is attenuated by the tissue present, according to its electron density.

CT scan is the most widely used advanced imaging modality in the evaluation of the fascial infections.

CT shows the extent of soft tissue involvement, for example: ① showing complete extent of inflammatory process. ② epicenter of inflammatory process. ③ differentiating between myositis-fasciitis, and abscess formation. ④ accurately demonstrating the status of airway and involvement of various group of lymph nodes.

CT shows extent of osseous involvement adjacently, and demonstrates early periosteal reaction associated with osteomyelitis. CT findings, associated with fascial space involvement include edema and ill-definition of various muscles (myositis) and fascial planes (fascitis), airway displacement or deformity of the soft tissues, air from gas forming pathogens, enhancing the inflammatory masses, fluid collection within involved space, abscess formation evidenced by a hypodense area representing an accumulation of exudates or necrotic tissue surrounded by an enhancing wall and osteomyelitis of involved bone.

Interventional procedures like:

(1) Fine needle aspiration of fluid collection: to obtain material for microbial analysis.

(2) Abscess drainage and drain placement can be done with CT guidance.

10.6　General Principles of Therapy for the Management of Acute Extensive Orofacial Infection

The management of acute odontogenic/orofacial infection comprises of the following: ①immediate hospitalization. ②aggressive medical treatment (supportive treatment along with antibiotic therapy). ③aggressive surgical intervention (including intubation and tracheostomy) should be done.

Surgical management: it consists of extraction of the offending tooth or teeth, incision and drainage or a combination of both.

10.6.1　Antibiotic therapy

Recent reports have shown, that on the basis of the recent changes in the antibiotic sensitivity patterns of the most frequent pathogens of orofacial infections, penicillin may no longer be the empiric antibiotic of choice for serious cases requiring hospitalization. Many recent studies, in outpatients, however, have confirmed that there is no difference in ultimate therapeutic success between penicillin and clindamycin, amoxicillin, with or without clavulanic acid and cephradine.

Indications for use of antibiotics: ①cute onset of infection. ②diffuse infections. ③compromised host defenses. ④involvement of fascial spaces. ⑤severe pericoronitis. ⑥osteomyelitis.

Selection of antibiotics: for treating odontogenic infections are as follows.

(1) In case, there is no exudates available for culture and antibiotic sensitivity of organism(s) involved before initial therapy, then the initial selection is made on empiric basis.

(2) When pus is present, a smear can be Gram stained to provide the basis for a presumptive diagnosis and selection of antibiotic.

In general, bactericidal antibiotics should be preferred to bacteriostatic antibiotics; as these can independently destroy the invading organisms. On the other hand, bacteriostatic antibiotics, only prevent multiplication of bacteria; and depend on host's defence mechanisms for eradication of organisms.

Spectrum: It is preferable to use antibiotic with the narrowest spectrum, which are effective against the organisms involved in the infection. The use of a broad spectrum antibiotic should be avoided; as it increases risk of development of resistant microbial strains; and also increases risk of superinfections, by disrupting the normal bacterial flora in various body cavities; and permit nonpathogenic bacteria to proliferate and cause disease.

Supportive therapy: It involves those modalities which aid the patient's own body defences. It consists of the following: ①dministration of antibiotics. ②hydration of patient through iv route, maintain adequate nutritional status—high protein intake through ryle's tube feeding. ③analgesic. ④bed rest. ⑤application of heat in the form of moist pack and/or mouth rinses. ⑥opening the tooth for drainage.

10.6.2　Principles of surgical management

Determination of severity of infection: it is necessary to do a thorough examination of a patient with severe infection, such as evaluation of the airway in the form of difficulty in breathing, swallowing, speaking, or handling secretions, etc. A change in quality of voice indicates a swelling in or near glottis, such as in parapharyngeal spaces (both lateral and retropharyngeal), or epiglottis. Other findings that may be obscured are as follows, which are usually indicative of parapharyngeal infection.

(1) Occasionally, the patient may exhibit an abnormal head posture, or a lateral deviation of head, in an attempt to position upper airway over the deviated trachea, as in a lateral pharyngeal space infection.

(2) In case of increased upper airway resistance, the patient may use the accessory muscles of respiration such as platysma and intercostals. Ability to protrude the tongue past the vermilion border of the upper lip is a fairly reliable sign that the sublingual space is not severely involved.

10.6.3　Determination of the anatomical location of infection

It is necessary to determine the precise location and involvement of different oral, fascial and cervical swelling associated with each of the superficial and deep fascial spaces involved.

Evaluation of the host defenses: the most common diseases that compromise immune system are as follows.

(1) Diabetes mellitus.

(2) Steroid therapy within the past two years: ①asthma. ②autoimmune or inflammatory disease. ③organ transplant therapy. ④cancer chemotherapy within the past year. ⑤renal dialysis. ⑥HIV seropositivity. ⑦primary immunodeficiencies.

It is important for the surgeon to recognize the situation of immune compromise in patient with orofacial infection and modify the treatment accordingly. Some of the modifications include use of bactericidal antibiotics, such as beta-lactams, high doses of clindamycin, metronidazole, vancomycin, and aminoglycosides. The antibiotics to be avoided in immunocompromised patients include macrolides and tetracyclines.

10.6.4　Secure the airway

The first step in the management of such a patient is to secure the airway. The commonly used airway management techniques appropriate for the infected patient are listed below: ①Tracheotomy under local anesthesia. ②Cricothyroidotomy under local anesthesia. ③Fiberoptic intubation. ④Blind awake intubation. ⑤Bullard laryngoscopic intubation. ⑥Transtracheal jet ventilation. ⑦Inhalation induction with asleep intubation.

The techniques have their advantages and disadvantages; and should be appropriate for individual infected patient.

10.6.5　Surgical drainage

Some authors advocate that drainage of all spaces involved by cellulitis or abscess caused by odontogenic infection, should be done, as soon as possible after diagnosis.

The rationale for the more aggressive approach includes the following, however, final resolution requires further investigations.

(1) It is impossible to diagnose deep space infections either by clinical or radiological examination with 100% accuracy.

（2）Drainage of cellulitis seems to abort the spread of infection into neighboring deep fascial spaces.

（3）Adequate culture specimen can be obtained from cellulitis fluid.

（4）Physical debridement and irrigation of infected space may hasten healing by decreasing the size of bacterial inoculum and the amount of necrotic tissue present.

（5）Early drainage may prevent later colonization of the site by more highly antibiotic resistant micro-organisms.

（6）Length of stay in the hospital may be decreased.

Guidelines for placement of incisions in infected cases.

（1）Incisions should be placed in the most dependent areas.

（2）Incisions should be parallel to the skin creases.

（3）Incisions should lie in an esthetically acceptable site as far as possible.

（4）Incisions should be supported by healthy underlying dermis and subcutaneous tissue.

Placing the incision through the thin, often shiny skin directly overlies the abscess, which normally gets undermined by an abscess burrowing its way to the surface; results in a puckered contracted scar which gets collapsed into abscess cavity.

（5）Incisions placed intraorally should not cross frenal attachments, and should be placed parallel to nerve fibers in the region of mental nerve.

（6）The removal of the cause, such as an infected tooth, a segment of necrotic bone, a foreign body, if not already done, then should be done at the time of incision and drainage procedure.

▶▶ *Summary*

Severe odontogenic infections can be the most challenging cases that an oral and maxillofacial surgeon will be called on to treat. Often the patient with a severe odontogenic infection has significant systemic or immune compromise, and the constant threat of airway obstruction due to infections in the maxillofacial region raises the risk of such cases incalculably. Furthermore, the increasing rarity of these cases and the ever-changing worlds of microbiology and antibiotic therapy make staying abreast of this field difficult for the busy surgeon. Therefore, the eight steps in the treatment of severe odontogenic infections, first outlined by Dr. Larry Peterson, remain the fundamental guiding principles that oral and maxillofacial surgcons must use in successful management of these cases. The application of the eight steps must be thorough and the surgeon's mind must always remain open to the possibility of treatment failure, an error in initial diagnosis. Antibiotic resistance, and previously undiagnosed medically compromising conditions. Although adherence to these principles can not always guarantee a successful result, it can assure the oral and maxillofacial surgeon that he or she is practicing at the highest standard of care.

Han Bo

Chapter 11

Injuries of Oral and Maxillofacial Region

As the exposed part of the human body, oral and maxillofacial region could easily get damaged. Injury is a common disease of this region. Due to the anatomical and physiological characteristics of the region of being the anterior end of the respiratory tract and digestive tract, where concentrate the body's important sense organs, damage at this region will result in not only reaction and dysfunction of the organs at different level, but also defects or even destruction in the face, causing serious psychological trauma. Therefore, the correct treatment of oral and maxillofacial trauma has great significance, the aim of which is not only to save lives, but also to restore the function and appearance of the injured person to the pre−injury level as far as possible. This is the basic principle of "equal stress on function and appearance" in the treatment of oral and maxillofacial injuries.

11.1　Overview

There are many causes of maxillofacial injuries. In peacetime, the main causes include traffic accidents, work − related injuries, and also accidental injuries in daily life and social interaction. In wartime, firearm injuries are the predominant cause. It is worth mentioning that in high−tech wars and terrorist incidents, there is a significant rise in firearm injuries of civilians, particularly injuries due to explosions in mines, which is a notable change.

The human body is a unitary system, therefore any topical damage can cause systemic reactions of different degrees. Multiple site injuries, associated injuries and combined injuries caused by different factors in the oral and maxillofacial regions further complicate the injury condition. For the fear of delaying the chance of the treatment and causing undue consequences, a comprehensive and systematic examination must be conducted to prioritize the situation, first to save lives, and then to introduce the intervention of specialists as soon as possible.

For the treatment of oral and maxillofacial trauma, aside from the generality of traumas and the common principles of management, it is still necessary to master the characteristics of oral and maxillofacial injuries, as well as the unique principles and skills of treatment.

The characteristics of oral and maxillofacial injuries are as follows.

(1) Oral and maxillofacial has abundant blood flow and strong capacity of tissue regeneration, repair and

anti-infection. Therefore, after debridement, injury initial suturing can still be applied to wounds within or over 48 hours, as long as there is no obvious purulent infection. However, also due to the abundant blood flow, the massive bleeding after injury is more likely to form hematoma, while tissue swelling as a traumatic response occurs early and obviously. The obstruction of hematoma, edema, tissue displacement, retraction of the tongue, blood clots, secretions or foreign bodies at the floor of the mouth, parapharyngeal site and the root of the tongue may affect the airway patency and even cause asphyxia, to which special attention must be paid.

(2) On the oral and maxillofacial region there locate many cavities and sinuses, such as nasal cavity, oral cavity, and nasal sinus. These cavities and sinuses often contain a considerable amount of pathogenic bacterium. The wounds and these cavities are open to each other, which could easily cause the infection. Therefore, during the debridement, wounds connected with these sinuses and cavities should be closed as soon as possible to reduce the chance of infection.

(3) The teeth are located on the jawbone. When the fracture segment of the jawbone is displaced, the occlusal relationship is disordered, leading to chewing dysfunction. Occlusal disorder is one of the important diagnostic bases of jaw fractures. Therefore, in the treatment of jaw fractures, restoring the normal occlusion relationship is an important standard. And the teeth, are often used as a basis for fixing jaw fractures. In addition, in injuries caused by high-speed crash, discounted or dislocated teeth and broken bone pieces may act like "the second shrapnel", which increases the damage to surrounding tissues and the chance of infection.

(4) The oral cavity is the entrance to the digestive tract, the injury of which often interferes with normal eating, therefore both eating methods and food ingredients should be carefully chosen to maintain the nutrition of the patient. After eating, it is necessary to clean the mouth, maintain the oral hygiene and prevent infection of the wounds.

(5) The oral and maxillofacial regions are also the upper end of the respiratory tract, where the injury is most likely to cause a mechanical obstruction. Therefore, when rescuing the injured the respiratory tract should be kept open to prevent asphyxia and aspiration.

(6) When there is open injury on the nose, lips, tongue, palate, ankle and cheeks, if improperly handled, displacement and deformation of tissues and organs or deformed scars may appear after the wound has healed. Therefore, in the treatment of maxillofacial wounds it is very important to retain tissues that might survive and perform precise alignmentsuture.

(7) The maxillofacial region is where parotid gland, facial nerve, and trigeminal nerve are located. If the parotid gland is injured, the salivary fistula may be concurrent; if the facial nerve is damaged, facial paralysis may occur; if the trigeminal nerve is injured, it may cause numbness in the relevant area.

(8) The maxillofacial region is adjacent to the brain. Severe maxillofacial injuries are often associated with craniocerebral injuries such as skull fractures, concussion, brain contusion, intracranial hematoma, and cervical vertebra fractures. When there is a concurrent basilarskull fracture, cerebrospinal fluid rhinorrhea and otorrhea becomes possible, and attention must be paid to identify it when giving rescue.

11.2　Emergency Treatment of Oral and Maxillofacial Injuries

11.2.1　Anapnea

11.2.1.1　Etiology

It can be classified into obstructive asphyxia and inspiratory asphyxia.

(1) Obstructive asphyxia

① Foreign body obstruction. Blood clots, bone fragments, tooth debris, and other sorts of foreign bodies can obstruct the respiratory tract and cause asphyxia. ② Displacement of tissue. For example, in the case of mandibular symphysis comminuted fracture or mandibular fractures of both sides, since the fractured segment of the mandibular body is subject to the traction by the depressor jaw muscle group (genioglossal muscle, geniohyoid muscle, and mandibular hyoid muscle, etc.), the tongue will move downwards and backwards as a whole, compressing the epiglottis and causing suffocation [Figure 11 - 1 (1)] When the maxilla suffers an open transverse fracture, affected by factors including gravity, impact force and traction of soft palate, it will move downwards and backwards to block the pharyngeal cavity, causing asphyxia [Figure 11-1 (2)]. ③ Airway stenosis: if the floor of mouth, root of tongue or the neck is injured, hematoma and severe reactive tissue swelling formed in this part may oppress the upper respiratory tract and cause asphyxia. For patients with facial burn, we shall also pay attention to the possibility of edema of the inner wall of the trachea caused by inhaled hot gas, which will lead to narrow lumen, and then asphyxia. ④ Valve-like obstruction. Injured mucosa covers the laryngopharynx, obstructing the inspiration.

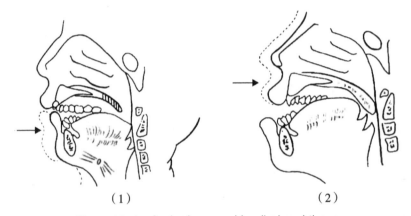

(1) (2)

Figure 11-1　Asphyxia caused by displaced tissue

(1) The tongue moves downwards and backwards in the mandibular fracture; (2) The soft palate blocks the pharyngeal cavity in the maxilla fracture.

1) Displacement of the mandible and retraction of the tongue blocking the pharyngeal cavity.

2) The maxillary fracture segment moving downward and backwards, with the soft palate sinking to block the pharyngeal cavity.

(2) Inspiratory asphyxia

The coma wounded directly inhales blood, saliva, vomit, or foreign matter into the trachea, bronchi, or even alveoli.

11.2.1.2　Clinical symptoms and signs

The prodromal symptoms are irritability, sweating, nasal ala flap, longer inspiration than exhalation, or laryngeal stridor. When the situation turns severe, we may witness cyanosis, the three depression sign (fossa of sternum, fossa of clavicle and sucken intercostal space), rapid and superficial breathing, followed by weak and rapid pulse, fall of blood pressure, and dilated pupils. Without timely rescue, it will lead to coma, respiratory heartbeat, cardiorespiratory arrest, and finally, the death.

11.2.1.3　Treatment

Asphyxia is a critical complication after oral and maxillofacial injuries, which is a huge threat to the lives of the wounded. The key to first aid is early detection and timely management. If the patient already has difficulty on breathing, we should make full use of every minute to implement rescue.

For asphyxial patient whose throat is choked by foreign bodies, we should immediately remove the blockage with fingers(wrapped with gauze or no), or extract it with a plastic tube. At the same time, change their position to the lateral or prone position, and then clear the secretions to relieve asphyxia. For asphyxia caused by retraction of tongue, open the dentition quickly and pull the tongue out of the mouth with tongue forceps or towel forceps. Even after the asphyxia is relieved, it is still necessary to pull the tongue out the mouth. To do this, penetrate the full layer of tongue tissue at 2 cm behind the apex of the tongue by using a thick silk thread or pins(Figure 11-2). The traction wire can be fixed at bandage or clothes. At the same time, hold forward the mandibular angle, keep the position with head to one side or prone position to facilitate the outflow of secretions. When the maxillary bone fractures and soft palate fall downwards, we can use pliers, sticks and chopsticks, with the help of maxillary molars on both sides, to lift the falling maxillary jaws and fix them on the bandages on the head. For swellings of the oropharynx of varying degrees, we can place different types of ventilation tubes. If the situation is urgent and there is no proper ventilation tube, we shall pierce the trachea through cricothyroid membrane with No. 15 or larger needle to relieve asphyxia, and then perform a tracheotomy. If the breathing has already stopped, an emergency endotracheal intubation or an emergency cricothyroid membrane puncture must be performed to rescue the patient. When the patient is in stable condition, the tracheotomy can be performed. For valve-like obstruction, the drooping mucosal flaps should be spliced back to the original site or cut of. If necessary, perform tracheotomy. For inhalation asphyxiation, the tracheotomy should be performed immediately, and the tracheal secretions and other foreign bodies should be quickly aspirated to restore airway patency. For such patients, we must be careful to prevent lung complications.

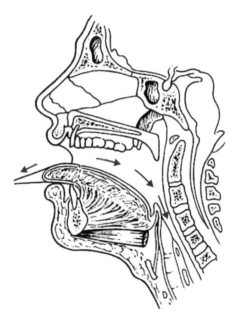

Figure 11-2   Using a thick silk thread
to pull the tongue out the mouth

11.2.2   Hemostasis

When implementing emergency treatment for hemorrhage, the appropriate treatment measures should be taken according to the site of the injury, the characteristics of the bleeding(blood capillary bleeding, venous bleeding, arterial bleeding) and site conditions.

11.2.2.1 Hemostasis by finger pressing

If urgent, press the proximal end of the main artery of the bleeding site to the nearby bone with fingers to temporarily stop the bleeding, and then further hemostasis methods are required. For example, press the superficial temporal artery and the zygomatic arch roots in front of the tragus with fingers to reduce the bleeding on the top of the head and the tempus. Press the facial artery on the mandible at the anterior edge of the masseter to reduce the facial bleeding; at the place below the junction of the anterior edge of the mastoid muscle and the greater horn of hyoid bone, press the arteria carotis communis onto in the 6 cervical vertebrae to reduce head and neck bleeding. However, such actions may cause bradycardia and arrhythmia, therefore will not be adopted for non-emergency situation.

11.2.2.2 Bandage hemostasis

It is suitable for bleeding of capillaries, small arteries and veins on the scalp, face, etc. First, roughly restore the displaced tissue, place a dressing on the wound surface, and then bandage with pressure. The power of pressing should be carefully controlled, or it may affect the airway patency.

11.2.2.3 Packing hemostasis

For patients who suffer from issue defects and penetrating wounds, fill the wounds with gauze and then bandage it with pressure. However, when dealing with wounds at the neck or floor of mouth, be careful to keep the airway open while to preventing asphyxia caused by pressure on the trachea. For patients with nasal bleeding, after excluding the situation of cerebrospinal fluid leakage, use gauzes to fill the nasal passages; if does not work well, add nasal orifice hemostasis.

11.2.2.4 Ligation hemostasis

Ligaturing the bleeding vessel inside the wound or ligaturing the proximal end of the bleeding artery at a distance will bring real effect of hemostasis. For serious bleeding in the maxillofacial region, if hemostasis in this particular region is not easily achieved, we could ligature the external carotid artery, and in case of emergency, hemostatic forceps can be used to clamp blood vessels to deliver the wounded.

11.2.2.5 Hemostasis with drugs

Apply hemostatic powder, glue, sponge and fiber or the thrombin to local body parts. The drugs should contact directly with the bleeding wound, and be dressed by gauze. Systemic chemical hemostatic agents such as etamsylate(dicynone), aminomethylbenzoic acid and carbazochrome(adrenobazonum) can be used as auxiliary drugs to accelerate blood coagulation.

11.2.3 Wound dressing

Bandaging is a very important step in the process of first aid. It is used to compress hemostasis, temporarily fix it, protect the wound, reduce the wound area, reduce pollution, reduce saliva outflow, and relieve pain. Traditional methods commonly used after maxillofacial injuries include bandage hooded dressing, triangle bandage dressing, cruciate bandage dressing, and four-tail bandaging.

11.2.4 Transportation of the wounded

When transporting the wounded, be careful to keep the airway open. For a wounded person in coma, put him/her in the prone position, raise the forehead so that the mouth and nose can be left open, which will facilitate the drainage and prevent the glossocoma. General wounded person can be placed in a lateral position to avoid accumulation of blood clots and secretions in the pharynx. During transportation, the body and local conditions should be closely observed to prevent the occurrence of critical situations such as asphyxiation and shock.

11.2.5   Infection prevention

The wounds of oral and maxillofacial injuries are often contaminated and even embedded with sandals, rags, and other foreign materials, as well as autologous soft and hard tissue fragments. The harm to the wounded by the infection is sometimes more serious than the original injury. Therefore, timely and effective prevention of infection is of utmost importance. If conditions permit, the debridement should be done as soon as possible; if not, wounds should be timely bandaged to isolate sources of infection. Antibiotics should be used to control infections of the wounds as soon as possible. While using antibiotics, dexamethasone can also be given to a small number of wounded at the same time to prevent excessive local swelling. For patients with brain injury, especially when there is leakage of cerebrospinal fluid, use drugs that can easily penetrate the blood – brain barrier and can reach effective concentrations in brain tissue, such as sulfadiazine, large−dose penicillin, etc. In case of wounded contaminated by soil, it is necessary to inject with tetanus antitoxin in time. For emergency treatment of shock and craniocerebral injury, please refer to related textbooks.

11.3   Management of Maxillofacial Trauma

11.3.1   Rigid fixation

Internal fixation simply implies the placement of wires, screws, plates, rods, pins, and other hardware directly to the bones to help stabilize a fracture. Internal fixation can be rigid or nonrigid depending on the nature of the fracture, and the type, strength, size, and location of the hardware placed. Since various degrees and many types of nonrigid fixation exist, it is useful to first define rigid internal fixation. By default any technique that does not satisfy this definition can then be considered nonrigid.

11.3.1.1   Rigid internal fixation

The term rigid internal fixation has many definitions. For instance, one definition is "any form of bone fixation in which otherwise deforming biomechanical forces are either countered or used to advantage to stabilize the fracture fragments and to permit loading of the bone so far as to permit active motion." This definition, although admittedly long and perhaps confusing, encompasses the essence of the technique as practiced today and includes clues to the methods of applying the appropriate hardware. A more basic definition which includes the same objectives is "any form of fixation applied directly to the bones which are strong enough to prevent interfragmentary motion across the fracture when actively using the skeletal structure." Most of the differences in technique are in the application of the fixation.

Examples of rigid fixation in the mandible are the use of two lag screws or bone plates across a fracture, the use of a reconstruction bone plate with at least three screws on each side of the fracture, and the use of a large compression plate across the fracture. Properly applied, these fixation schemes are of sufficient rigidity to prevent interfragmentary mobility during the healing period.

An inseparable corollary to the prevention of interfragmentary mobility by rigid fixation is a peculiar type of bone healing where no callus forms. The bones instead go on to heal by a process of haversian remodeling. Histologically, osteoclasts cross the fracture gap and are followed by blood vessels and osteoblasts.

New bone is laid down by the osteoblasts, forming osteons which cross the gap and impart microscopic points of bony union to the fracture. A remodeling phase then converts the entire area to morphologically normal bone. This type of bone healing is termed primary or direct bone union, and it requires absolute immobilization between the osseous fragments, that is, rigid fixation, and minimal distance (gap) between them.

11.3.1.2 Nonrigid internal fixation

Any form of bone fixation that is not strong (rigid) enough to prevent interfragmentary motion across the fracture when actively using the skeletal structure is considered nonrigid. The basic difference between rigid and nonrigid fixation centers on interfragmentary mobility. If there is mobility of the osseous fragments during active use of the skeletal structure following application of internal fixation devices, internal fixation is nonrigid. An example of nonrigid fixation is a transosseous wire placed across a mandibular fracture. The wire can only provide stability by virtue of its (limited) ability to prevent spreading of the gap, but by itself, the wire can not neutralize torsion and/or shear forces. Additional fixation measures then become necessary, such as the use of maxillomandibular fixation (MMF).

However, various forms of nonrigid fixation are recognized, and there is a continuum between rigid fixation and no fixation at all. There are some forms of nonrigid fixation that are strong enough to allow active use of the skeleton during the healing phase but not of sufficient strength to prevent interfragmentary mobility. These types of fixation have been called functionally stable fixation, indicating that there is adequate stability to allow function even though there is not adequate stability to allow direct bone union. Many of the fixation schemes that are being used clinically in the maxillofacial area are not truly rigid fixation, but functionally stable fixation.

Functionally stable fixation in maxillofacial surgery is a spectrum that varies from one region of the facial skeleton to another, from one fracture to the next, and from one patient to the next. Examples of functionally stable fixation include the single miniplate technique of treating mandibular angle or body fractures. In spite of the interfragmentary motion that these techniques may permit, the clinical outcomes are excellent, indicating that absolute immobility of the fragments is unnecessary for satisfactory recovery.

In the late 1950 s the Swiss Association for the Study of Internal Fixation (AO/ASIF) promulgated four biomechanical principles in fracture management:

(1) Accurate anatomic reduction.

(2) Atraumatic operative technique preserving the vitality of bone and soft tissues.

(3) Rigid internal fixation that produces a mechanically stable skeletal unit.

(4) Avoidance of soft tissue damage and "fracture disease" by allowing early, active, pain-free mobilization of the skeletal unit.

These principles had as their aim the rigid fixation of fractures. In recognition of the finding that functionally stable fixation is very effective clinically, in 1994, the AO/ASIF changed its third biomechanical principle from rigid internal fixation to functionally stable fixation.

Bone healing under the condition of mobility between the osseous fragments is termed indirect or secondary bone healing. In such circumstances there is deposition of periosteal callus, resorption of the fragment ends, and tissue differentiation through various stages from fibrous to osseous.

11.3.2 Management of maxilla fractures

11.3.2.1 Surgical anatomy

Fractures of the maxilla are usually the result of direct force and range from simple alveolar fractures to extensive injuries to the bones of the nose, orbit, palate, skull, etc.

Displacement is usually the result of the traumatic force. Muscle contraction plays an unimportant role in the displacement of maxillary fractures, except in those extending into the region of the pterygoid plates, in which displacement of maxilla may be in a downward and posterior direction due to the action of the pterygoid muscles. In complete craniofacial disjunction associated with fractures of the zygoma, action of the masseter muscle may be a factor in displacement.

11.3.2.2 Classification of fractures of middle third of facial skeleton

Classification is mainly helpful for communication purpose. The present precise knowledge of the lines of fracture in the middle third of the facial skeleton, which are produced following injury, is largely due to the experimental studies carried out by a French surgeon, Rene LeFort in 1901 in Paris. Following experimental trauma to the cadaver head and removal of the soft tissues, LeFort discovered that the complex fracture patterns could be broadly subdivided into three groups: LeFort I, LeFort II and LeFort III (Figure 11-3).

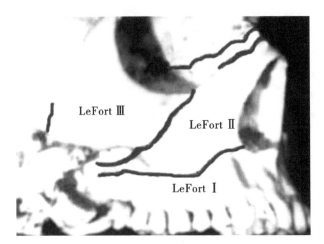

Figure 11-3 LeFort's classification for middle third of the facial skeleton

Clinically, the identical solitary lines may not be seen, but the direction and description of the lines will help in planning the reduction and fixation. Otherwise, at many places like anterior wall of the maxillary sinus, multiple fragmentation will be seen.

(1) Lefort I fracture

It is also called as horizontal fracture of the maxilla or Guerin's fracture. It is also known as floating fracture, as there is a separation of complete dentoalveolar part of the maxilla (pterygomaxillary dysjunction) and the fractured fragment is held only by means of soft tissues.

The fractured fragment is freely mobile and the resultant displacement will depend on the direction of the force. Depending on the displacement of a fragment, variety of occlusal disharmony can be seen in this type of fracture (anterior open bite, cross bite, reverse overjet, etc.).

A violent force applied over a more extensive area, above the level of the teeth will result in a LeFort I fracture, which is not confined to smaller section of the alveolar bone. Here, the horizontal fracture line is seen above the apices of the teeth, which detaches the tooth bearing portion of the maxilla from the rest of the facial skeleton. The fracture line commences at the point on the lateral margin of the anterior nasal aperture, passes above the nasal floor, and it passes laterally above the canine fossa and traverses the lateral antral wall, dipping down below the zygomatic buttress and then inclines upward and posteriorly across the pterygomaxillary fissure to fracture the pterygoid laminae at the junction of their lower third and upper two thirds.

At the same time, from the same starting point, the fracture also passes along the lateral wall of the nose and subsequently joins the lateral line of fracture behind the tuberosity. The typical LeFort Ⅰ fracture is always bilateral, with the fracture of the lower third of the nasal septum. But it can be unilateral also. The displacement will depend on the direction and severity of the force. Posterior, lateral displacement or rotation around its axis can be seen. The LeFort Ⅰ fracture may occur as a single entity or in association with LeFort Ⅱ and Ⅲ fractures.

Clinical signs and symptoms of LeFort Ⅰ fracture

1) Slight swelling and edema of the lower part of the face along with the upper lip swelling(gross edema or facial disfigurement is not present).

2) Ecchymosis in the labial and buccal vestibule, as well as contusion of the skin of the upper lip may be seen. Laceration of upper lip and intraoral mucosa may be seen.

3) Bilateral epistaxis or nasal bleeding may be observed.

4) The most common significant feature is the mobility of the upper dentalveolar portion of the jaw, which is frequently mobile to digital pressure.

5) Occlusion may be disturbed. Patient will not be able to masticate the food.

6) Pain while speaking and moving the jaw.

7) Sometimes there will be upward displacement of the entire fragment, locking it against the superior intact structures, such a fracture will be called as impacted or telescopic fracture. A classical anterior open bite may be seen in this case.

8) Percussion of the maxillary teeth produces dull "cracked cup" sound.

(2) Lefort Ⅱ fracture

Violent force, usually from an anterior direction, sustained by the central region of the middle third of the facial skeleton over an area extending from the glabella to the alveolar margin results in a fracture of a pyramidal shape. The force may be delivered at the level of the nasal bones.

The fracture line runs below the frontonasal suture from the thin middle area of the nasal bones down on either side, crossing the frontal process of the maxillae and passes anteriorly across the lacrimal bones, immediately anterior to nasolacrimal canal. From this point the fracture line passes downward, forward and laterally crossing the inferior orbital margin, in the region of zygomaticomaxillary suture. It may or may not involve the infraorbital foramen. The fracture line now extends downward and forward and laterally to traverse the lateral wall of the antrum, just medial to the zygomaticomaxillary suture line.

Clinical signs and symptoms of Lefort Ⅱ fracture

1) There is a gross edema of the middle third of the face known as ballooning or moon face. Edema sets in within a short time of injury.

2) Presence of bilateral circumorbital edema and ecchymosis(black eye). Rapid swelling of the eyelids makes examination of the eyes difficult.

3) Bilateral subconjunctival hemorrhage confined to medial half of the eye.

4) The bridge of the nose will be depressed(flat face). Nasal disfigurement.

5) If there is impaction of the fragment against the cranial base, then shortening of the face with anterior open bite will be seen.

6) If there is gross downward and backward displacement of the fragment, then elongation or lengthening of the face will be seen with posterior gagging of the occlusion with anterior open bite(dishshaped face).

7) Bilateral epistaxis may be present.

8)Difficulty in mastication, and speech.

9)Loss of occlusion may be seen.

10)Airway obstruction may be seen due to posterior and downward displacement of the fragment impinging on the dorsum of the tongue.

11)Surgical emphysema—crackling sensation transmitted to the fingers due to escape of air from the paranasal sinuses is seen.

12)CSF leak may be present.

13)Step deformity at the infraorbital margins may be seen.

14)Anesthesia and/or paresthesia of the cheek is noted.

(3)Lefort III fracture

It is also known as high level fracture. The line of fracture extends above the zygomatic bones on both sides as a result of trauma being inflicted over a wider area, at the orbital level. The force is usually applied from the lateral direction with a severe impact. Here the initial impact is taken by the zygomatic bone resulting in depressed fracture and then because of the severe degree of the impact, the entire middle third will then hinge about the fragile ethmoid bone and the impact will then be transmitted on the contralateral side resulting in laterally displaced zygomatic fracture of the opposite side(craniofacial dysjunction).

In a typically high level LeFort III fracture, the line commences near the frontonasal suture, causes dislocation of the nasal bones and disruption of cribriform plate of the ethmoid bone with tearing of dura mater and consequent CSF rhinorrhea. In such cases, the line of fracture crosses both the nasal bones and the frontal process of the maxilla, near the frontonasal and frontomaxillary sutures and then traverses the upper limit of the lacrimal bones. Continuing posteriorly, the line crosses the thin orbital plate of the ethmoid bone constituting part of the medial wall of the orbits. As the medial orbital wall is very thin, comminution of the fracture line is seen in this region. As the optic foramen is surrounded by a dense ring of bone, the fracture line gets deflected downward and laterally to reach the medial aspect of the posterior limit of the inferior orbital fissure. From this point, the fracture descends across the upper posterior aspect of the maxillae in the region of the sphenopalatine fossa and upper limit of the pterygomaxillary fissures and fractures the roots of the pterygoid laminae at its base.

Clinical signs and symptoms of Lefort III fracture

Clinically this fracture appears similar to the LeFort II fracture, but close examination will demonstrate a more serious condition. After stabilizing the head and then gripping of the maxillary teeth with one hand and simple manipulation, will confirm complete movement of the middle third of the face. Mobility of whole skeleton as a single block can be felt.

1)Gross edema of the face, ballooning. "Panda facies", within 24－48 hours.

2)Bilateral circumorbital/periorbital ecchymosis and gross edema "Racoon eyes". Gross circum orbital edema will prevent eyes from opening.

3)Bilateral subconjunctival hemorrhage, where posterior limit will not be seen, when patient is asked to look medially.

4)There may be tenderness and separation at the frontozygomatic sutures. This will produce lengthening of the face and lowering of the ocular level. Unilateral or bilateral hooding of the eyes is seen.

5)Characteristic "dish face" deformity.

6)May be enophthalmos, diplopia or impairment of vision, temporary blindness, etc.

7)Flattening and widening, deviation of the nasal bridge.

8)Epistaxis, CSF rhinorrhea.

11.4 Treatment of Midfacial Fracture

The principles of treatment of midfacial fracture consist of the reduction and fixation of the fractured bones to one another and to the skull. Restoration of the occlusion is a must for the correct reduction of the dentulous jaw segments. The bony framework and buttresses of the mid face must also be repositioned or restored and fixed. Resto ration of the form will also restore the function. Reduction and fixation can be achieved by either conservative or operative methods. It should be undertaken as early as possible following injury. The sooner the treatment is carried out, the greater the prospects for restoration of normalcy.

After the availability of minibone plate system, the conservative methods have largely been replaced by surgical methods. Common to both methods is splinting of both jaws in all cases, in which the alveolar process of the maxilla is involved in the fracture. Fixation of the midface must be maintained by external or internal skeletal fixation until consolidation is achieved. The immobilization to stable skeletal segments of the skull should be maintained for approximately 6 – 8 weeks. IMF is maintained until occlusal disturbances can no longer result, that is, 3 – 4 weeks. In case miniplate osteosynthesis has been performed, then there is no need for IMF.

11.4.1 Management of mandibular fractures

The mandible is the second most commonly fractured part of the maxillofacial skeleton because of its position and prominence. The location and pattern of the fractures are determined by the mechanism of injury and the direction of the vector of the force. In addition, the patient's age, the presence of teeth, and the physical properties of the causing agent also have a direct effect on the characteristics of the resulting injury.

Bony instability of the involved anatomic areas is usually easily recognized during clinical examination. Dental malocclusion, gingival lacerations, and hematoma formation are some of the most common clinical manifestations.

In the management of any bone fracture, the goals of treatment are to restore proper function by ensuring union of the fractured segments and reestablishing preinjury strength; to restore any contour defect that might arise as a result of the injury; and to prevent infection at the fracture site. Restoration of mandibular function, in particular, as part of the stomatognathic system must include the ability to masticate properly, to speak normally, and to allow for articular movements as ample as before the trauma. In order to achieve these goals, restoration of the normal occlusion of the patient becomes paramount for the treating surgeon.

11.4.2 Classification of mandibular fractures

The following classification of mandibular fractures was divided based on their anatomic location.

Dentoalveolar fracture: any fracture that is limited to the tooth–bearing area of the mandible without disruption of continuity of the underlying osseous structure.

Symphysis fracture: any fracture in the region of the incisors that runs from the alveolar process through the inferior border of the mandible in a vertical or almost vertical direction.

Parasymphysis fracture: a fracture that occurs between the mental foramen and the distal aspect of the lateral mandibular incisor extending from the alveolar process through the inferior border.

Body fracture: any fracture that occurs in the region between the mental foramen and the distal portion of the second molar and extends from the alveolar process through the inferior border.

Angle fracture: any fracture distal to the second molar, extending from any point on the curve formed by the junction of the body and ramus in the retromolar area to any point on the curve formed by the inferior border of the body and posterior border of the ramus of the mandible.

Ascending ramus fracture: a fracture in which the fracture line extends horizontally through both the anterior and posterior borders of the ramus or that runs vertically from the sigmoid notch to the inferior border of the mandible.

Condylar process fracture: a fracture that runs from the sigmoid notch to the posterior border of the ramus of the mandible along the superior aspect of the ramus; fractures involving the condylar area can be classified as extracapsular or intracapsular, depending on the relation of the fracture to the capsular attachment.

11.4.3   Management of mandibular fractures

Basic principles of orthopedic surgery also apply to mandibular fractures including reduction, fixation, immobilization, and supportive therapies. It is well known that union of the fracture segments will only occur in the absence of excessive mobility. Stability of the fracture segments is key for proper hard and soft tissue healing in the injured area. Therefore, the fracture site must be stabilized by mechanical means in order to help guide the physiologic process toward normal bony healing.

Reduction of the fracture can be achieved either with an open or closed technique. In open reduction, as the name implies, the fracture site is exposed, allowing direct visualization and confirmation of the procedure. This is typically accompanied by the direct application of a fixation device at the fracture site.

A closed reduction takes place when the fracture site is not surgically exposed but the reduction is deemed accurate by palpation of the bony fragments and by restoration of the functioning segments, for example, restoration of the dental occlusion by wiring the teeth together, using splints, or employing external pins

Fixation must be able to resist the displacing forces acting on the mandible. It can take two forms: direct or indirect. When direct fixation is used, the fracture site is opened, visualized, and reduced; then stabilization is applied across the fracture site. The rigidity of direct fixation can range from a simple osteosynthesis wire across the fracture (i. e. , nonrigid fixation) to a miniplate at the area of fracture tension (i. e. , semirigid fixation) or a compression bone plate (i. e. , rigid fixation) to compression screws alone (lag screw technique).

Indirect fixation is the stabilization of the proximal and distal fragments of the bone at a site distant from the fracture line. The most commonly used method for mandibular fractures is intermaxillary fixation (IMF). A further example of indirect fixation is the use of external biphasic pin fixation in combination with an external frame.

Over the past three decades many different techniques and approaches have been described in the literature to surgically correct facial fractures. More recently the use of internal fixation utilizing plates has shown the highest success rates with the lowest incidence of nonunions and postoperative infections. The origin of plating as a treatment option for fractures can be traced to Dannis and colleagues, who reported the successful use of plates and screws for fracture repair in 1947. Later refinement of this technique is credited to Allgower and colleagues at the University of Basel, who successfully used the first compression plate for extremity fracture repair in 1969. However, it was not until 1973 that Michelet and colleagues reported on the use of this treatment modality for fractures of the facial skeleton.

In 1976 following Michelet's success, a group of French surgeons headed by Champy developed the protocol that is now used for the modern treatment of mandibular fractures. But it was not until 1978 that these findings were published in the English literature.

Basically, there are two categories of plating systems: rigid compression plates such as the AO/ASIF and the semirigid miniplates. The advantages and disadvantages of each system have been extensively discussed; however, the question remains: does compression of fractures really offer a clinically significant advantage in terms of better bone healing and fewer complications?

Proponents of the AO system state that primary or direct bone healing is the main advantage offered by this system. When a fracture is compressed, absolute interfragmentary immobilization is achieved with no resorption of the fragment ends, no callus formation, and intracortical remodeling across the fracture site whereby the fractured bone cortex is gradually replaced by new haversian systems. However, in other studies it has been shown that absolute rigidity and intimate fracture interdigitation is far from mandatory for adequate bony healing. Compression is not necessary at the fracture site for healing, and it is questionable whether compression stimulates osteogenesis.

Han Bo, Xu Yingying

Chapter 12

Diseases of Temporomandibular Joint

The temporomandibular joint (TMJ) is one of the most complex diarthrodial joint of the human body. It is made up primarily of articular fossa of the temporal bones, condyle of the mandible, capsule, ligaments and related chewing muscles. Each part will be manifested various diseases just like other joints. There are no unified globally accepted standards for the classification of TMJ diseases. The following are common definitions in the textbooks of oral maxillofacial surgery: the temporomandibular joint disorders (TMD), TMJ dislocation, ankylosis, congenital or developmental disease, trauma, infection and tumors of this system. The chapter mainly discuss TMD, TMJ dislocation, ankylosis, infection and tumors of this system. Functional anatomy must be understood before disorders can have meaning.

12.1　Functional Anatomy of the Temporomandibular Joint

Anatomy of the TMJ is complex and important in understanding the pathology and treatment of temporomandibular joint diseases. TMJ anatomy comprises the bones, ligaments, tendons and muscles of the region. The TMJ is the most complex joint in the body. It provides for hinging movement in one plane (a ginglymoid joint), and provides for sliding movements (an arthrodial joint). Therefore, it is technically a ginglymo-arthrodial joint. The TMJ is classified as a compound joint, i. e. , requiring the presence of at least three bones.

12.1.1　Articular disc and retrodiscal tissues

12.1.1.1　Articular disc

The articular disc is composed of dense fibrous connective tissue devoid of any blood vessels or nerve fibers. Functionally it serves as a non-ossified bone that permits the complex movements of the joint. The articular disc can be divided into central, anterior and posterior regions. The central area, as the intermediate zone, is the thinnest. The anterior border is generally slightly thinner than the posterior border. From an anterior view, the disc is generally thicker medially than laterally, which corresponds to the increased space between the condyle and the articular fossa toward the medial aspect of the joint. On opening, the superior surface of the articular disc has a sigmoid shape. The disc is firmly attached downward to the medial and lateral poles of the condylar head. The retrodiscal tissue is the primary storage site for synovial fluid.

12.1.1.2 Retrodiscal tissues

The retrodiscal tissue, or posterior attachment, consists of an area of loose connective tissue that is attached to the posterior aspect of the articular disc. It is highly vascularized and innervated, and is bordered superiorly by the superior retrodiscal lamina. The superior retrodiscal lamina consists of connective tissue containing many elastic fibers. It attaches the articular disc posteriorly to the tympanic plate. Its function is to counter the forward pull of the superior belly of the lateral pterygoid muscle on the articular disc. When the mouth is fully opened, the retrodiscal tissue is fully stretched. The superior retrodiscal lamina prevents the disc from dislocating anteriorly and also results in posterior rotation of the meniscus, allowing the thin intermediate portion of the disc to remain between the articular surfaces of the condyle and eminence of joint.

The inferior retrodiscal lamina consists mainly of collagenous fibers. It is located at the lower border of the retrodiscal tissues. It attaches the inferior border of the posterior aspect of the disc to the posterior margin of the articular surface of the condyle. Posteriorly, the remaining body of the disc is attached to a large venous plexus that fills with blood as moving the condyle forward. Anteriorly, the superior and inferior aspects of the disc are attached to the capsular ligament, which surrounds most of the joint. The superior and inferior attachments are to the anterior margins of the articular surface of the temporal bone and condyle respectively. The disc is also attached by tendinous fibers to the superior lateral pterygoid muscle, between the attachments of the capsular ligament.

The articular disc is attached to the capsular ligament anteriorly and posteriorly, as well as medially and laterally. This divides the joint into two distinct cavities. The internal surfaces of the cavities are surrounded by specialized endothelial cells that form a synovial lining. This lining, along with a specialized synovial fringe located at the anterior border of the retrodiscal tissues, produces synovial fluid that fills both joint cavities.

The articular surfaces of the mandibular fossa and condyle are lined with dense fibrous connective tissue rather than hyaline cartilage, as in most mobile joints. The fibrous connective tissue in the joint affords several advantages over hyaline cartilage; it is generally less susceptible to the effects of aging and therefore less likely to break down over time, and has a much greater ability to repair.

12.1.2 Articular, or glenoid fossa

The TMJ is composed of the condyle (mandible) and the articular (or glenoid) fossa of the temporal bones, bilaterally. The temporal bone consists of five parts: squamous, petrous, internal acoustic meatus, zygomatic, and middle cranial fossa. The facial nerve (motor control over the facial muscles) and the vestibulocochlear nerve (balance and hearing) both travel the course of the internal acoustic meatus. The middle cranial fossa is the floor, which supports the brain stem from which the cranial nerves originate. The connection between the TMJ and the middle ear is through the petro-tympanic fissure. This runs the length of the glenoid fossa.

The TMJ is referred to as a synovial joint. The articular disc is the primary source of synovial lubricant within the TMJ. The synovial fluid acts as a medium for providing metabolic requirements to these tissues. There is free and rapid exchange between the vessels of the capsule, the synovial fluid, and the articular tissues. The inferior joint space contains about 0.9 mL of synovial fluid, and the superior joint space contains about 1.2 mL of synovial fluid. The synovial fluid also serves as a lubricant between articular surfaces during function. The articular surfaces of the disc, condyle, and fossa are very smooth—this minimizes friction during movement. The synovial fluid helps to minimize the friction further. This lies on the condylar head like a cap and drapes over all surfaces, extending most caudad to the condylar neck in its posterior aspect. When the mandible is depressed, the inferior joint space opens to a great extent posteriorly, giving the appearance in lateral view of a teardrop in the inferior joint space posterior to the condylar head. The anterior portion of the inferior joint space forms a small fossa where the fibers of that capsular ligament and the anterior band of the disc form a concretion. This sling–like structure helps to stabilize the disc against the condylar head during function.

12.1.3   Capsule and superior and inferior joint space

Superior joint space is larger and more anteriorly placed than the inferior joint space. Its shape in the cephal aspect corresponds closely to the glenoid fossa. On the caudal aspect, the concavity of the intermediate zone can be noted. The separation of the retrodiscal tissue from the posterior band is clearly differentiated when viewed from the superior joint space. The anterior fossa of the superior joint space forms a concavity in front of the condylar head. The medial fossa forms a concavity medial to the condylar head.

The precise shape of the disc is determined by the morphology of the condyle and mandibular fossa. During movement, the disc is somewhat flexible and can adapt to the functional demands of the articular surfaces. However, flexibility and adaptability do not imply that the morphology of the disc is reversibly altered during function. The disc maintains its morphology unless destructive forces or structural changes occur in the joint.

12.1.4   Synovial membrane

The joint is enclosed by a browse capsule, which is lined by a synovial membrane. This membrane is highly vascular and is continuous with the connective tissue of the capsule. Both upper and lower joint compartments are lined with their own synovial membrane.

The synovial membrane allows diffusion of a plasma filtrate and components of its own to produce synovial fluid that fills both joint compartments. Its shape is altered during functional movement. The largest area of synovial tissue is on the superior and inferior retrodiscal lamina. It forms small folds, or villi, that stretch on translation of the condyle and disc. The articulating surfaces of the temporal bone, the condyle, and the disc are not covered. The synovial tissue can be divided into three layers.

(1) The synovial lining, or intima, is the most intimate with the functional joint surfaces.

(2) The subsynovial tissue, which is like the intima but with a more developed connective tissue network.

(3) The capsule, which is a relatively acellular layer with thick bands of collagen that forms the outer boundary of the joint.

Synovial surfaces are nonadherent. The cells on the surface bind to the underlying matrix but not to the opposing tissue. Constant movement against opposing surfaces is thought to break down any forming cross–links. Collagenase secretion by the synovial lining cells also helps prevent the formation of surface adhesions and ensures that fragmented collagen on the tissue surface does not activate the coagulation cascade.

Synovial tissue has the ability to regenerate when damaged. Synovial fluid is a filtrate of plasma that passes through fenestrations in the sub–endothelial capillaries into the intercellular spaces. Because there is no epithelium, no basement membrane, no barrier exists between the synovium and the fluid present in the joint spaces. Movement is mainly by passive diffusion.

12.1.5   Proteoglycans and glycosaminoglycans

These are within the articular tissues on the anterior part of the condyle, in the central part of the disc, and on the lateral portion of the articular eminence.

The presence and amount of proteoglycans, specifically glycosaminoglycans(GAGs) relative to the collagen matrix in articular tissues is a measure of the resilience of the tissue and, therefore, determines the amount of compressive loading that the joint can withstand. Proteoglycans are macromolecules found in all connective tissues, extracellular matrices and on the surface of many cells. They contain a core protein to which one or more GAG polysaccharide chains are covalently bonded.

The insufficient concentration GAGs may cause the cartilage tissue to imbibe extracellular water, thus producing a cushion against compressive loads. The flexible, hydrophilic nature of the GAG chains and their high concentration of negatively charged fixed groups leads to a high swelling pressure, while the macromolecular mesh of collagen ensures a low hydraulic permeability. GAGs are ideal as a load–bearing material with low surface coefficient of friction.

A reduction in collagen concentration or an increased disorder in collagen orientation would lead to a decrease in the degree of cartilage reinforcement and an increase in local hydraulic permeability. There are three requirements for healthy cartilage.

(1) Plenty of water for diffusion of nutrients and for lubrication.

(2) Proteoglycans, due to their anionic nature, are tremendously hydrophilic, serving to attract and maintain water molecules.

(3) A collagenous mass in which these proteoglycans can bind together.

12.1.6　Boundary and weeping lubrication

Synovialfluid lubricates the articular surfaces by way of two mechanisms: boundary lubrication and weeping lubrication. Boundary lubrication occurs when the joint is moved and synovial fluid is forced from one area of the cavity into another. The synovial fluid located in the border regions is forced upon the articular surface, thus providing lubrication. Boundary lubrication prevents friction in the moving joint.

Weeping lubrication refers to the ability of the articular surfaces to absorb a small amount of synovial fluid. When the articular surfaces are placed under compressive forces, this small amount of synovial fluid is released. Weeping lubrication helps eliminate friction in the compressed without moving joint. Only a small amount of friction is eliminated because of weeping lubrication and prolonged compressive forces to the articular surfaces will exhaust this supply.

12.1.7　Ligaments and tendons

The function of ligaments is to hold the skeleton together. Ligaments attach to bone and are made up of collagenous connective tissue, which does not stretch. They act as passive restraining devices to limit and restrict joint movement. They prevent joint laxity. They transfer tensile strength from bone to bone. They are virtually identical to tendons. They have a poor vascular supply. The three functional ligaments that support the TMJ are as follows.

(1) The collateral or discal ligaments.

(2) The capsular ligament.

(3) The temporomandibular ligament.

There are two accessory ligaments of the TMJ.

(1) The sphenomandibular ligament.

(2) The stylomandibular ligament.

The collateral, or discal, ligaments attach the medial and lateral borders of the articular disc to the poles of the condyle. The medial discal ligament attaches the medial edge of the disc to the medial pole of the condyle. The lateral discal ligament attaches the lateral edge of the disc to the lateral pole of the condyle.

The collateral ligaments are composed of collagenous connective tissue fibers, and therefore do not stretch. They divide the joint mediolaterally into the superior and inferior joint cavities. They function by restricting movement of the disc away from the condyle and causing the disc to move passively with the condyle as it glides anteriorly and posteriorly. These ligaments permit the disc to be rotated anteriorly and posteriorly on the articular surface of the condyle, and are responsible for the hinging movement of the TMJ. They are vascularly supplied and are innervated; this innervation provides information regarding joint position and movement. Strain on these ligaments produces pain.

The entire TMJ is surrounded and encompassed by the capsular ligament. The fibers of the capsular ligament are attached superiorly to the temporal bone along the borders of the articular surfaces of the mandibular fossa and the articular eminence.

Inferiorly, the fibers of the capsular ligament are attached to the neck of the condyle. The capsular ligament acts to resist any medial, lateral, or inferior forces that tend to separate or dislocate the articular surfaces. A significant function of the capsular ligament is to encompass the joint, thus retaining the synovial fluid. The capsular ligament is well innervated and provides proprioceptive feedback regarding position and movement of the joint.

The lateral aspect of the capsular ligament is reinforced by strong, tight fibers that make up the lateral ligament or the temporomandibular ligament. The temporomandibular ligament is composed of two parts.

(1) The outer oblique portion, which extends from the outer surface of the articular tubercle and zygomatic process posteroinferiorly to the outer surface of the condylar neck.

(2) The inner horizontal portion, which extends from the outer surface of the articular tubercle and zygomatic process posteriorly and horizontally to the lateral pole of the condyle and posterior part of the articular disc.

The oblique portion of the TM ligament resists excessive dropping of the condyle and therefore limits the extent of mouth opening. This portion of the ligament also influences the normal opening movement of the mandible. During the initial phase of opening, the condyle can rotate around a fixed point until the TM ligament becomes as tight as its point of insertion on the neck of the condyle. When the ligament is taut, the neck of the condyle can not rotate further. If the mouth were to be opened wider, the condyle would need to move downward and forward across the articular eminence.

The inner horizontal portion of the TM ligament limits posterior movement of the condyle and disc. When force applied to the mandible displaces the condyle posteriorly, this portion of the ligament becomes tight and prevents the condyle from moving into the posterior region of the mandibular fossa. The TM ligament protects the retrodiscal tissues from trauma created by the posterior displacement of the condyle. The inner horizontal portion also protects the lateral pterygoid muscle from over lengthening or extending.

Sphenomandibular ligament arises from the spine of the sphenoid bone and extends downward to a small bony prominence on the medial surface of the ramus of the mandible called the lingula. It does not have any significant limiting effects on mandibular movement.

The second accessory ligament is the stylomandibular ligament. It arises from the styloid process and extends downward and forward to the angle and posterior border of the ramus of the mandible. It becomes taut when the mandible is protruded and is most relaxed when the mandible is opened. The stylomandibular ligament therefore limits excessive protrusive movements of the mandible.

Tendons are the connective tissues that attach muscle to bone. They are composed primarily of collagen. Tendons are nonelastic but flexible. They have a poor vascular supply. Tendons are attached to bone via either periosteum or fasciculi of fibers. Golgi tendon organs are tension sensors located in the tendons.

12.1.8　Muscles of the TMJ region

The position of the mandible and its craniomandibular articulation in space are mainly determined by the activity of the masticatory muscles that attach the jaw:Temporalis muscle elevate and retrude the mandible coordinating the closing movements. Masseter muscle elevate and protrude the mandible. Medial pterygoid,protracts and elevates the mandible. Superior lateral pterygoid,stabilize the disc during mouth opening and closing. Inferior lateral pterygoid,pull the condyle down along the eminence and the mandible is lowered and protruded. Anterior and posterior digastric,depress the mandible and coordinate mandibular function.

12.1.9　TMJ disc movement

When the mouth is opened the condyle rotates and,at the same time,moves down the posterior slope of the articular eminence. The superior head of the lateral pterygoid muscle then moves the disc forward. This enables the disc to remain between the two bones,thus providing a cushion which keeps the two bones from rubbing together. As the jaw closes, the condyle moves back up into the glenoid fossa and the disc follows,being guided by the lateral ligament. The biconcave shape of the disc, which is thicker at both ends,helps keep the disc in its proper relationship on the head of the condyle during opening and closing of the jaw.

12.1.10　Features that are unique to the TMJ

There are several features that are unique to the TMJ.

(1)It is a bilateral diarthrosis;the left and right side must function together.

(2)The articulating surfaces are covered with fibrocartilage rather than hyaline cartilage.

(3)The TMJ has a close relation to the teeth which making occlusal contact.

(4)The TMJ is a compound joint which combined with hinging and sliding forms.

(5)The TMJ is a remodeling joint during one's lifetime.

12.2　Temporomandibular Disorders

Temporomandibular disorders (TMD) is a symptom complex that covers pain and dysfunction of the muscles of mastication and the temporomandibular joints (TMJ). The most important features are pain,restricted mandibular movement and noises from the TMJs during jaw movement. TMD is thought to be caused by multiple factors. There are many treatments available,and no widely accepted treatment protocol. 20% – 30% of the adult population are affected. It is more common in females than males.

12.2.1　Definitions of the TMD

TMD,is described as a clinical term that refer to musculoskeletal disorders affecting the TMJ and their associated musculature. It is a collective term which represents a diverse group of pathologies involving the TMJ,the muscles of mastication,or both.

12.2.2　Signs and symptoms

Signs and symptoms of TMJ disorder vary in their presentation. The symptoms will usually involve more than one of the various components of the masticatory system, muscles, nerves, tendons, ligaments, bones, connective tissue, or the teeth. The three classically described, cardinal signs and symptoms of TMD are listed below.

(1) Pain and tenderness on palpation in the muscles of mastication, or of the joint itself. Pain is usually aggravated by manipulation or function, such as chewing, clenching, or yawning, and often worse upon waking. The character of the pain is usually dull or aching, poorly localized, and intermittent, although it can sometimes be constant. The pain is more usually unilateral.

(2) Limited range of mandibular movement, which may cause difficulty eating and even talking. There may be locking of the jaw, or stiffness in the jaw muscles and the joints. There may also be incoordination, asymmetry or deviation of mandibular movement.

(3) Noises from the joint during mandibular movement, which may be intermittent. Joint noises may be described as clicking, popping, or crepitus.

Other signs and symptoms have also been described, although these are less common and less significant than the cardinal signs and symptoms listed above.

(1) Headache, e. g. , pain in the occipital region, or the forehead; or other types of facial pain including migraine, tension headache. or myofascial pain.

(2) Pain elsewhere, such as the teeth or neck, shoulders, and back.

(3) Diminished hearing and loss, tinnitus, dizziness, etc.

12.2.3　Etiology

TMD is a symptom complex, that is thought to be caused by multiple but the exact etiology is unknown. Overall, two hypotheses have dominated research into the causes of TMD, namely a psychosocial model and a theory of occlusal disharmony. TMJ disc displacement, degenerative joint disease, psychosocial factors, bruxism and other parafunctional habits such as pen chewing, lip and cheek biting, trauma, occlusal factors, genetic factors such COMB, hormonal factors as estrogen are also suggested to contribute to the development of TMD.

A possible link between some chronic pain conditions and TMD has been hypothesized to be due to shared pathophysiological mechanisms, and they have been collectively termed "central sensitivity syndromes". These conditions include obstructive sleep apnea, rheumatoid arthritis, systemic joint laxity, chronic back pain, irritable bowel syndrome, headache, chronic neck pain, interstitial cystitis, regular scuba diving.

12.2.4　Diagnosis

Various diagnostic systems have been described. Some consider the Research Diagnostic Criteria method as the gold standard. Abbreviated to "RDC/TMD", this was first introduced in 1992 by Dworkin and LeResche try to classify temporomandibular disorders by etiology and apply universal standards for research into TMD. The Research Diagnostic Criteria(RDC/TMD) categorizes temporomandibular disorders into two axes: axis I is the physical aspects, and axis II involves assessment of psychological status, mandibular function and TMD–related psychosocial disability. Axis I is further divided into three general groups. Group I is muscle disorders, group II is disc displacements and group III is joint disorders, although it is common for people with TMD to fit into more than one of these groups.

McNeill 1997 described TMD diagnostic criteria as follows.

(1) Pain in muscles of mastication, the TMJ, or the periauricular area, which is usually made worse by manipulation or function.

(2) Asymmetric mandibular movement with or without clicking.

(3) Limitation of mandibular movements.

(4) Pain present for a minimum of 3 months.

12.2.5 Management

TMD can be difficult to manage, and since the disorder transcends the boundaries between several health-care disciplines—in particular, dentistry and neurology, the treatment may often involve multiple approaches and be multidisciplinary.

(1) Psychosocial and behavioral interventions: cognitive behavioral therapy, hypnosis, relaxation techniques, including progressive muscle relaxation, yoga, and meditation are helpful.

(2) Devices: occlusal splints are often used to treat TMD. Types of occlusal splint are stabilization splint, soft stabilization appliances, anterior positioning appliances, and anterior bite appliances. These appliances should be monitored in their use.

(3) Medication: many drugs have been used to treat TMD pain, such as (pain killers), benzodiazepines (e. g. , clonazepam, prazepam, diazepam), anticonvulsants (e. g. , gabapentin), muscle relaxants (e. g. , cyclobenzaprine), and others. Other drugs described for treating in TMD include glucosamine hydrochloride/chondroitin sulphate and propranolol. Botulinum toxin solution, local anesthetic may provide temporary pain relief. However, evidence in support of the effectiveness of these drugs is lacking.

(4) Physiotherapy, biofeedback and similar non – invasive measures, acupuncture, TENS, ultrasound, massage, low level laser therapy, are sometimes used as an adjuvant to other methods of treatment in TMD.

(5) Occlusal adjustment and orthodontic treatment: occlusal adjustment can be very complex, involving orthodontics, restorative dentistry or even orthognathic surgery.

(6) Surgery: just a few patients need to proceed to surgery, include arthrocentesis, arthroscopy, meniscectomy, disc repositioning, condylotomy or joint replacement.

12.2.6 Prognosis

It has been suggested that the natural history of TMD is benign and self-limiting, with symptoms slowly improving and resolving over time. Therefore the prognosis is good. However, the persistent pain symptoms, psychological discomfort, physical disability and functional limitations may detriment quality of life.

12.3 Dislocation of TMJ

TMJ dislocation involves a non self-limiting displacement of the condyle, outside of its functional positions within the glenoid fossa and posterior slope of the articular eminence. Although the most common condylar dislocation is anterior to the articular eminence, onto the pre-glenoid plane, there have also been reports of medial, lateral, posterior, and intracranial dislocations. Subluxation refers to a condition in which the joint is transiently displaced without complete loss of the articulating function, and is usually self-reduced by the patient.

12.3.1 Classification of the TMJ dislocation

TMJ dislocation is divided into three categories: acute, chronic, and chronic recurrent. Acute dislocations may be associated with any number of etiologies, including prolonged mouth opening during a lengthy dental procedure, vomiting, yawning, or singing. There have also been reports of acute dislocation secondary to epileptic seizures, acute facial trauma, and direct laryngoscopy. Frequent dislocation may also be seen in patients with connective tissue disease, such as Ehlers-Danlos Syndrome(EDS) or muscular dystonias.

(1) Acute dislocation is the most common and is defined as a sudden onset of the condyle being displaced anteriorly beyond the articular eminence, which can not be reduced by the patient.

(2) Chronic recurrent TMJ dislocation may occur as a result of everyday activities such as yawning laughing, or during events that require mouth opening for a continuous amount of time (such as during dental treatment). Chronic recurrent TMJ dislocation is distressing because it is painful and it interferes with daily routine activities. The pathogenesis of chronic recurrent TMJ dislocation is attributed to a combination of factors including laxity of the TMJ ligaments, weakness of the TMJ capsule, an unusual eminence size or projection, muscle hyperactivity or spasms, trauma, and abnormal chewing movements that do not allow the condyle to translate back. Recurrent dislocation of the TMJ may cause injury to the disc, the capsule, and the ligaments, leading to progressive TMJ internal derangement.

(3) Long-standing dislocation or protracted dislocation is rare, and is defined as dislocation not reduced immediately.

12.3.2 Clinical manifestations

Signs and symptoms are the same for acute and chronic dislocation.

(1) Inability to close mouth.

(2) Severe pain over TMJ.

(3) Preauricular skin depression, which is palpable.

(4) Excessive salivation.

(5) Tense, spasm of the masticatory muscles.

12.3.3 Diagnosis

Clinical history and examination are the most important tools in diagnosing TMJ dislocation. Other confirmatory diagnostic aids include plain and panoramic radiographies, showing the location of the condylar head anterior to the articular eminence. Three-dimensional computed tomography is the best in terms of its perfection to show this entity.

12.3.4 Management

12.3.4.1 Acute dislocation

It is a very painful clinical condition, but easy to manage. The conservative methods in its management include symptomatic pain relief with analgesics and manual reduction. The manual reduction method is performed by first pressing the mandible downward, then backward, and finally upward as described by Hippocrates. In 1987, Awang described another simple, safe, and rapid method in managing acute dislocation. According to him, induction of the gag reflex by probing the soft palate creates a reflex neuromuscular action that resulted in the reduction.

12.3.4.2　Chronic dislocation

If this condition is long-standing or recurrent, it poses a challenge to the treating clinician. The management is divided into two stages, the conservative methods are opted; if the results are not satisfactory, then we go for the surgical methods.

12.3.4.3　Chronic recurrent dislocation

The conservative method includes the use of various sclerosing agents like alcohol, sodium tetradecyl sulfate, sodium psylliate, morrhuate sodium, and platelet-rich plasma that has been injected into the joint space. In case of chronic protracted dislocation, elastic rubber traction with arch bars and ligature wires or intermaxillary fixation(IMF) with elastic bands are useful to achieve the reduction. The use of autologous blood in recurrent dislocation was reported by Brachmann in 1964 and is very popular nowadays. The volume of blood to be used ranges 2-4 mL in the upper joint space and 1-1.5 mL in the pericapsular structures, repeated twice a week for 3 weeks. To further enhance the fibrosis, restriction of the mandibular movement with a head bandage is required for the period of 3-4 weeks.

Another newer conservative method is the application of Botulinum Toxin A(BTX-A) in recurrent TMJ dislocation. BTX injection therapy is also an option in those patients who suffer from recurrent dislocation of the TMJ because of impaired muscle coordination, secondary to oromandibular dystonia, neuroleptically-induced early and late dyskinesias, epilepsy, and brainstem stroke syndromes. The adverse effect involves diffusion into the adjacent tissues, transient dysphagia, nasal speech, nasal regurgitation, painful chewing, and dysarthria. It is contraindicated in a few conditions like hypersensitivity to BTX and myasthenia gravis in pregnant and lactating women.

12.3.4.4　Chronic long standing dislocation

The surgical methods are indicated in those cases where the patients have not responded well to the conservative methods. Various other methods like condylotomy, modified condylotomy, and myotomy had been tried. Few authors have suggested surgical procedures that either remove the mechanical obstacle in the condylar path or create a mechanical obstacle by augmenting the articular eminence. Augmentation of the articular eminence can be done by autogenous bone grafts like the iliac crest or the calvarial bone. Total joint replacements should be considered when all the appropriate treatments fail in chronic protracted and chronic recurrent dislocations, especially those with associated degenerative joint diseases.

12.4　Ankylosis of TMJ

Ankylosis of the TMJ is referred to difficulties in opening mouth or complete restraint from injury or infection of the TMJ and adjacent tissues that tether condyle movement within the capsule. According to the site of the lesion, it is divided into the intra-articular ankylosis, the extra-ankylosis and the mixed joint ankylosis. Intra-articular ankylosis refers to the fibrous or osseous adhesions within the joint, also known as the true joint ankylosis. The extra-articular ankylosis is located outside the joint. Fibrous or bony adhesions are in the skin, mucosa or deep tissues between the upper and lower jaws, also called pseudo ankylosis or intermaxillary contracture. Mixed ankylosis refers to the conditions that true ankylosis and pseudo ankylosis co-exist.

12.4.1 Etiology

The most common etiological factor is trauma and infection. The joint trauma, condylar fracture, and the mandible injuries will lead to the condyle fracture or intra-articular hemorrhage that results in the ankylosis.

Primary infection of the TMJ, such as tuberculosis, gonorrhea, syphilis, scarlet fever, typhus fever, actinomycetes, etc., can appear rare joint ankylosis. Hematogenous infection, such as sepsis, is also rare. It can cause hematogenic pyogenic arthritis and eventually lead to joint ankylosis. Secondary infection of adjacent tissue is common, such as otitis media, papillomitis, temporal bone osteomyelitis and parotid infection. Most of the pathogens are hemolytic streptococcus, and pus can directly spread to the joints. Noninfectious inflammation, such as rheumatoid arthritis, can also cause joint ankylosis, usually bilateral fibrous ankylosis. Radiation therapy can also lead to joint ankylosis.

12.4.2 Classifications

Ankylosis of temporomandibular joint can be divided into congenital and acquired, congenital is extremely rare. Many congenital cases are caused by a forceps delivery or an injury in early infancy.

Depending on the location of the cause of restraint, the joint ankylosis are also classified as contracture of elevator muscles, capsular fibrosis, and ankylosis.

12.4.3 Clinical manifestations

Most of the joint ankylosis occurs in children and appears progressive limitation of opening mouth with age. In the early stage is characterized by fibrous ankylosis and further developed into osseous ankylosis. The fibrous ankylosis has no pain in the joint area and the patient can gently open the mouth because of the elasticity of the fibrous tissue. Later, the lateral movement is obviously limited and the opening type is deflected toward the affected side. The condyle activity of the affected side is obviously weakened.

Osseous ankylosis is characterized by a complete inability to open the mouth. It is usually accompanied difficulties in speech and eating and the activity of the condyle disappears.

Children with ankylosis of temporomandibular joint are often characterized by facial asymmetry and micrognathia, leading the chin moved to the affected side. Bilateral ankylosis, especially with bony ankylosis, because of the mandibular developmental disorder caused by mandibular retraction, will reflect a special facial profile and most of patients are associated with sleep apnea.

12.4.3.1 Contracture of elevator muscles

The identifying characteristics of muscular contracture involving elevator masticatory muscles are as follow:

(1) History of prolonged myositic activity in the muscle or protracted restriction of mouth for any reason.

(2) No pain, unless the muscles are injured by abusive efforts to open the mouth.

(3) Restriction of mandibular movement, extracapsular in type, and involving opening movement only.

(4) No interference during mandibular movements.

(5) No acute malocclusion.

(6) Radiographic confirmation of extracapsular restriction of mandibular movement.

12.4.3.2 Capsular fibrosis

It results from inflammation of the capsule, usually due to trauma. The identifying characteristics of capsular fibrosis are as follow:

(1) history of prior trauma, surgery, or capsulitis.

(2) No pain, unless the capsular ligament is abused by excessive translatory movements.

(3) Restriction of mandibular movement that restricts condylar movement, protrusion and lateral extrusion to the same degree as in opening.

(4) No interference during mandibular movements.

(5) No acute malocclusion.

(6) Radiographic confirmation of capsular restriction of mandibular movement.

12.4.3.3　Ankylosis

Intracapsular adhesions or actual ossification that tether condylar movement within the capsule is termed ankylosis. It results from trauma that causes hemarthrosis, which may organize and form a matrix for cicatrization. Ankylosis is usually unilateral because trauma is more likely to occur in a single joint affliction. It should be noted that when one joint is immobilized, degenerative change may take place in the opposite joint, due to unnatural movements imposed. The identifying characteristics of TMJ ankylosis are as below:

(1) History of prior injury or infection of the joint.

(2) No pain, unless the joint is abused.

(3) Intracapsular restriction of mandibular movement.

(4) No interference during mandibular movements.

(5) No acute malocclusion.

(6) Radiographic confirmation, with condylar restraint in open and lateral positions being identical and remaining fairly closed to the closed joint position.

12.4.4　Therapy

12.4.4.1　Contractured elevator muscle

Extracapsular chronic mandibular hypomobility due to muscular contracture may become inflamed due to excessive opening efforts. As such, it should be treated as myositis, until acute symptoms subside.

It should be noted that myofibrotic contracture of long standing may be complicated by other elevators.

12.4.4.2　Capsular fibrosis

The usual problem during this period is that of injury induced by excessive force used to extend condylar movement. The injured capsule becomes inflammed, and the condition should be treated as a capsulitis.

12.4.4.3　Ankylosis

As fibrous ankylosis is the usual form, forceful movements may injure the adhesions, which causes pain and inflammation. Treatment consists of voluntary restraint of joint use until the inflammatory condition subsides. Anti-inflammatory medications and deep-heat therapy are usually beneficial. Exercises are contraindicated. Good postsurgical care and followup are essential to satisfactory results.

12.5　Infection of TMJ

Inflammatory disorders of the TMJ have pain as their chief symptom—more or less continuous inflammatory arthralgic pain. Usually it is aggravated by the demands of function. The chief features that cause these conditions to be grouped together for classification are the following:

(1) History of trauma, infection, polyarthralgia, or noninflammatory degenerative condition of the joint.

(2) To some degree, continuous arthralgia related to the demands of function, manual palpation of the joint proper, and functional manipulation.

(3) Frequently complicated by referred pains, secondary hyperalgesia, and muscle-spasm activity in the masticatory muscles.

12.5.1   Classifications

Inflammatory disorders of the TMJ may be classified as:

(1) Synovitis and capsulitis.

(2) Retrodicitis.

(3) Inflammatory arthritis.

The inflammatory disease of the TMJ is less than that of other joints in the whole body. Due to no antibiotics, infection of the temporomandibular joint caused by odontogenic infection and ear infection were common in the nineteenth century and early twentieth century. With the widespread use of antibiotics, the incidence of TMJ infection is significantly reduced.

12.5.2   Diagnosis

12.5.2.1   Synovitis

Inflammation of the synovial membrane and capsular ligament causes swelling and palpable tenderness over the involved joint. It may result from localized trauma, abusive use, and specific infection. It is difficult clinically to distinguish between synovitis and capsulitis. The identifying characteristics of synovitis and capsulitis are as follow:

(1) History of prior trauma or some preexisting condition that could secondarily involve the capsule in an inflammatory process.

(2) Pain is continuous and of the capsular arthralgic type.

(3) Restriction of the mandibular movement, if any, is of capsular type.

(4) Usually, no interference during mandibular movement is present other than from a preexisting or coexisting condition.

(5) Acute malocclusion, of any, is due to inflammatory effusion within the joint cavity, causing a sensation of disocclusion of the ipsilateral posterior teeth.

(6) Radiography may confirm capsular restriction of mandibular movement, if any, may also be confirmed by comparing the width of the articular disc space in the unclenched and clenched occluded positions.

12.5.2.2   Retrodiscitis

Injury sustained by the retrodiscal tissues, cither as a result of direct external trauma or due to condular encroachment from any cause, may induce inflammation of the retrodiscal tissues, attended by intracapsular pain and swelling. Swelling of the tissue and effusion of inflammatory exudate in the joint cavity may displace the condyle anteriorly, thus causing acute malocclusion. This is sensed as disocclusion of the ipsilateral posterior teeth and premature striking of the contralateral anterior teeth. Pain occurs especially when maximum intercuspation forces the condyle back against the retrodiscal tissue. This pain can be reduced by biting against a separator to prevent intercuspation. If hemathrosis takes place, ankylosis may result.

The identifying characteristics of retrodiscitis are the following:

(1) History of extrinsic trauma. Chronic retrodiscitis may related to preexisting chronic occlusal, sleletal disharmonies or to protracted functional anterior dislocations.

(2) Pain is arthralagic type and of the retrodiscal variety.

(3) No restriction of the mandibular movement.

(4) No interference during mandibular movement is present other than preexisting symptoms.

(5) Acute malocclusion is due to displacement of the condyle anteriorly as a result of inflammatory effusion within the joint cavity, this is sensed as disocclusion of the ipsilateral posterior teeth and premature striking of the contralateral anteriors.

(6) Acute malocclusion may be confirmed radiographically by comparing the unclenched and clenched occluded positions of the joint. The unclenched position shows the condyle to be anteriorly displaced.

12.5.2.3 Inflammatory arthritis

The identifying characteristics of inflammatory arthritis are as below:

(1) History of trauma, infection, systemic illness, involvement of other joints, prior noninflammatory disc-interference disorder, ankylosis, or structural aberration.

(2) Pain is arthralagic.

(3) Restriction of the mandibular movement may be negligible. At other times, capsulitis and secondary muscle effects may immobilize the joint.

(4) Interference during mandibular movement is consistent with preexisting etiologic conditions.

(5) Acute malocclusion results from inflammatory effusion within the joint cavity.

(6) Radiographic studies may be decisive.

Infection of the TMJ is divided into acute infection and chronic infection. According to the type of infection, it can be divided into acute suppurative arthritis, traumatic arthritis, degenerative arthritis, infectious arthritis, rheumatoid arthritis, osteoarthritis, psoriatic arthritis, ankylosing spondylitis and so on.

12.5.2.4 Traumatic arthritis

(1) Chronic occlusal harmony, especially aggravated by bruxism and clenching.

(2) All sorts of functional abuse or overloading that lead to the joint injury.

(3) Localized pain and swelling over the joint.

(4) Restriction of TMJ function.

(5) Interference during mandibular movement.

(6) Coexisting muscle effects.

(7) Radiographic evidence confirmed.

12.5.2.5 Infectious arthritis

Although synovitis may occur in conjunction with systemic infection as a nonspecific or immunologic response, actual purulent bacterial invasion of the joint may take place. This may be due to penetrating wounds, trauma, or the spreading of infection from adjacent tissues. Occasionally, infectious arthritis may be the result of bacteremia from systemic infection (gonorrheal arthritis). The diagnosis is made from the history, clinical symptoms, examination of fluid aspirated from the joint cavity, and blood examines.

12.5.2.6 Rheumatoid arthritis

The TMJs frequently are involved rheumatoid arthritis. The symptoms may be mild and go unnoticed. Rheumatoid arthritis (RA) is an inflammatory condition of unknown etiology in which the inflamed and hypertrophic synovial membrane grows onto the articulating surfaces. RA is variable in incidence, severity, and clinical course. Diagnosis of RA requires medical confirmation.

12.5.2.7　Hyperuricemia

An excessive level of serum uric acid causes a type of inflammatory arthritis in which pain with functional movements of the joint may be the chief complaint. High levels may show deposits of urates in and about the joint. It is seen more frequently in older people. The diagnosis is confirmed by blood examines.

12.5.3　Treatment

12.5.3.1　Therapy for capsulitis and synovitis

Most cases displaying symptoms of capsulitis are secondary to other inflammatory conditions arising as the result of injury to the discal collateral ligament or the temporomandibular ligament. Some are secondary to inflammatory arthritis, periarticular conditions, or injury to a preexistent capsular fibrosis. In general, the treatment for capsulitis and synovitis includes the following:

(1) Restriction of condylar movement.

(2) Deep-heat therapy using diathermy or ultrasound.

(3) Anti-inflammatory medications.

(4) Special considerations are needed if the capsulitis is secondary to other disorders; if the capsulitis is due to periarticular inflammation, active treatment of the primary condition, including antibiotics supportive medical and surgical care, may be needed. If the capsulitis is a manifestation of inflammatory arthritis, treatment should be directed primarily toward the arthritic condition.

12.5.3.2　Therapy for retrodiscitis

Many inflammatory conditions of the retrodiscal tissue result from extrinsic trauma of a type that could have caused a mandibular fracture. The diagnosis usually is made only after a futile radiographic search for a fracture line. Since hemarthrosis may be present, treatment should be taken into account the prevention, if possible, of ankylosis. The treatment for this kind of retrodiscitis entails the following:

(1) Intermaxillary fixation to establish normal occlusal relations.

(2) Periodic release of the fixation and active movement of the joint for 5-10 minutes at least twice daily.

(3) As soon as the occlusion will remain stabilized without the aid of intermaxillary fixation, active movement of the joint should be encouraged until resolution is complete.

If the retrodiscitis occurs insidiously as a result of injury to the retrodiscal tissue (due to posterior overclosure), occlusal correction is needed. If due to protracted functional dislocation, surgical intervention may be required.

12.5.3.3　Therapy for inflammatory arthritis

The symptoms of generalized inflammation of the joint are much the same, regardless of cause.

Therefore, certain general principles of treatment may apply to all types. As the specific kind of arthritis becomes evident, special considerations are needed. The following therapeutic principles are usually indicated:

(1) Functional demands should be reduced voluntarily to bring them well within the capabilities of the inflamed joint.

(2) Nonpainful movements of the joint should be maintained on a periodic schedule of 5-10 minutes two to three times daily to keep the joint mobile. This should not be carried out to the point of pain or other sign of aggravation of the inflammatory condition.

(3) Acute malocclusion and other obvious discrepancies in occlusal function should be corrected by

occlusal disengagements. If an occlusal splint is used, it should be corrected periodically as resolution or other further deterioration takes place.

(4) Medically supervised anti-inflammatory medications and other supportive medical treatment are indicated.

(5) Judicious physiotherapy in the form of deep heat should be used unless it seems to aggravate the condition.

(6) Degenerative arthritis may require special management of the dentition according specific condition. RA is essentially a medical problem. Progressive loss of contact of the anterior teeth may require occlusal splinting, adjusted periodically as further change takes place. Reconstructive arthroplasty may be needed.

(7) Traumatic and infectious arthritis may require antibiotic therapy as well as general supportive medical and surgical care.

(8) Hyperuricemia is a medical problem requiring active treatment and follow-up.

(9) Corticosteroid therapy may have a place in the treatment program. But considerable judgement should be exercised in its use. It is frequently part of RA treatment. Injection of sodium hyaluronate (HA) into the joint is considered to be useful in improving the functional condition of the joint.

12.6 Tumors of TMJ

Neoplastic involvement of a TMJ is relatively rare. Tumors of cartilage and osseous structure are reported most frequently. Osteoma of the condyle may be extremely difficult to distinguish from hyperplasia. Chondroma, osteochondroma, giant cell granuloma, and hemangioma have been reported. All such tumors involving the mandibular condyle are extremely rare.

12.6.1 Importance of early recognition of neoplasms and pseudotumors of TMJ

Although primary malignant disease of the TMJ proper has been reported, direct invasion from surrounding structures is considerably more frequent. When this occurs, the initial joint complaint is usually painless restriction of joint movement, which is highly suggestive of fibrous ankylosis. It is only when the disorder expresses itself as a progressively worsening condition with an increasing component of pain that malignancy may be suspected. Needle biopsy can help make a positive diagnosis.

Early recognition of neoplasms and pseudotumors of the temporomandibular joint will prevent therapeutic delay and may have a dramatic impact on patient morbidity and mortality.

12.6.2 Rare TMJ lesions

(1) Synovial chondromatosis.

(2) Osteochondroma.

(3) Osteoma.

(4) Osteoblastoma.

(5) Pigmented villonodular synovitis.

(6) Ganglion.

(7) Synovial cyst.

(8) Simple bone cyst.

(9) Aneurysmal bone cyst.

(10) Epidermal inclusion cyst.

(11) Hemangioma.

(12) Nonossifying fibroma.

(13) Langerhans cell histiocytosis.

(14) Plasma cell myeloma.

(15) Sarcoma.

12.6.3　Diagnosis and differential diagnosis

Certain clinical manifestations can help us distinguish between TMD and tumor disease: numbness of the territories innervated by the trigeminal nerve branches, hearing loss, constant pain not influenced by mandibular movements, increased severity of symptoms, a lack of response to treatment, alterations in dental occlusion, the presence of swelling, unexplained weight loss, ear suppuration or swallowing difficulties. However, these manifestations are not present in all cases, and many patients with TMJ tumors are initially diagnosed and treated as cases of TMD. The resulting delay in establishing the correct diagnosis causes increased suffering, a greater risk of treatment complications and, in the case of malignant tumors, an increased threat to patient survival. It is necessary to identify the symptoms, signs and radiological alterations advising the inclusion of TMJ tumors in the differential diagnosis.

Many tumors show no radiological alterations in the panoramic X-Ray. Radiotransparencies were more frequent in the tumors than in the pseudotumors. In contrast, radiopacities were significantly more common in the pseudotumors than among the tumors. Radiotransparency, and especially a poorly defined tumor contour, are suggestive of malignancy. Treatment usually involves surgery, and relapse is observed in 10% of the cases, particularly among malignant tumors.

Kang Hong

Chapter 13

Tumors of Oral and Maxillofacial Regions

Oral and maxillofacial regions is an important part of head and neck tumor. According to the clinical classification of International alliance against cancer(UICC), the head and neck tumor is divided into seven anatomical parts: lip、oral、maxillary sinus, swallow, salivary gland, throat and thyroid, most of them are in the oral and maxillofacial region. Quasi-tumors and tumor-like lesions quasl is not a true tumor, but there are some biological characteristics and clinical manifestations of tumors, so this is a discussion with the tumor.

13.1 Overview

13.1.1 General situation

Oral and maxillofacial regions are the concentration areas of many important organs in the human body. The anatomical structure is complex, and the tissue occurs from multiple layers of embryonic leaves. In this case, the tumors that occur are of various types and biological characteristics, and are prone to early invasion of adjacent vital organs(such as eyes, skull base and neck). The characteristics of odontogenic and salivary gland derived tumors are specific tumors of oral and maxillofacial features. The name of the oral and maxillofacial tumor is also includes three aspects, for example location, tissue origin and biological characteristics, such as ameloblastoma of the mandible, squamous cell carcinoma of the tongue, and maxillary osteosarcoma, malignant lymphoma, etc. According to this clinical nomenclature, there is a general understanding of the tumor, some tumors are benign.

But it has local infiltration growth and malignant tendency, clinically referred to as "borderline tumor". Such as ameloblastoma, pleomorphic adenoma. For these tumors, the right surgical treatment must be used for these tumors.

In our country, there is no accurate information about the incidence of oral and maxillofacial tumors. According to the report of Parkin in 1993, the mouth and pharynx, the estimated incidence of malignancy was 8. 7/100,000 (male) and 6. 0/100,000 (female). According to 1997 Shanghai tumor registration data, the incidence of head and neck cancer was about 12. 7(standard 10. 5)/100,000(women) and 15. 4 (standard 12. 7)/100,000 (men); the incidence of oral maxillofacial facial cancer is about 3. 3(1. 8)/

100,000 (female) and 3. 8 (standard 2. 4)/10 between ten thousand men. In prevalence (prevalence rate), the Xinjiang region of oral and maxillofacial tumors survey is 8. 10/100,000. The prevalence of oral cancer was (1. 06 – 1. 09)/100,000, according to the guangzhou survey. The above information indicates the oral and maxillofacial features of our country. The incidence and prevalence of cancer are not high, but due to the large population in our country, the absolute number of patients is very large.

In general tumors, the ratio of benign to malignant is about 1 : 1. However, in oral and maxillofacial tumors, there is more benign than malignant, according to the ninth affiliated hospital of Shanghai Jiao Tong University. In 1991, there were 15,983 cases were gathered statistic, malignant tumors accounted for 32. 08%. The benign endothelial neoplasm of the face is the most common, and the malignant nectar is the most important. In recent years, there has been a significant increase in oral cancer in women.

So far, there have been few reports on the overall survival rate of oral cancer. In the case of reclining facial cancer, The 5–year survival rate reported in China in the 1990s was about 64%, and the key to improving the survival rate was early detection, early diagnosis and early treatment. Although the oral and maxillofacial position is located in the superficial, it can be seen that the diagnosis should not be difficult, but there are reports of clinical misdiagnosis, the rate is up to 30%, probably due to lack of knowledge and attention to the oral cavity. Therefore, effective measures should be taken to make non oral major medical workers have better knowledge of oral and maxillofacial tumors.

13.1.2　Clinical manifestation and diagnosis

Early detection, correct diagnosis is the key to cure malignant tumor. In clinical practice, oral and maxillofacial malignant tumors are easily misdiagnosed as gingivitis, traumatic ulcer, maxillary sinusitis, mandibular osteomyelitis, tuberculosis, etc. , thus causing the patient to delay or lose the opportunity to cure. In the course of tumor diagnosis, it is important to distinguish between tumor or non–tumor diseases (such as inflammation, parasites, deformity or tissue hyperplasia).

13.1.2.1　Medical history collection

The emphasis should be on the timing of the initial symptoms, the exact location, the rate of growth, and the recent sudden acceleration of growth. It is helpful to distinguish benign tumor from malignant tumor and determine the primary site of advanced malignant tumor. If you have suspicious symptoms, you should catch them, Do not ignore any of the patient's chief complaints (Table 13–1).

Table 13–1　To identify the benign tumors and malignant tumors

	Benign tumour	Malignant tumor
Age of onset	At any age	Cancer is more common in old age, sarcomas more in middle age
Growth speed	Generally slow	A fast
Growth pattern	Expanded growth	Invasive growth
Relationships with surrounding organizations	There is an envelope that does not infringe on the surrounding tissue, the boundaries are violated, the surrounding	Infringe, destroy the surrounding organization, the limit is unclear, the activity is restricted
Symptoms	No	Often local pain, numbness, headache, opening. Limit, facial paralysis, bleeding and other symptoms

Continue to Table 13-1

	Benign tumour	Malignant tumor
Transfer	No	Constant transfer
Impact on the body	Generally, it has no effect on the body, but it can be life-threatening due to rapid development and metastasis	When the key part or occurrence complication, also with invading important organ and occurrence cachexia. life-threatening death
Histological structure	Cell differentiation is good, the structure is similar to normal tissue	cell morphology and cell differentiation are poor, cell morphology and structure are atypical

13.1.2.2 Clinical examination

Visual diagnosis and palpation are important in clinical examination. Visual can understood morphology, growth location, size and presence of the tumor. Palpation can understand the boundaries, texture, activity and relationship with adjacent tissues. For the tumor of mouth, tongue, etc. it should be palpated with both hands. Auscultation is helpful to the diagnosis of angiogenic tumors. When suspicion is a malignant tumor, the cervical lymph node was also examined to determine whether the lymph nodes were metastatic or not. Meanwhile, the patients should be examined with important organs. To remove distant metastasis from the tumor.

X-ray examination is mainly used to understand the nature of bone tissue tumors and the invasion of bone tissue by soft tissue tumors.

13.1.2.3 Imaging examination

For example, in the primary jaw bone cancer, the X-ray plate of the jaw bone is characterized by a small, worm-like bone destruction zone in the middle of the jaw bone. As for the gingival cancer is characterized by a small basal ganglia, with alveolar bone at the bottom. For malignant neoplasms, the chest radiographs should be routinely performed to check for metastasis angiographic examination, such as salivary gland contrast, carotid artery. Angiography, tumor(sinus) and angiography can help determine the nature and extent of the tumor and provide reference for treatment.

Computed tomography(CT), magnetic resonance imaging(MRI) and digital subtraction angiography (DSA)were used for oral and maxillofacial depth tumor examination. The diagnosis of a tumor, especially MRI, is very accurate in the resolution of deep soft tissue tumors, and it also provides an accurate surgical scope.

Ultrasonography is usually performed by ultrasound probe. Oral and maxillofacial cystic tumors and soft tissue tumors, it is more accurate to indicate whether there is a mass or not. In addition, the boundary definition of the sound image and the distribution of points of light in the tumor are even. Whether or not, is to judge the tumor benign and malignant evidence. It can be applied to the examination of lumps with undulating or deep soft boundary in the diagnosis of lumps. For example, deep hemangioma puncture can be inhaled.

13.1.2.4 Puncture and cytological examination

The puncture of the cyst can suck out the fluid, sometimes smear to see congealed blood or cholesterol crystallization. In recent years, the salivary glands or some deep tumors may also be used for puncturing cytological examination, or fine needle aspiration biopsy. The accuracy of this method is 95%, but it is difficult to be completely certain of the histological type of tumor.

13.1.2.5   Living organization inspection

The morphology and structure of the cells were observed under the microscope to determine the degeneration of the cells, quality, tumor type and degree of differentiation. This is more accurate and reliable at present, and is also a conclusive diagnostic method. But it should be combined comprehensive analysis of the bed and other examination methods that can make the diagnosis more accurate. The biopsy must be properly handled because inappropriate biopsy can not only increases the patient's pain, but also promotes tumor metastasis and affects the therapeutic effect. Patients with malignant melanoma are should not be done, the cryopathology can be used to help diagnose and minimize iatrogenic diffusion.

13.1.2.6   Examination of tumor markers

With the development of biological chemistry, immunology, molecular biology, cell engineering and genetic engineering, specific chemicals are found in the blood, urine, or other body fluids of patients with malignant tumors, which are usually antigenic and stimulated. In the form of elements, receptors, enzymes, proteins, and various oncogenes, these products are produced, secreted and released by tumor cells. It is called a "tumor marker". Therefore, sometimes according to the blood and urine test, not only can understand the patient general condition, but also can assist in the diagnosis of tumor. Patients with malignant tumor, the blood sedimentation rate and the viscosity increase. The blood of patients with advanced osteosarcoma, the alkaline phosphatase can be increased. Plasma globulin increased in patients with multiple plasma cell sarcoma, and thrombin was found in urine(also known as Bence-Jones protein); in the whole body metastasis of malignant melanoma, the melanin test can be positive.

13.1.3   Treatment

For the treatment of tumor, it is necessary to establish comprehensive treatment. According to the nature and clinical manifestation of the tumor, patients should be combined physical condition with specific analysis, and determine to adopt corresponding treatment principle and method, make a more reasonable treatment plan.

13.1.3.1   Principles of treatment

(1)Benign neoplasms are usually treated with surgical treatment, such as a borderline tumor, which should be excised. Resection tissue for frozen section examination. If there is a change, the scope of resection should be extended.

(2)Malignant tumor should be based on the tumor tissue source, growth site, differentiation degree, development speed, clinical stage, patient's machine. After comprehensive study, the appropriate treatment method should be selected.

13.1.3.2   Treatment

(1)Surgical treatment is still the main and effective method for the treatment of oral and maxillofacial tumors, which is suitable for benign tumors, especially for those therapy and chemotherapy can not cure malignant tumors. For malignant tumors that may be metastatic to the neck, Neck lymph node dissection should be performed.

The main reason for the failure of oral and maxillofacial malignant tumors is local recurrence and(or) distant metastasis. Therfore, in surgery, strictly abide by the principle of "no tumor"; Surgical excision of tumor is performed in normal tissue, avoid cutting the tumor and contaminating the surgical field.

Crush the tumor to avoid spreading. It should be excised as a whole, not to be cut apart. The exposed part of the tumor should be covered with gauze and suture. The surface of the ulcer can be treated with electrocautery or chemotherapy to avoid contamination during the operation. Before suture, a large number of hypotonic saline could used. Study drug(5% mg nitrogen mustard) to wash wet application; gloves and instruments must be replaced when the wound is stitched. In order to prevent the tumor from spreading, it is still available. The use of electric knife can also be used in intraoperative and postoperative intravenous or regional arterial injection.

(2) Radiotherapy, in addition to early and minor, and lymphatic, hematopoietic tissue source of tumor, etc. It can be treated as part of the treatment, preoperative or postoperative radiotherapy can be done. Preoperative radiotherapy can shorten the tumor, inhibit the rapid growth of tumor, create conditions for the operation, and put more after wooding. It is used for surgical resection and some recurrent carcinomas to reduce local recurrence.

Preparation before radiotherapy: before radiotherapy, removal of the adjacent teeth of the tumor, and the metal crown and crown bridge should be removed. In this way, the possibility of infection and mandibular necrosis can be reduced, and the tumor can be directly irradiated by radiation. In addition, notice oral hygiene. After radiotherapy, there should be further treatment of the mandibular necrosis or osteomyelitis.

(3) Chemotherapeutic treatment is a part of comprehensive treatment for middle and advanced oral and maxillofacial malignancies, usually first. With chemotherapy, the reduction of tumor reoperation can increase the chance of surgical treatment, which is called neoadjuvant chemotherapy or induction chemotherapy.

In clinical application, the first choice is pingyangmycin (PYM), methotrexate (MTX), cisplatinum (CDDP), It is usually administered by intravenous injection or drip. It can also be used for regional chemotherapy with arterial intubation to improve local drug concentration, reduce systemic toxicity and improve curative effect.

At present, chemotherapy can be combined with heat therapy(thermal chemotherapy), immunotherapy (immunotherapy) and traditional Chinese medicine, as well as surgery and radiotherapy. Combination of drug therapy improve the long-term efficacy of malignant tumor therapy.

(4) The role of biological therapy surgery, radiotherapy and chemotherapy in the comprehensive treatment of head and neck cancer has been recognized. And certainly, the treatment of cancer has not been completely successful. With the progress of molecular biology research in recent years. The biological therapies that mobilize the body's own anticancer function to achieve clinical therapeutic goals are widely favored and are expected to be in the near future. It is the fourth conventional method to treat cancer. In a broad sense, biological treatment includes immunotherapy, cytokine therapy, and gene therapy, etc.

(5) In order to improve the therapeutic effect of the tumor, the treatment of advanced tumor is more likely to be comprehensive treatment or multidisciplinary treatment. Because any kind of treatment has two sides, has its advantages, also has its deficiency. Comprehensive treatment can be taken long, and short, complementary, to get the best results, but must be based on concrete analysis.

At present, there is a combination of surgical, radiotherapy and chemotherapy in the homophobia and the native place emphasis on surgical treatment. It should be pointed out that the comprehensive treatment is not hard, its purpose is to improve the curative effect. The relevant oncology professionals will discuss and discuss the different stages of tumor and development in different natures according to the general situation of the patients.

A reasonable individualized treatment plan should be developed in a systematic and rational way. Its characteristic individual's synthesis, and should also be the treatment methodical arrangement. To this end, more accurate should be called "integrated sequence therapy".

13.1.4 Prevention of oral and maxillofacial tumors

13.1.4.1 Elimination or reduction of carcinogenic factors

Removing the cause is the best way to prevent it. For the prevention of oral and maxillofacial tumors, the external chronic stimulants should be eliminated, such as timely treatment of residual roots, crowns, dislocation teeth, and sharpening sharp teeth, removal of defective prostheses and defective partial or complete denture, in order to avoid the frequent injury and irritation of the oral mucosa, it will avoid causing cancer, especially tongue, cheek and gum cancer. Pay attention to oral hygiene, avoid ironing and stimulating foods. In addition, abstinence from cigarettes and alcohol; exposure to outdoor or in hazardous industries. The protection measures should be strengthened when the material contact works. Avoid excessive stress and depression, maintain an optimistic spirit, and prevent swelling. The occurrence of tumor has certain significance.

13.1.4.2 Timely treatment of precancerous lesions

The most common precancerous lesions in oral and maxillofacial features are white and erythema. Oral mucosa is considered to be the most common precancerous lesion. The incidence of leukoplakia was reported in the literature, with less than 1% of the low and 60% higher. The common precancerous condition of the cheek part of the mouth is considered to be planar lichen, submucosal fibrosis, discoid lupus erythematosus.

Dermal hyperkeratosis, congenital keratosis and syphilis, pigmented xeroderma, etc. For flat moss, especially erosion and atrophy. The flat moss has a long cure, should heighten vigilance. According to the literatures, the malignant rate of lichen is 1%–10%. Early malignant tumors can be cured, but the treatment of advanced tumors is very poor. Early tumors are often unclear due to symptoms.

13.1.4.3 To carry out surveillance of cancer screening or susceptible population

It is similar to the symptoms of certain diseases and is easily overlooked. Cancer screening can be detected early, early diagnosis, and thus obtained. Early effective treatment. The occurrence and development of tumors takes a certain amount of time, usually a few years or more. Tumors tend to develop slowly in the early stages and develop rapidly later in life, indicating that most cancers can be detected early. Timely diagnosis and early treatment are necessary.

13.2 Cysts of Oral and Maxillofacial Regions

13.2.1 Soft tissue cyst

13.2.1.1 Sebaceous cyst

Sebaceous cyst in traditional Chinese medicine is called powder tumor. The main reason is the sebaceous gland excretory duct obstruction, sebaceous cystic epithelium. A retention cyst formed by the expansion of an increasing amount of internal content. The cyst is the secretion of the white tufted sebaceous glands.

(1) Clinical manifestations

It often happened on the face, small as the size of a bean, big as the size of a small like village orange sample. The cyst is located in the skin and protrudes to the surface of the skin. The skin is closely adhered to, and there is a small pigment spot in the center. Clinically, it can be distinguished from epidermoid cyst by this main characteristic.

(2) Treatment

Surgical excision was performed under local anesthesia. A spindle incision along the skin of the face should be excised to include the skin that adheres to the wall of the cyst.

13.2.1.2 Dermoid cyst or epidermoid cyst

Dermoid cyst or epidermoid cyst(epidermoid cyst) is the dermoid cysts resulting from trapped embryonic epidermis and present as a rounded mass. It contains keratinizing squamous epithelium, sweat glands, and other associated skin appendages.

(1) Clinical manifestations

Dermatoid or epidermoid cysts are more common in children and young adults. The dermoid cyst is good at the mouth and submental area, the epidermoid cyst is good at the eyelid, forehead, nose, outer part of the orbit, and lower ears. The growth is slow and circular. The mucosa on the surface of the cyst or the skin is smooth, cyst and week. There is no adhesion to the surrounding tissue, skin or mucous membrane. The cyst is tough and elastic.

The puncture examination can extract the milky white bean residue sample secretion, sometimes the gross specimen can be seen the hair.

(2) Treatment

Excision to prevent recurrent infections, with attention to the facial nerve, is the most successful treatment.

13.2.1.3 Thyroglossal duct cyst

At the 6th week of the embryo, the thyroglossal duct disappeared, leaving at the starting point only a superficial four or tongue blind hole. If the thyroglossal duct does not disappear, in the absence of time, the residual epithelial secretions accumulated and formed a congenital thyroglossal duct cyst.

(1) Clinical manifestations

Thyroglossal cysts are commonly seen in children between 1 and 10 years old, and can also be seen in adults. Cysts can occur in the midline of the neck. Any part of the incision between the hole and the sternum, but is most common in the upper and lower hyoid bone. Cysts grow slowly, round and clinically common. Such as walnut, located in the middle of the neck, sometimes slightly laterally. Soft, clear boundary, no adhesion to surface skin and surrounding tissues.

In the case of a cyst below the hyoid bone, the hyoid bone and the cyst may be in the form of a bond with the hyoid bone, so it can be swallowed and protruded.

The thyroglossal duct cyst can be diagnosed according to its location and the movement of swallowing, and sometimes the puncture can be used to extract the transparent and slightly mixed.

The puncture can draw out a transparent, slightly turbid liquid. For the thyroglossal fistula, it is possible to make an iodide oil contrast to clarify the fistula.

(2) Treatment

Surgical excision of the cyst or fistula, and should be thorough, otherwise easy to relapse. The key to surgery is, in addition to the cyst or fistula, It should be excised from the hyoid bone.

13.2.1.4 Branchial cleft cyst

Branchial cleft cyst may result from branchial cleft anomalies, these anomalies are subdivided into type I and type II cysts. There are lymphoid tissues, usually covered with stratified squamous epithelium, and a few are columnar epithelium.

(1)Clinical manifestations

Branchial cleft cyst is often located in the upper part of the neck, mostly in the lingual bone level, and is near the anterior margin of the sternocleidomastoid. Sometimes it is attached to the neck.

The surface of the cyst is smooth, which from the posterior portion of the scabbard, or from the internal jugular to the external carotid, and to the side of the pharynx, but sometimes lobular. Bump big small and uncertain, slow growth. Patients who have no conscious symptoms, such as an upper respiratory tract infection can suddenly increase, but feel uncomfortable. Branchial cleft after perforation of the cyst, the branchial fistula can be formed for a long time.

(2)Treatment

Radical resection, if residual tissue, can lead to recurrence.

13.2.2   Jaw cyst

13.2.2.1   Odontogenic jaw swelling

Odontogenic cyst occurs in the jaw bone but is related to the formation of a tooth or tooth. Depending on the source. It is divided into the following:

(1)Radicular cyst is caused by periapical granuloma and chronic inflammation.

Skin residual hyperplasia. The hyperplasia of the epithelium is denaturation and liquefaction, and the surrounding tissue fluid is constantly seeping and gradually forming cysts. It is called periapical cyst.

(2)A primordial cyst (periapical cyst) is the most common type odontogenic cysts. Small radicular cysts do not usually become acutely infected, are frequently asymptomatic, and can be identified on routine dental X-rays. Larger cysts may produce expansion of the bone, displacement of tooth roots. Infected radicular cysts are painful, the involved tooth is sensitive to percussion, and there may be swelling of the overlying soft tissues and lymphadenopathy. Dental X-rays show a cyst around the end of the root that can extend beyond the bounda ries of the involved tooth. Treatment of radicular cysts involves endodontic therapy for small cysts(<5 mm), endodontic therapy plus periapical surgery and cyst enucleation for larger lesions. Or tooth extraction combined with cyst enucleation. The prognosis is excellent following the appropriate treatment.

(3)Dentigerous cyst is the second most common type of jaw cyst associated with the crown of an impacted, unerupted, or developing tooth. Small dentigerous cysts rarely produce clinical symptoms. Larger cysts can produce a bony expansion, which creates an intraoral swelling, an extraoral swelling, or both. They also can result in facial tries or become secondarily infected, which results in pain. The most common radiographic appearance of a dentigerous cyst is that of a well-defined, radiolucent lesion. Aspirationa light, straw-colored fluid is characteristic of a dentigerous cyst. The treament consists of enucleation of the cyst and removal of the associated tooth.

(4)Odontogenic keratocyst, 3%-10% odontogenic cysts are keratocysts and can occur at any age; however, 60% of patients are between 10 and 40 years of age. The mandible is involved in 60%-80% of odontogenic keratocysts, with a tendency to involve the posterior mandible and ascending ramus. These cysts have a locally aggressive clinical behavior. Small odontogenic keratocysts usually are asymptomatic and are identified during routine dental examination and imaging. Larger odontogenic keratocysts may produce pain, drainage, swelling from secondary infection, and asymmetries from bony expansion. The adjacent teeth are vital, but can be displaced. Panoramic X - rays for large, expansile lesions reveal an ocally destructive, multilocular lesion that can displace teeth, resorb tooth roots, deflect the mandibular canal inferiorly, and displace the floor of the maxillary sinus superiorly. Aspiration of an odontogenic keratocyst produces a whitish or pale yellow, inspissated, cheese-like material. Enucleation or decompression and marsupialia tion are the treatments of choice. Most recurrences become evident within 5 years of the initial treatment

13.2.2.2 Non-odontogenic

Non-odontogenic developmental cysts are found in regions of epithelial embryonic remnants, pseudo-cysts usually present in site-specific regions.

(1) Globulomaxillary cyst occurs between the maxillary lateral incisors and the fangs, and the teeth are often displaced. The X-ray shows the cyst shadow on the root, not the root tip. The tooth has no decay and discoloration, and the pulp has vitality.

(2) Nasopalatine cyst is located in or near the incisor(from the residual epithelium of the incisors). X-ray film can be seen that the cyst shadow enlarged by the incisor.

(3) Median cyst is located at any part of the palate after the incisor. There is a circle on the X-ray. Shape cyst shadow. It can also occur in the middle of the mandible.

(4) Nasolabial cyst is located in the upper lip and nasal vestibule. It may come from the epithelium of the nasolacrimal duct cyst. On the surface of the bone. There is no bone damage on the X-ray film. The presence of a cyst on the outside of the oral vestibule. Cysts are common in adolescents. The initial symptoms were unconsciousness. If it continues to grow, the bones gradually swell around and form facial deformity.

(1) Clinical manifestations

Cysts are common in adolescents. The initial symptoms were unconsciousness. If it continues to grow, the bones gradually swell around and form facial deformity. And that comes with is it to different parts can appear corresponding local symptom.

(2) diagnostic

According to the history and clinical manifestations. X-ray examination is of great help in diagnosis. The cyst is shown as a clear circle on the X-ray. The transparent shadow of the shape or oval, with neat edges, is often presented with a clear white bone reaction line, but sometimes the edges of keratinized cysts.

(3) treatment

After diagnosis, surgical treatment should be performed in time so as to avoid further displacement and malocclusion of teeth. Surgery in the mouth, if accompanied by infection, must be treated with antibiotics or other antimicrobial agents before surgery.

13.3 Benign Neoplasms and Tumor-like Lesions

13.3.1 Tumor samples lesions

13.3.1.1 Nevus(nevi)

(1) Intradermal nevus is differentiated into large nevus cells, which is a more mature nevus cell, and into the dermis. It's surrounded by connective tissue.

(2) At the junction of the epidermis and dermis, the nevus cells of junctional nevus show multiple nests, with clear boundaries and distribution. The distance is even, the upper half of each cluster is in the lower layer of the epidermis, while the lower half is within the superficial layer of the dermis. These cells are

small moles, the pigment is deeper.

(3)Compound nevus is often accompanied by endothelial lamentation and residual at the same time when the mole cells enter the dermis. The mole is a mixture of these two moles.

1) Clinical manifestations: borderline nevus is light brown or dark brown macules, papules or nodules, generally small, surface smooth, hairless, flat or slightly above the skin. There is no conscious symptom. Protruding on the surface of the skin, the mole is easily stimulated by washing, shaving, friction and injury. It may cause a malignant change: mild itching, burning or pain. The volume of moles increases rapidly; color burn. On the surface of the current infection, rupture, hemorrhage, or the presence of the skin around the nevus with satellite dot, radiation black line, melanin ring. And the drainage of the mole. Regional lymph node enlargement and so on. Malignant melanoma often comes from the junction of moles.

It is believed that nevus, freckle-like nevus are all skin nevus or compound nevus. This type of mole is rarely malignant, if it has a malignant transformation.

2)Treatment: there is no evidence that the facial expression is large, but it can be taken into consideration for partial resection, good appearance and function preservation, but not applicable for malevolent. It can also be resected, adjacent flap transfer or free skin grafting. If there is any doubt, surgery should be taken. The biopsy was performed at one time. The operation should be made on normal skin outside the boundary of the mole. Smaller moles were removed. After the skin has been removed, the skin can be removed directly to the suture.

13.3.1.2 Gingival tumor

The odontoma(epulis)is derived from the non-true tumor of the periodontal membrane and the connective tissue of the jaw bone.

(1)Clinical manifestations

There are more women with gingival tumors, which are common in young and middle-aged people. Most of them are in the gingival papilla. It is located on the lips and chin and the tongue and palate. The most common site is the premolar area. The tumor is more circumscribed, circular or elliptic, sometimes lobular. They are not of uniform size. The diameter is several millimeters to several centimeters. Some of the lumps are like polyps, some are unattached, and the base is broad. Usually grows slowly, but in female gestation, it may rapidly increase, the larger tumor can cover part of the tooth and the alveolar process, the surface can be seen the tooth indentation, easily be bitten by the bite. Ulcer and infection may occurs with the growth of the mass, the alveolar bone wall can be damaged. The X-ray films show that the bone absorbe the periodontal membrane to widen. Teeth may be loose and displaced.

(2)Treatment

Surgical removal can be performed under local anesthesia. Resection must be complete, otherwise it is easy to relapse. The teeth involved in the lesion should be removed at the same time.

13.3.2 A benign tumour

13.3.2.1 Ameloblastoma

The ameloblastoma is the most common clinically significant and potentially lethal the odontogenic tumor.

(1)Clinical manifestations

Ameloblastoma is more common in young people, Mandibk body and mandible angle are more common. Slow growth is the rule with untreated tumors leading to tremendous facial disfigurement. The most common diographic feature is that of a multilocular radiolucency. Resorption of adjacent tooth roots is common. Owing to the highly infiltrative and aggressive nature of the solid or multicystic ameloblastoma, it is recommended resection of the tumor with 1. 0 cm linear bony margins. Unicystic ameloblastomas are most commonly seen in young patients with about 50% of these tumors being diagnosed during the second decade of life, usually in the molar/ramus region. A unilocular radiolucency found in the mandimimicking a dentigerous cyst, is the most common radiographic presentation.

(2) Diagnostic

According to the history, clinical manifestation and X-ray characteristics, preliminary diagnosis can be made. X-ray manifestation of typical ameloblastoma: early be the room shape, after the formation of multiple atrial cyst shadow, single room relatively few. Ameloblastoma is due to multiple localities and a certain degree of local.

Infiltration, so the edge of the cystic wall is often irregular, with a half-moon cut. The root tip of the capsule has irregular absorption.

(3) Treatment

The ameloblastoma is most appropriately treated with a wide local excision. Because ameloblastoma has the characteristics of local infiltration surrounding bone, the bone surrounding the tumor should be at least 0. 5 cm excision, otherwise, the treatment will not completely lead to recurrence, and relapse can turn malignant.

13.3.2.2 Hemangioma

Hemangioma is absent at birth or history of small premonitory mark at birth and rapid neonatal growth of the lesion. Cutaneous lesions develop either a typical "strawberry" appearance or a bluish. Most commonly, the diagnosis of hemangioma is determined by the history and physical examination. The history typically reveals that more than 50% of hemangiomas are seen at birth as a prominent cutaneous mark. A superficial hemangioma assumes the typical "strawberry" appearance, making the diagnosis obvious. In a subcutaneous, intramuscular, or viscera tumor, the diagnosis may be uncertain. In these instances, various radiologic modalities can be very helpful. MRI is diagnostic when the diagnosis is uncertain or when serial exam is not possible. Visceral involvement is suspected if there are more than three cutaneous lesions. Progressive stridor in the appropriate age group(2-9 months) is suspicious for airway hemangioma.

The decision to intervene and attempt to treat the patient without an active or inevitable complication from hemangioma must be weighed against the fact that most hemangiomas resolve completely or with minimal long-term sequelae. For hemangiomas with active or inevitable complications, multiple treatment options exist. The most appropriate treatment depends on the location and the nature of the impending complication as well as the childs specific medical and social situation. For example, if follow-up is not possible, early definitive surgical management may be more strongly considered.

Steroids are the usual first line of treatment. Typical initial doses are 2-5 mg/(kg · d) of prednisolone or prednisone. Interferon alfa-2a is a comparatively new agent for the treatment of hemangiomas. Vincristine is gaining popularity as another efficacious treatment for complicated or refractory hemangiomas. There are relatively few side effects compared with interferon. Laser therapy for hemangiomas is becoming widely practiced to combat mucosal lesions and cutaneous lesions with or without ulceration. It is common to consider excision in a completely involuted lesion when the residum causes a functional or esthetic problem.

13.3.2.3 Vascular malformation

(1) Venous malformations cause symptoms dependent on location. They are almost always a cosmetic problem, and thrombosis often makes these lesions painful, impairing basic activities. It usually presents at birth, but not detected. As they become apparent, venous malformations are bluish-purple, raised, and easi-

ly compressible. Enlarge it when dependent. Gradually dilate, giving the appearance of the sclerotherapy is the mainstay of treatment for craniofacial lesions and for extensive extremity lesions. Sderosants are effective for these lesions because the sclerosant stays in the lesion or can be made to stay in the lesion with compression of the outflow pathway.

Alcohol-based sclerotherapy are the most commonly used type of sclerosing agent. Complications of sclerotherapy can occur, most commonly skin necrosis with alcohol-based agents, alcohol is typically not used in and around the eye to avoid complications leading to damaged vision.

(2) Venular malformation is a common wine stain. Multiple in facial skin, often along distribution of trigeminal nerve. Oral mucosa is less. It is bright red or purplish red, with smooth surface and clear boundary. Its shape is irregular, they are not of uniform size, from small spots to a few centimeters, big can be extended to the department or the center line to the contralateral side profile. With finger pressing disease. Loss of surface color. After relieving the pressure, the blood immediately fills the lesion area, restoring the original size and color. The so-called mediu microvenous malformation is mainly caused by the lesion in the middle line, the most common part, and the second can occur between the forehead and the brow. And upper lip medium. Unlike wine stains, it can go away on its own.

(3) Arteriovenous malformations(AVMS), excluding in tracranial lesions, are uncommon and are most often found in the head and neck. Commonly noted at birth and confused with a hemangioma or a capillary malformation. Eventually, local warmth and pulsation lead to diagnosis. Not easily compressible. Overlying skin changes usually precede heart failure.

Ligating a large feeding vessel is always contraindicated. This procedure shifts the blood flow to collateral vessels and serves only to accelerate the growth of the malformation. Complete surgical excision is the only way to ensure a permanent, successful treatment. With early diagnosis surgical excision of a stage I malformation is possible. Early lesions have a greater chance for complete and successful surgical excision, super-selective arterial embolization with permanent material can be used palliatively to relieve pain or other symptoms, or as part of a combined treatment plan intended to completely eliminate the lesion.

(4) Lymphatic malformations. 50%-60% of lymphatic malformatto recognized at birth; 90% are recognized by the second year. 80% of all lymphatic malformations are located in the head and neck. A lymphatic malformation tends to be slowly progressive, growing with the child. In some instances, it is apparent that the lymphatic malformation rapidly increases in size. In these cases, it is likely that the lesion has either hemorrhaged into itself or has become infected. There are reports of spontaneous regression, although they are far from typical. An MRI scan is the typical and best means for evaluating patients with a presumed lymphatic malformation. Based on the radiographic appearance of the size of the lymphatic spaces located within the lesion, lymphatic malformations are then broadly categorized as either macrocystic or microcystic.

1) Microcystic type: the old classification is called capillary type and cavernous lymphangioma, which is expanded by lymphatic vessels lined with endothelial cells. The lymphatic tube is extremely dilated and bent, forming a multilocular cyst, which is similar to spongiform. Lymphatic vessels are filled with lymph. The mucosa presents isolated or multiple scattered cystic nodular or punctiform lesions, colorless, soft, and generally incompressible. The lesion boundary is not clear. The lymphatic malformation of oral mucosa is sometimes associated with microvenous malformation, and yellow and red vesicular processes appear. This is called lymphatic microvenous malformation. Occurs in the lips, lower jaw, and the frequency division, sometimes can make the affected area significantly hypertrophic deformity. It occurs in the tongue and is often caused by giant tongue disease. Jaw deformity, open, anti-almost, tooth displacement, occlusion disorder and so on. The surface of the tongue mucosa is rough, nodular or veined, with yellow blister fluid. On the ba-

sis of chronic inflammation, the tongue can harden.

2) Large cystic type: the old classification is called cyst type or cystic water tumor. It occurs mainly in the neck supraclavicular area and also occurs in the lower jaw, lower and upper neck. It is usually multilocular cyst with clear, pale yellow liquid. The lesion size varies. The skin color is normal and filling, and the palpation is soft and fluctuating. Different from deep venous malformation is the position movement test, but sometimes the light test is positive. Many treatments have been used for the management of the lesions, which indicates that none has been completely effective. The treatment of localized malformations relies essentially on sclerosis or surgery, except in some specialized locations. Both surgery and sclerosis are very effective for localized lesions, the management of diffuse cases is much more complex and may be a lifelong endeavor. Surgical management is the mainstay of treatment for these lesions, sometimes it is impossible.

(5) There is a type of vascular malformation with a type of vascular malformation, which can be referred to as a mixed vascular anomaly, such as the aforementioned, microvenous malformation and microcystic lymphatic malformation coexist. Arteriovenous malformation accompanied by localized microvenous malformation. Naturally, the venous deformity is also possible. It also exists with large cystic lymphatic malformation.

13.3.2.4　Neurofibroma

Neurofibroma is a benign tumor composed of nerve sheath cells and fibroblasts. There are two types of neurofibromatosis, or neurofibromatosis.

It manifests that nerve fibroma (neurofibroma) grows slowly in young people, slow growth. It is rare in the mouth. Facial nerve fibroma, the main clinical manifestations are brown spots with different sizes of surface skin, or small black spots or patchy lesions. When you are palpating, your skin will note that there are multiple tumor nodules, and they are hard to touch. Multiple tumor nodules may follow the skin. The nerve distribution, in the form of a rosary, can also appear from to form, such as rice. Sensory nerve can have obvious tenderness. In regions along the nerve distribution, there are sometimes connective tissue with heterotactic hyperplasia, skin flabby or fold.

Fold down, cover the eyes, malfunction, facial deformity. The tumor is soft, although the tumor is rich in blood, but generally can not be pressed. Deformity may occur when adjacent bone is infringed. Head facial multiple neurofibroma can be accompanied by congenital occipital defect. Neurofibromatosis has a genetic predisposition to autosomal dominant inheritance. Therefore, the family of the patients, especially the immediate family members. A thorough physical examination can determine whether there is a family history.

Treatment: surgical removal. The small and localized neurofibromatosis can be completely resected at one time; but it can only be partially cut for large tumors, in addition to correct deformity and alleviate dysfunction.

13.3.2.5　Ossifying fibroma

Ossifying fibroma for maxillofacial benign tumors of bone are common.

(1) Clinical manifestations

Ossified fibroma is common in young people, mostly single disease, can occur in upper and lower jaw bone, but the following jaw bone is more common, Female more sex than men. This tumor growth is slow, early unconscious symptom not easy to be detected. As the tumor grows, it can cause the expansion of the jaw bone. Enlargement causes facial deformity and tooth displacement. Occurs in the upper maxillary bone, often affecting the frontal bone, and may affect the maxillary sinus and the palate, making the eye socket. Deformity, eyeball protrusion or shift, or even produce diplopia. In addition to facial deformities, the mandibular ossifying fibroma can lead to occlusion.

Disorder,sometimes secondary infection,accompanied by osteomyelitis.

(2)Diagnostic

On the X-ray film,it is characterized by localized dilatation of the jaw bone. The lesion is developed in the surrounding area. The boundary is clear,round or oval,and the density is reduced. The lesion can be seen with an uneven and irregular calcification shadow.

(3)Treatment

Because ossified fibroma is a true tumor,surgical excision should be performed in principle.

13.4 Oral and Maxillofacial Malignant Tumors

It is the most common form of squamous cell carcinoma and less form of sarcoma in oral and maxillofacial regions. Cancer squamous cell origin in oral and maxillofacial, include the carcinoma of oral cavity,carcnoma of the facial skin, carcinoma of oropharynx, carcinoma of the maxillary sinus and entral carcinoma of the jaws. We also discuss soft tissue sarcomas,sarcoma osin,lymphoma,plasma cell sarcoma,midline lethal granuloma and malignant melanoman this chapter.

13.4.1 Tongue cancer

Carcinoma of tongue is the most common oral cancer. According to the ninth people's hospital of Shanghai Jiao Tong University, 1954. The statistical data of 1751 cases of oral cancer treated in 1990 years,551 cases of tongue cancer(31.6%), ranked first. More than 85% of tongue cancer occurs. At the tongue,with advancing disease,local pain,ipsilateral referred otalgia,and jaw pain are experienced by the patient. Most carcinoma of tongue occurs on the lateral border of tongue at the junction between middle and posterior thirds. Approximately 30% of patients present with pilate cervical node metastasis. When carcinomas are in the midline,bilateral neck metastasis would occur.

13.4.1.1 Clinical manifestations

In the early stage of tongue carcinoma,there are three types of ulcer,exogenous and infiltration. In some cases,the first symptom is only tongue pain,sometimes it can be reversed.

Carcinoma of tongue is often asymptomatic. Frequently carcinoma of tongue presents as painless mass or ulcer that fails to heal alter a minor trauma. With advancing disease, local pain, ipsilateral referred otalgia,and jaw pain are experienced by the patient. Most carcinoma of tongue occurs on the lateral border of tongue at the junction between middle and posterior thirds. Approximately 30% of patients presents with pilate cervical node metastasis. When carcinomas are in the midline,bilateral neck metastasis would occur. The tongue movement can be severely restricted and fixed,and the salivary fluid can be overflowed,but cannot control,eating,swallowing and speaking will feel difficult.

13.4.1.2 The diagnosis

The diagnosis of tongue carcinoma is generally easier, but it is important to be vigilant for early tongue cancer,especially invasive type. Diagnosis of tongue carcinoma by palpation notes. This is especially important. Pathological biopsy should be sent for a definite diagnosis.

13.4.1.3 Treatment

Early highly differentiated tongue carcinoma consider to be treated with radiotherapy,simple surgical resection or cryotherapy. Advanced tongue cancer should be treated with comprehensive treatment, root, primary focus

According to different conditions, radiotherapy plus surgery or triplet(chemotherapy, surgery, radiotherapy) or quadruple(Chinese traditional medicine or immunotherapy) are used.

(1)Radiotherapy can be used as adjuvant therapy for advanced tongue cancer cases before and after surgery.

(2)Surgical treatment is the main method to treat tongue cancer. T1 case can be row distance from the lesion outside LCM, straight. After suture; T2–T4 cases should be resected to complete tongue resection.

The tongue is an important organ for chewing and speech. Tongue reconstruction is required for more than half of tongue defects.

(3)Chemotherapy for advanced cases can be preoperatively induced by chemotherapy. Chemotherapy has a better effect on tongue cancer, and it is expected to improve patient's survival rate.

Cryotherapy treatment for tongue carcinoma of T1 and T2 may be treated with cryotherapy.

(4)Treatment of metastases.

Therefore, in addition to T1 case, the selective cervical lymph node dissection should be considered. In patients with positive bed lymph nodes, the treatment of cervical lymph node dissection should be performed in the same period.

13.4.1.4　The prognosis

According to the data of our country, the 5-year survival rate is more than 60% in the treatment of surgery. Case of T1 can reach up to 90%.

13.4.2　Carcinoma of gingival

Carcinoma of the gingival is second cancer of oral cancer, but has decreased year by year in recent years.

13.4.2.1　Clinical manifestations

The clinical manifestations of gingival cancer can be ulcerated or exogenous. It is starts with the interdental nipples.

Transparent area, ulcer is superficial, reddish, can appear proliferation later. Because of the sticky periosteum and alveolar protrusion, it is easy to infringe teeth early. Alveolar periosteum and bone, and then the tooth looseness, and can fall off. X-ray films could show the destructive characteristics of malignant tumors – irregularly absorbed.

Gingival cancer often occurs secondary infection, the tumor companion with necrotic tissue, the touch is easy to bleed. When the volume is too large, the face can be swollen and soaked, embellish skin. Carcinoma of gingival quickly spread to invade the alveolar, mandible and maxilla. Invasion may spread along the ramus of mandible to lingual and is suggested by ipsilateral numbness of the lower teeth and lip. The common nodal basins for metastasis include the superior deep jugular node(level Ⅱ), followed by level Ⅲ.

13.4.2.2　Diagnosis

The diagnosis of gingival cancer is not difficult, it is convenient to send pathological biopsy.

13.4.2.3　Treatment

Even early gingival cancer, in principle, should be resected, not just gingivectomy. Surgery involves at least marginal mandibulectomy or maxillectomy to obtain clear margins. Patients with no neck lymph node metastasis should also undergo at least elective ND and with palpable metastatic lymph node are best managed with therapeutic ND.

13.4.2.4   Prognosis

The 5-year survival rate of gingival cancer is higher, according to the 1970s statistics of the ninth people's hospital affiliated to Shanghai Jiao Tong University is 62.5%.

13.4.3   Carcinoma of buccal mucosa

The cancer that originated in the mucous membrane is called buccal carcinoma. The ninth people's hospital affiliated to Shanghai Jiao Tong University medical school of the 1,751 cases of oral cancer, 365 cases were recorded, accounting for 20.85%.

13.4.3.1   Clinical manifestations

Carcinoma of buccal mucosa may commonly appear as the middle differential squamous cell carcinoma. Mucosal squamous cell carcinoma usually has ulceration, accompanied by deep infiltration, and only a few of them appear as verrucous or mastoid gland. There are few ulcers in the carcinogenic buccal cancer, mainly manifested as external or infiltration of hard-knot masses. The frequency cancer often develops from white spot. You could find spots in the affected area. There is no obvious pain in the early stage of frequency cancer, so patients often delay medical treatment, when the cancer is infiltrated by deep tissue or merge infection.

When there is obvious pain, the opening is limited to varying degrees until the jaws are closed. After periodontal tissue is tired, could appear toothache or tooth is loose. Due to cancer infiltration, ulcer formation, especially with infection, can cause local secondary hemorrhage, pain aggravation. In patients with often submandibular lymph node enlargement, may also involve the neck deep lymph node group.

13.4.3.2   Diagnosis

The diagnosis of frequency cancer is mainly based on the history, clinical manifestation and pathological examination.

13.4.3.3   Treatment

Currently, the predominant treatment for carcinoma of buccal mucosa is surgical excision. Early cancer (T1 and T2) can also be effectively treated with primary radiation. Therapeutic ND should be performed in all patients, with clinically positive lymph node.

(1) Preoperative or postoperative radiotherapy

The dose of 40-50 Gy was used in 4 weeks. If preoperative radiotherapy, after radiotherapy, usually rest 4-6 weeks. The surgical removal of cancerous tumors can be performed without special conditions.

(2) Preoperative chemotherapy

Preoperative chemotherapy, also known as induction chemotherapy, is the most commonly used and effective measure in the comprehensive treatment of buccal cancer. The drug can be used as a single drug and can be used in combination with the drug. The drug can be administered intravenously or through the external carotid branch.

(3) Surgical treatment

The principles and main points of surgical treatment of buccal carcinoma are as follows.

Adequate depth, even in early cases, must include submucosal fat and fascia.

Adequate boundaries should be excised at the normal tissues of 2 cm beyond the clinical boundary where cancer can be judged.

Cervical lymph node dissection (including submandibular lymph node), or the primary lesion at T3 or above. Cancer Ⅱ magnitude; or buccal cancer grows fast; be located in frequency hind part, should routine do the same side neck lymphatic dissection technique.

13.4.3.4 Prognosis

Due to the different combination of cases, the 5-year survival rate of frequency cancer reported by the literature was very different. The 5-year survival rate was 62.29%.

13.4.4 Palate carcinoma

The carcinoma of the palate is rare. At Shanghai Jiao Tong University medical school affiliated to the ninth people's hospital statistics. In 1751 cases of oral cancer, palatal cancer was ranked 4th, 186 cases, accounting for 10.2%.

13.4.4.1 Clinical manifestations

The palatal cancer often begins on one side and spreads quickly to the gum side and to the other side. Most of them are exogenous, and the edges are turned out to bleed and bleed. Callus, the bleeding of touch, sometimes ulcerated. The mucous membranes surrounding the palatal cancer can sometimes be seen in the presence of tobacco stomatitis or leukoplakia. The mucous membrane and palatine bone are close to the bone. So it is easy to invade the bone early. The lymph node metastasis of palatine carcinoma mainly invaded the lymph nodes of the lower jaw and the deep cervical lymph nodes. Post – pharyngeal lymph node metastasis is difficult clinically. Judgment is more found in surgery.

13.4.4.2 Diagnostic

The diagnosis of palatal cancer is not difficult, but it can be obtained directly from pathology.

13.4.4.3 Treatment

(1) Treatment of the original oven

The treatment of cancer is mainly operated by surgery. The operation of palatal cancer is usually performed with a lesion of the palatine bone. For the larger disease, the upper clavicle should be completely cut.

(2) Treatment of metastases

For the larger disease, the lymphatic metastasis rate of cancer is around 40%; in advanced cases, bilateral neck metastases often occur, and bilateral selective neck may be considered. Lymphatic dissection can be performed by one side modified radical or bilateral modified radical neck dissection.

13.4.4.4 Prognosis

The prognosis of palatine squamous carcinoma is worse than that of the palatal salivary gland carcinoma. Statistically, the 5-year survival rate was 66%. The prognosis of late and lymph node metastases was poor, and the 5-year survival rate was only about 25%.

13.4.5 Carcinoma of the floor of mouth

Carcinoma of the floor of mouth refers to squamous cell carcinoma that occurs in the mucosa of the mouth.

13.4.5.1 Clinical manifestations

Oral cancer is common on both sides of the tongue, with ulcerations or lumps. Carcinoma of the floor of mouth is often asymptomatic in the early stages of disease. As the tumor enlarges, bleeding, ulceration, pain, and submandibular duct obstruction become more common. The clinically apparent cervical metastasis occurs at early stage with multiple levels of nodal involvement.

13.4.5.2   Diagnostic

As tongue cancer, the palpation of the mouth, especially the hands, is very important, and the nature and reality of the tumor can be understood by palpation.

Infiltration part. In case of bone destruction, X-ray film can be used to assist in the diagnosis(early occlusal tablet is appropriate and late stage is optional Oral panoramic tablet.

13.4.5.3   Treatment

Early carcinoma of the floor to mouth can be effectively treated with either surgery or radiation. For carcinoma of advance stage, the primary cancer resection, segmental mandibulectomy and ND should be performed.

13.4.5.4   Prognosis

The prognosis of early oral cancer is better and the late stage is worse. The ninth people's hospital affiliated to Shanghai Jiao Tong University medical school in eighty, for data, the annual survival rate was about 61%.

13.4.6   Maxillary sinus carcinoma

The carcinoma of the maxillary sinus is often treated in otolaryngology due to its different location and clinical manifestations. And stomatology, which is common in squamous cell carcinoma.

13.4.6.1   Clinical manifestations

In the early stage, because cancer is confined to the maxillary sinus, the patient can be asymptomatic without detection. When the tumor develops to a certain extent. After that, obvious symptoms appear and the patient is noticed. Clinically, different symptoms can be observed according to the different primary sites of the tumor. When the tumor occurs from the lower wall of the maxillary sinus, it is first causes that the tooth to loosen, the pain, the buccal groove is swollen, if the toothache is thought to be periodontitis and so on and so on the tooth extraction, the tumor is protruding in the tooth groove, the wound. The failure to heal formed a festering surface. When the tumor occurs in the upper maxillary sinus, it usually begins with nasal obstruction, nasal bleeding, and an increase in nasal secretion. More, Nasolacrimal duct obstruction, there are tears. When the tumor arises from the upper wall, it usually causes the eyeball to protrude and shift upward, which may cause diplopia and swollen. When the tumor arises from the outer wall, it is shown as swelling of the face and groove, and then the skin is broken, the tumor is exposed, and the suborbital nerve is affected.

To be insensitive or numbness. When the tumor occurs from the posterior wall, it can invade the fossa and cause the opening to be restricted. The maxillary sinus carcinoma is often metastasized to the lower mandibular and cervical lymph nodes, sometimes to the anterior and posterior pharyngeal lymph nodes. Distant metastases is rare.

13.4.6.2   Diagnosis

Conventional X-ray films, with a certain reference value, are far inferior to the diagnosis of primary tumor and location CT, therefore, the imaging examination of maxillary sinus carcinoma, CT should be the first choice.

13.4.6.3   Treatment

The treatment of maxillary sinus carcinoma should be based on the comprehensive treatment, especially the combination therapy combined with radiotherapy.

(1) Radiation therapy

The confirmed cases of maxillary sinus carcinoma can be preoperatively preoperative radiotherapy and 3-4 weeks after radiotherapy.

(2) Surgical treatment

Total maxillectomy is indicated for treatment early stage of carcinoma of the maxillary sinus. Extensive maxillectomy and combined cranio-facial resection is recommended for the advanced disease. The palpable cervical metastasis should be performed a therapeutic ND.

(3) Chemical treatment

The method of regional chemotherapy with arterial intubation was used. The drug can be used with methotrexate, pingyangmycin or fluorouracil. Perfusion, operation after the end of chemotherapy.

13.4.6.4　Prognosis

The prognosis of maxillary sinus cancer remains unsatisfactory so far, according to the literature, the 5-year survival rate is mostly within 50%. Its failure main reason is local recurrence after treatment, and rarely die from metastasis.

13.4.7　lip cancer

Carcinoma of the lip is a carcinoma of the lip red mucosa, mainly squamous cell carcinoma. The medial mucosa of the lip should be frequency. Mucosal carcinoma, occurs in the lips of the skin, due to skin cancer.

13.4.7.1　Clinical manifestations

Lip cancer often occurs Lip cancer can occur anywhere along the upper or louer lip, but is most common on the lower lip. Early herpes, scabs of the mass, followed by a volcano. Oral ulcer or cauliflower mass. Later, the tumor spreads to the surrounding skin and mucosa, and infiltrates the deep muscle tissues. Terminal can wave oral vestibular and maxillary bone. Lower lip cancer often metastases to submental and submandibular lymph nodes. The upper lip cancer is metastatic to the anterior, submandibular and cervical lymph nodes.

13.4.7.2　Diagnosis

According to the history and clinical manifestations, it is not difficult to make a diagnosis. It is necessary to do a biopsy to clarify the tumor nature.

13.4.7.3　Treatment

The early cases were treated with surgery, radiation, laser or hypothermia. But for advanced cases, surgical-based comprehensive treatment should be used.

13.4.7.4　Prognosis

The prognosis of lip cancer is better. The 5-year survival rate of the ninth people's hospital affiliated to Shanghai Jiao Tong University medical school is 85.7%.

13.4.8　Carcinoma of the oropharynx

The malignant tumor of mouth pharynx refers to the level between soft palate and hyoid bone, including tongue root, soft glue, tonsil, pharynx, and posterior pharyngeal wall. A malignant tumor in the surrounding area. The oropharyngeal carcinoma can be divided into tongue root cancer, tongue, pharyngeal arch (pharynx), tonsillar carcinoma and soft palate cancer.

13.4.8.1   Clinical manifestations

There are some differences in the clinical manifestations of oropharyngeal carcinoma, but the main clinical manifestations are similar. It include ulcerationtype, exogenous type and infiltration type. The initial symptoms of oropharyngeal cancer are not obvious, but the pharynx is uncomfortable and foreign. The tumor broke and became infected. Now pharyngeal pain, fixed at the lesion side, can also have glossopharyngeal reflex of the ear pain. If the tumor is in the flat tonsil pharynx lateral wall, upward and nasopharynx, can cause a side ear stuffy, hearing loss. If tumor invasion and the pharynx side, infringe the internal muscle, can appear the difficulty of opening mouth. After the deep infiltration of tongue tumor can appear the tongue deviation and the sound barrier, and often saliva blood, halitosis, the breath is not smooth. Obstruction caused by the grawth of tumor cam lead to the difficulty in obstruction can cause difficulty in breathing and swallowing.

13.4.8.2   Diagnosis

Partial detailed examination of oral pharynx, turmors had actually been clearly visible. Biopsy is a necessary means of diagnosis.

13.4.8.3   Treatment

Surgical treatment is the main treatment.

13.4.8.4   Prognosis

Due to the dissection of the mouth pharynx, the adjacent relationship is complicated, so the long-term effect is poor.

13.4.9   Skin cancer

According to the malignant degree and pathological type, the facial skin malignant tumor is generally divided into melanoma and non-melanoma. It can come from skin epidermis, also can come from skin accessory, for example sweat gland cancer. In China, the proportion of basal cell carcinoma is higher than cell carcinoma.

13.4.9.1   Clinical manifestations

Carcinoma of the facial skin is frequently found at the nose, wrinkled nose, eyelid, lip skin, cheek and ear. It can be shown as a central depression with a cirrus edge. It can also cause bleeding due to trauma and ulcer, and it can break down. It can also appear as ulcer and the scar forms a nest patch.

13.4.9.2   Diagnosis

The diagnosis of skin cancer is relatively easy, once the clinical suspicion, can do pathological examination diagnose.

13.4.9.3   Treatment

The preferred treatment is surgery. In addition, the primary focal point for the removal of difficult areas and multiple primary skin cancer may be low temperature or light therapy excitation.

13.4.9.4   Prognosis

The effect of skin cancer is generally better, especially basal cell carcinoma, with a 5-year survival rate of over 95% Squamous cell carcinoma. The annual survival rate is also above 90%. The prognosis of sweat adenocarcinoma is worse than that of the first two, and the 5-year survival rate is only about 50%. So skin cancer is treated follow up after treatment.

13.4.10　Fibrosarcoma

Fibrosarcoma is a malignant tumor of the oral and maxillofacial fibroblasts(fibroblasts).

13.4.10.1　Clinical manifestations

In young adults, the tumor is spherical or lobular, which occurs in the mouth, and grows rapidly. It is found in the teeth and the jaw bone. Occurred in the skin can be nodular. Late stage results in maxillofacial deformity and dysfunction. It can also be transferred to the lungs by circulation.

13.4.10.2　Diagnosis

The diagnosis is mainly based on biopsy.

13.4.10.3　Treatment

Surgical treatment is the main, should adopt partial radical excision. If there is lymph node metastasis, the cervical lymph node dissection should be performed. Chemical treatment was used before surgery. Such as cyclophosphamide 600 – 800 mg/m, normal saline 40 mL, intravenous injection, once a week.

13.4.10.4　Prognosis

The prognosis is usually worse than that of cancer.

13.4.11　Osteosarcoma

It is composed of neoplastic osteoblasts and osteoid tissues, and is a malignant tumor originating from osteoclast.

13.4.11.1　Clinical manifestations

Clinically, it is often occurs in adolescents, the mandible is more common than the maxillary bone, and has a history of injury. Early symptoms are intermittent in the affected part. Numbness and pain, which can then be turned into persistent severe pain with reflex pain. The tumor grows rapidly and destroys the alveolar process and jaw bone. The tooth is loose, shift, facial deformity, still can occurrence pathological fracture. The X–ray shows irregular damage, from the inside to outside. The extender is the osteolytic type; bone cortical destruction, replaced by hyperplasia of the bone, radiated by the solar radiation is osteogenic. It can also be seen in clinic. There is a mixture of the above two forms. In advanced patients, serum calcium and alkaline phosphatase can be increased, and the tumor is easily transferred to the lung along the blood circulation.

13.4.11.2　Diagnosis

In addition to the clinical manifestations, the primary diagnosis depends on the X–ray and CT, and finally the pathological examination can be determined.

13.4.11.3　Treatment

Comprehensive treatment based on surgery. Large radical resection is required, especially the concept of organ resection to avoid. Local recurrence due to the propagation of pipe or cavity.

13.4.11.4　Prognosis

According to the literature, the 5–year survival rate of osteosarcoma is 30% – 50%.

13.4.12　Malignant lymphoma

Malignant lymphoma is broadly subclassified as Hodgkins lymphoma and non–Hodgkins lymphoma.

Hodgkins lymphoma very rarely present with extronodal disease whereas non-hodgkins lymphoma may present with extranodal masses as their primary disease presentation. The incidence of the ratio of NHL to HL is about 5 : 1. Shanghai Jiao Tong University medical school affiliated to the ninth people's hospital oral disease department oral and maxillofacial of the 127 malignant lymphomas in the neck, NHL accounted for 86. 6% (110 cases) ,6. 5 times higher than that of HL.

13. 4. 12. 1　Clinical manifestations

It could occur at any age, especially in the middle age. It originated in the nodes of the lymph node and is the most common in the cervical lymph nodes. It originates from the outside of the lymph node, and can occur in the gums, palate, frequency, oropharynx, jawbone and so on. The internal type of the neck is early. The lymph nodes in the department, armpit, groin and so on are enlarged. The texture is firm and elastic, without tenderness, size, movement, and future. The phase is fused into a block, and the motion is lost. The clinical manifestations were diverse, including inflammation, necrosis and mass. In the late stage, it is universal, such as fever, big liver, big brand, body wasting, anemia.

13. 4. 12. 2　Diagnosis

In the case of malignant lymphoma, timely disease detection is very important. The intracellular cytology can be used for biopsy, and it can also be removed. A lymph node for disease detection; for the junction type, the clamp or excise biopsy can be considered. Immunohistochemical staining can be used to improve the diagnosis. Malignant lymphoma is systemic disease, except oral and maxillofacial, neck disease, should exclude mediastinal, chest, liver, spleen, hind.

In addition to conventional X-ray films, CT or MRI is a necessary means of examination.

13. 4. 12. 3　Treatment

Malignant lymphoma is sensitive to radiotherapy and chemotherapy, so it is a combination of radiotherapy or chemotherapy. It may also be considered for malignant lymphoma of oral and maxillofacial and maxillofacial and maxillofacial lymphoma after radiotherapy. Local radical resection was expanded, and chemotherapy was considered after surgery.

13. 4. 12. 1　Prognosis

The prognosis of HL in malignant lymphoma is better than that of NHL, but in general, the prognosis is not satisfactory.

He Xiaoyong

Chapter 14

Maxillofacial Nervous Disease

The trigeminal nerve and the facial nerve are the main cranial nerves which control oral and maxillofacial sensation and motor function. Trigeminal neuralgia is a syndrome of neuropathic pain characterized by severe paroxysmal lancinating pain in one or more distributions of the trigeminal nerve. Facial paralysis is a common problem that involves the paralysis of any structures innervated by the facial nerve. The most common of facial paralysis is Bell's palsy, however Frey's syndrome is rare. In this chapter you can learn about trigeminal neuralgia, Bell's palsy and Frey's syndrome. You can also learn about glossopharyngeal neuralgia which has paroxysmal pain in areas innervated by cranial nerves IX and X. The emphasis of the chapter should be handled for a qualified physician.

14.1 Trigeminal Neuralgia

14.1.1 Definition

Trigeminal neuralgia(TN) is a syndrome of neuropathic pain characterized by severe paroxysmal lancinating pain in one or more distributions of the trigeminal nerve. The trigeminal nerve is a paired cranial nerve that has three major branches: the ophthalmic nerve(V_1), the maxillary nerve(V_2), and the mandibular nerve(V_3). One, two, or all three branches of the nerve may be affected. TN most commonly involves the middle branch(the maxillary nerve or V_2) and lower branch(mandibular nerve or V_3) of the trigeminal nerve. TN is characterized by sudden severe and intense attacks of stabbing or electrical–shock–like pain that are typically brief, lasting for a few seconds up to several minutes. TN pain is mostly unilateral, involving the innervation area of the trigeminal nerve. Each pain attack may come on spontaneously or be triggered by certain stimuli, usually in the affected areas of the face. Common triggers may include simple touch, talking, eating, drinking, chewing, tooth brushing and hair combing. In contrast, pinching or pressing these trigger points will not usually cause TN pain.

14.1.2 Classification

TN is classified in three etiologic categories. Idiopathic TN occurs without apparent cause. Classical TN is caused by vascular compression of the trigeminal nerve root. Secondary TN is the consequence of a major neurologic disease, e. g. , a tumor of the cerebellopontine angle or multiple sclerosis.

14.1.3   Epidemiolgy

The prevalence of TN is rare and accounts for 100–200 per 100,000; the incidence is 5. 9/100,000 in women and 3. 4/100,000 in men. Despite its low incidence, TN is one of the more frequently seen neuralgias in the older adult population. The incidence increases gradually with age; most idiopathic cases begin after age 50, although onset may occur in the second and third decades or, rarely, in children.

14.1.4   Etiology

The pathogenesis of TN is uncertain. The disorder typically is idiopathic but may be due to a structural lesion. Several hypotheses have been stated, including traumatic compression of the trigeminal nerve by neoplastic(for example, cerebellopontine angle tumor) or vascular anomalies; infectious agents, including the human herpes simplex virus; and demyelinating conditions, such as multiple sclerosis. A popular explanation is that TN arises secondary to a vascular loop that cross–compresses the trigeminal nerve a few millimeters proximal to the pons. This vulnerable area, known as the nerve root entry zone, marks the transition from central to peripheral myelin. A substantial number of patients may have concomitant dental problems, such as microabscesses, which may exacerbate the symptoms of TN.

14.1.5   Pathophysiology

At the point just before it enters the brainstem, there is a short segment where nerve axons are still ensheathed in central myelin(produced by oligodendrocytes), but after a few millimeters, there is a transition to peripheral myelin(produced by Schwann cells). The region of this transition is called the Obersteiner–Redlich zone. It is thought that the area of the nerve containing the central form of myelin is especially susceptible to pathologic changes from vascular contact that result in demyelination and altered conduction. Pathologic studies from patients with TN have demonstrated severe damage to myelin as well as axon loss within the nerve adjacent to the site of compression. Radiographic and anatomic studies have demonstrated that vascular contact with the trigeminal nerve is common even in asymptomatic individuals but tends to be more severe and more proximal on the nerve ipsilateral to TN symptoms. Patients with TN are more likely to have contralateral arterial compression than asymptomatic people even though bilateral TN is distinctly rare. Symptomatic and asymptomatic arterial compression of the trigeminal nerve increases with age because of elongation of cisternal arteries, explaining why it is primarily a disease of older adults.

14.1.6   Clinical symptoms and signs

The typical pain that characterizes TN must meet the following criteria: unilateral affliction of the face limited to the distribution of one or more divisions of the trigeminal nerve; the pain is abrupt in onset and termination; high intensity of stabbing or burning character; evoked in trigger zones by trivial stimuli including washing, shaving and tooth brushing; pain–free intervals.

The pain of TN tends to occur in paroxysms and is maximal at or near onset. Facial muscle spasms can be seen with severe pain. This finding gave rise to the older term for this disorder, tic douloureux. The pain is often described as electric, shock–like, or stabbing. It usually lasts from one to several seconds, but it occur repetitively. A refractory period of several minutes during which a paroxysm can not be provoked is common. Some patients with longstanding TN may have continuous dull pain that is present between paroxysms of pain. Unlike some other facial pain syndromes, TN typically does not awaken patients at night.

TN is typically unilateral. Occasionally the pain is bilateral, though rarely on both sides simultaneously. The distribution of pain most often involves the V_2 and/or V_3 subdivisions of the trigeminal nerve. Autonomic symptoms, usually mild or moderate, can occur in association with attacks of TN in the V_1 trigeminal distribution, including lacrimation, conjunctival injection, and rhinorrhea.

Trigger zones in the distribution of the affected nerve may be present and are often located near the midline. Lightly touching these zones often triggers an attack, leading patients to protect these areas. Trigger zones can sometimes be demonstrated on physical examination. Other triggers of TN paroxysms include chewing, talking, brushing teeth, cold air, smiling, and/or grimacing.

Some patients have a history of "pretrigeminal neuralgia", a dull, continuous, aching pain in the jaw that evolves over time into TN. This brief, milder pain is sometimes suspected to have a dental origin, and unnecessary dental procedures have been performed in some cases. On the other hand, TN can be precipitated by dental procedures (e. g. , dental extraction), resulting in increased confusion about the precise etiology of this problem.

14.1.7　Diagnosis

The diagnosis of TN is based upon the characteristic clinical features described above, primarily paroxysms of pain in the distribution of the trigeminal nerve. Once the diagnosis of TN is suspected on clinical grounds, a search for secondary causes should be undertaken. For all patients with suspected TN or those with recurrent attacks of pain limited to one or more divisions of the trigeminal nerve and no obvious cause (e. g. , herpes zoster or trigeminal nerve trauma), the neuroimaging is recommended to help distinguish classical TN from secondary TN. Neuroimaging of the brain can be done with MRI or CT, though MRI with and without contrast is much preferred because its higher resolution enables imaging the trigeminal nerve and small adjacent lesions.

14.1.8　Differential diagnosis

The diagnosis of the disease remains a clinical diagnosis mostly dependent on a history of sudden shooting or stabbing pain, coming either as solitary sensations or paroxysms and separated by pain-free intervals. The huge list of differential diagnoses includes various dental diseases, temporomandibular joint disorders, paranasal sinus infections, ophthalmic pain syndromes, temporal arteritis, facial migraine, myofascial pain, idiopathic facial pain and psychological disorders. These disorders should all be excluded before defining TN as the responsible disease causing the pain syndrome.

Classical TN or secondary TN can sometimes be confused with dental causes of pain. Dental pain is usually continuous, intraoral pain that is dull or throbbing, whereas classic TN is typically intermittent pain and sharp. However, classic TN is often triggered by oral manipulations such as chewing and brushing the teeth, which can suggest a dental cause and lead patients to present for dental care prior to seeking a medical evaluation. Furthermore, some patients have a phase of "pretrigeminal neuralgia" characterized by atypical symptoms (e. g. , jaw or tooth pain) that might mimic dental pain.

14.1.9　Treatment

14.1.9.1　Medical treatment

Pharmacologic therapy is the initial treatment of most patients with classical TN. Surgery is reserved for patients who are refractory to medical therapy.

(1) Carbamazepine

Carbamazepine is a tricyclic imipramine first synthesized in 1961 and introduced for treatment of trigeminal neuralgia in 1962. Carbamazepine is the best studied treatment for classical TN and is established as effective. Side effects can be a problem but are generally manageable, particularly if low doses are prescribed initially with gradual titration. The usual starting dose of carbamazepine is 100–200 mg twice daily. The dose can be increased gradually in increments of 200 mg daily as tolerated until sufficient pain relief is attained. The typical total maintenance dose is 600–800 mg daily, given in two divided doses for tablets and extended release capsules, or four divided doses when for oral suspension. The maximum suggested total dose is 1,200 mg daily. Adverse effects of carbamazepine include drowsiness, dizziness, nausea, and vomiting; slow titration may minimize these effects. Carbamazepine–induced leukopenia is not uncommon, but it is usually benign; aplastic anemia is a rare side effect.

(2) Oxcarbazepine

Oxcarbazepine is a daughter drug of carbamazepine, but its pharmacokinetics are less complex. Oxcarbazepine can be started at a total dose of 600 mg daily, given in two divided doses. The dose can be increased as tolerated in 300 mg increments every third day to a total dose of 1,200–1,800 mg daily.

(3) Baclofen

The starting dose of baclofen is 15 mg daily given in three divided doses, with gradual titration to a maintenance dose of 50–60 mg/d. Sedation, dizziness, and dyspepsia can occur with treatment, and the drug should be discontinued slowly since seizures and hallucinations have been reported with upon withdrawal.

(4) Lamotrigine

In patients who are not taking other anticonvulsants, lamotrigine is typically started at 25 mg daily for the first 2 weeks, and then increased to 50 mg daily for 3 and 4 weeks. The dose is then titrated to effect, increasing by 50 mg daily every 2–3 weeks. The suggested total dose of 400 mg daily is given in two divided doses. For patients taking an anticonvulsant drug that induces hepatic enzymes(e. g. , carbamazepine, phenytoin, or primidone), the initial dose of lamotrigine is 50 mg once daily, titrating upward as needed to 100 mg once daily at week 3; 200 mg once daily at week 5; 300 mg once daily at week 6; and 400 mg once daily at week 7. For patients taking valproate, the initial dose of lamotrigine is 12. 5–25 mg every other day, with increases of 25 mg every two weeks as needed to a maximum of 400 mg per day.

14. 1. 9. 2　Surgical treatment

Patients with TN who are refractory to medical therapy are candidates for surgery. A variety of surgical methods have been employed to relieve the symptoms of TN. Although surgical therapy for TN is generally well – tolerated, a feared complication is painful posttraumatic trigeminal neuropathy (anesthesia dolorosa), a condition characterized by persistent, painful anesthesia or hypesthesia in the denervated region.

(1) Microvascular decompression

Microvascular decompression(MVD) is a major neurosurgical procedure that involves craniotomy and the removal or separation of various vascular structures, often an ectatic superior cerebellar artery, away from the trigeminal nerve. MVD is ideal for young healthy patients with TN. All patients should undergo MRI before MVD to verify that there is no intracranial mass lesion that may be responsible for the pain, such as a tumor, cyst, aneurysm, or arteriovenous malformation.

(2) Rhizotomy

Rhizotomy encompasses a number of percutaneous surgical techniques that are performed by passing a cannula through the foramen ovale, followed by lesioning of the trigeminal ganglion or root using one of several options: radiofrequency thermocoagulation rhizotomy, which creates a lesion by application of heat; mechanical balloon compression, which uses a Fogarty catheter to compress the gasserian ganglion; chemical(glycerol) rhizolysis, which involves the injection of 0.1 – 0.4 mL of glycerol into the trigeminal cistern.

(3) Radiosurgery

Gamma knife radiosurgery produces lesions with focused gamma radiation. The therapy is aimed at the proximal trigeminal root since targeting the gasserian ganglion produced poor results. The aiming of the beams is carried out with a stereotactic frame and MRI. The doses used are 70 – 90 grays (Gy). The beams cause axonal degeneration and necrosis. Pain relief with gamma knife surgery occurs after a lag time (of about 1 month).

(4) Peripheral neurectomy

Peripheral neurectomy can be performed on the branches of the trigeminal nerve, which are the supraorbital, infraorbital, alveolar, and lingual nerves. Neurectomy is accomplished by incision, alcohol injection, radiofrequency lesioning, or cryotherapy. Cryotherapy involves freezing of the nerve using special probes, in theory to selectively destroy the pain fibers.

14.1.10　Prognosis

The course of TN is variable. Episodes may last weeks or months, followed by pain-free intervals. Recurrence is common, and some patients have concomitant persistent background facial pain. Most often, the condition tends to wax and wane in severity and frequency of pain exacerbations. However, there are no pure natural history studies of TN, most likely because the severity of the pain leads to intervention.

14.2　Glossopharyngeal Neuralgia

14.2.1　Definition

Glossopharyngeal neuralgia(GN) is defined as paroxysmal pain in areas innervated by cranial nerves IX and X. GN is a rare condition in which there are repeated episodes of severe pain in the tongue, throat, ear, and tonsils. This can last from a few seconds to a few minutes. There are numerous analogies to TN, with which it occasionally coexists, although GN is much less common.

14.2.2　Epidemiology

GN, a rare disorder, usually begins after age 40 and occurs more often in men.

14.2.3　Etiology

Often, its cause is unknown. However, GN sometimes results from an abnormally positioned artery that compresses the glossopharyngeal nerve near where it exits the brain stem. Rarely, the cause is a tumor in the brain or neck.

14.2.4　Clinical symptoms and signs

GN is characterized by paroxysmal, severe, stabbing pain involving the ear, tonsillar fossa, base of the tongue, or beneath the angle of the jaw. Thus, the pain can occur in the distributions of the auricular and pharyngeal branches of the vagus nerve as well as of the glossopharyngeal nerve. Bilateral involvement has been reported in 12% of patients. Typical triggers include chewing, swallowing, coughing, speaking, yawning, certain tastes, or touching the neck or external auditory canal (rarely the pre-or postauricular areas). The pain typically radiates upward from the oropharynx toward the ear. The duration of the severe paroxysms is seconds to minutes, but there may also be a low grade, constant dull background pain. Several dozen attacks can occur per day, sometimes awakening the patient from sleep. Some episodes may also be associated with strenuous coughing and/or hoarseness.

Like trigeminal neuralgia, GN can occur in a pattern of episodes lasting weeks to months, alternating with longer periods of remission. Severe attacks have rarely been associated with bradycardia/asystole resulting in syncope, presumably because input from cranial nerve IX into the tractus solitarius has an effect upon the dorsal motor nucleus of the cranial nerve X.

14.2.5   Diagnosis

Diagnostic criteria for GN, according to the International Classification of Headache Disorders 3rd edition (ICHD-3), require all of the following: at least three attacks of unilateral pain; pain is located in the posterior part of the tongue, tonsillar fossa, pharynx, beneath the angle of the lower jaw and/or in the ear; pain has at least three of the following four characteristics (recurring in paroxysmal attacks lasting from a few seconds to two minutes; severe intensity; shooting, stabbing, or sharp in quality; precipitated by swallowing, coughing, talking, or yawning); no clinically evident neurological deficit; not better accounted for by another ICHD-3 diagnosis.

As with TN, there are idiopathic and secondary forms of GN. Secondary causes include demyelinating lesions, cerebellopontine angle tumor, peritonsillar abscess, carotid aneurysm, and Eagle syndrome (in which cranial nerve IX is compressed laterally against an ossified stylohyoid ligament). Vascular compression of cranial nerves IX and X can occur at the nerve root entry zone by the vertebral artery or posterior inferior cerebellar artery. The differential diagnosis of GN includes nervus intermedius neuralgia.

The evaluation of a patient suspected of suffering from GN includes a thorough history, especially inquiring about the presence of trigger factors and nocturnal awakening. A careful intraoral and neck examination (e. g. , done by a specialist in otorhinolaryngology) should be undertaken to help exclude local disease as a cause for the pain. MRI/MRA is indicated in virtually all patients to rule out a mass lesion or vascular pathology; plain skull films may reveal an ossified stylohyoid ligament (consistent with Eagle syndrome).

14.2.6   Treatment

Medical therapy of GN is essentially the same as for TN. In addition, application of local anesthetics to the oropharynx may prove both diagnostic and therapeutic. Surgical treatment is considered for patients who fail medical therapy. Possible procedures includ that it can section cranial nerve IX plus the upper three to four root lets of cranial nerve X at the jugular foramen intracranial, or drepress blood vessels. The latter is a relatively safe procedure with good short-term and long-term outcomes.

14.2.7   Prognosis

Some individuals recover from an initial attack and never have another. Others will experience clusters of attacks followed by periods of short or long remission. Individuals may lose weight if they fear that chewing, drinking, or eating will cause an attack.

14.3　Facial Paralysis

Facial paralysis is a common problem that involves the paralysis of any structures innervated by the facial nerve. The pathway of the facial nerve is long and relatively convoluted, and so there are a number of causes that may result in facial nerve paralysis. The most common is Bell's palsy, a disease of unknown cause that may only be diagnosed by exclusion.

14.3.1　Bell's palsy

14.3.1.1　Definition

Bell's palsy, described first by Charles Bell in the early 1800s, is defined as an acute peripheral facial palsy of unknown cause.

14.3.1.2　Epidemiology

The annual incidence rate is between 13 and 34 cases per 100,000 population. There is no race, geographic, or gender predilection, but the risk is three times greater during pregnancy, especially in the third trimester or in the first postpartum week.

14.3.1.3　Etiology

There is no known cause of Bell's palsy. It may be caused by a viral infection. Herpes simplex virus activation has become widely accepted as the likely cause of Bell's palsy in most cases. Herpes zoster is probably the second most common viral infection associated with facial palsy. Histopathology of the facial nerve in patients with Bell's palsy is consistent with an inflammatory and possibly infectious cause, and the appearance is similar to that found with herpes zoster infection, further supporting an infectious hypothesis. Specifically, the facial nerve has a thickened, edematous perineurium with a diffuse infiltrate of small, round, inflammatory cells between nerve bundles and around intraneural blood vessels. Myelin sheaths undergo degeneration. These changes are seen throughout the bony course of the facial nerve, although nerve damage is maximal in the labyrinthine part of the facial canal where edema causes compression. And the tenuous blood supply adds to the damage. Alternate postulated mechanisms of Bell's palsy include a genetic predisposition, diabetes, pregnancy and ischemia of the facial nerve.

14.3.1.4　Clinical symptoms and signs

Patients with Bell's palsy typically present with the sudden onset(usually over hours) of unilateral facial paralysis. Common findings include the eyebrow sagging, inability to close the eye, disappearance of the nasolabial fold, and drooping at the affected corner of the mouth, which is drawn to the unaffected side. Decreased tearing, hyperacusis, and/or loss of taste sensation on the anterior 2/3 of the tongue may help to site the lesion, but these findings are of little practical use other than as indicators of severity.

14.3.1.5　Diagnosis

The diagnosis of Bell's palsy is based upon the following criteria: ①There is a diffuse facial nerve involvement manifested by paralysis of the facial muscles, with or without loss of taste on the anterior 2/3 of the tongue, or altered secretion of the lacrimal and salivary glands. ②Onset is acute, over a day or two; the course is progressive, reaching maximal clinical weakness/paralysis within 3 weeks or less from the first day of visible weakness; and recovery or some degree of function is present within 6 months.

A thorough medical history and physical examination, including a neurological examination, are the first steps in making a diagnosis. Facial movement is assessed by observing the response to command for closing the eyes, elevating the brow, frowning, showing the teeth, puckering the lips, and tensing the soft tissues of the neck to observe for platysma activation. The evaluation also includes a general physical examination and neurologic examination. Particular attention is directed at the external ear to look for vesicles or scabbing (which indicates zoster), and for mass lesions within the parotid gland. Additional investigations may be pursued, including blood tests such as erythrocyte sedimentation rate for inflammation, and blood sugar levels for diabetes. If other specific causes, such as sarcoidosis or Lyme's disease are suspected, specific tests such as angiotensin converting enzyme levels, chest X-ray or Lyme's disease may be pursued. If there is a history of trauma, or a tumor is suspected, a CT scan may be used.

14.3.1.6 Differential diagnosis

Facial paralysis may be caused by a variety of disorders that can be confused with Bell's palsy, including herpes zoster infection, Guillain–Barré syndrome, otitis media, Lyme disease, HIV infection, and others discussed below. In addition, a "peripheral" pattern of facial weakness involving the forehead and all muscles of facial expression can be caused by a central lesion, such as a stroke, involving the ipsilateral facial nerve nucleus or facial nerve tract in the pons.

14.3.1.7 Treatment

The mainstay of pharmacologic therapy for Bell's palsy or facial nerve palsy of suspected viral etiology is early short–term oral glucocorticoid treatment. In severe acute cases, combining antiviral therapy with glucocorticoids may improve outcomes. Eye care is important for patients with incomplete eye closure.

(1) Glucocorticoid and antiviral therapy

Treatment should preferably begin within three days of symptom onset. The suggested regimen is prednisone(60–80 mg/day) for one week. The suspicion that Bell's palsy is caused by herpes simplex virus in most patients led to trials of antiviral therapy.

(2) Eye care

In severe cases of Bell's palsy, the cornea may be at risk because of poor eye lid closure and reduced tearing. Artificial tears are available without a prescription in liquid, gel, and ointment forms. Liquid or gel formulations of artificial tears should be applied every hour while the patient is awake, and ointment formulations, which contain mineral oil and white petrolatum, should be used at night.

(3) Physical therapy

Physical therapy encompasses a host of different interventions for Bell's palsy, including but not limited to exercises, mime therapy, massage, electrical stimulation, acupuncture, heat therapy, biofeedback, and combinations.

(4) Surgical decompression

The issue of surgical decompression of the facial nerve is mentioned only for discussion, as it is not a currently recommended treatment.

14.3.1.8 Prognosis

The prognosis of Bell's palsy is related to the severity of the lesion. A simple rule is that clinically incomplete lesions tend to recover.

14.3.2 Frey's syndrome

14.3.2.1 Definition

Frey's syndrome, also known as gustatory sweating syndrome, is a rare neurological disorder resulting from damage to or near the parotid glands responsible for making saliva, and from damage to the auriculo-temporal nerve often from surgery. The disorder was first reported in the medical literature by Baillarger in 1853. A neurologist from Poland, Dr. Lucja Frey, provided a detailed assessment of the disorder and coined the term "auriculotemporal syndrome" in 1923.

14.3.2.2 Epidemiology

The exact incidence of Frey syndrome is unknown. The disorder most often occurs as a complication of the surgical removal of a parotid gland (parotidectomy). The percentage of individuals who develop Frey's syndrome after a parotidectomy is controversial and reported estimates range from 30% to 50%. In follow-up examinations, approximately 15% of affected individuals rated their symptoms as severe. Frey syndrome affects males and females in equal numbers.

14.3.2.3 Etiology

Frey's syndrome often results as a side effect of surgeries of or near the parotid gland or due to injury to the auriculotemporal nerve, which passes through the parotid gland in the early part of its course. The Auriculotemporal branch of the Trigeminal nerve carries parasympathetic fibers to the sweat glands of the scalp and the parotid salivary gland. As a result of severance and inappropriate regeneration, the parasympathetic nerve fibers may switch course, resulting in "gustatory sweating" or sweating in the anticipation of eating, instead of the normal salivatory response. It is often seen with patients who have undergone endoscopic thoracic sympathectomy, a surgical procedure wherein part of the sympathetic trunk is cut or clamped to treat sweating of the hands or blushing. The subsequent regeneration or nerve sprouting leads to abnormal sweating and salivating. It can also include discharge from the nose when smelling certain food.

Rarely, Frey's syndrome can result from causes other than surgery, including accidental trauma, local infections, sympathetic dysfunction and pathologic lesions within the parotid gland. An example of such, rare trauma or localized infection, can be seen in situations where a hair follicle has become ingrown and is causing trauma or localized infection near or over one of the branches of the auriculotemporal nerve.

14.3.2.4 Clinical symptoms and signs

Symptoms and signs include erythema (redness/flushing) and sweating in the cutaneous distribution of the auriculotemporal nerve, usually in response to gustatory stimulation. There is sometimes pain in the same area, often of a burning nature. Between attacks of pain there is sometimes numbness or other altered sensations (anesthesia or paresthesia). This is sometimes termed "gustatory neuralgia".

14.3.2.5 Diagnosis

Diagnosis is made based on clinical signs and symptoms and a starch iodine test, called the Minor Iodine-Starch test. The affected area of the face is painted with iodine which is allowed to dry, then dry corn starch is applied to the face. The starch turns blue on exposure to iodine in the presence of sweat.

14.3.2.6 Treatment

Although Frey syndrome can be mild and well-tolerated, in some individuals, it can cause excessive discomfort. Treatment is symptomatic and directed toward relief of symptoms. Until recently, most treatment measures have generally been unsatisfactory. Treatment options include drug therapy or surgery.

Topical application of drugs that block certain activities of the nervous system (anticholinergics) or drugs that hinder sweating (antihidrotics) have been used. Surgical removal (excision) of the affected skin and the insertion (interposition) of new tissue to the affected area (muscle flaps) has been described, but are considered risky because of the presence of facial nerve fibers right below the skin after parotidectomy.

In the last decade botulinum A toxin has become established as a therapy for individuals with bothersome Frey syndrome. The therapy consists of local injections of botulinum A toxin in the affected skin. Initial results have demonstrated that this therapy results in the suppression of sweating and causes no significant side effects. Another advantage of botulinum A toxin is that it is minimally invasive compared to other therapies. As in other indications, the effect of botulinum toxin is not permanent, lasting on average 9–12 months.

Gao Zhen

Chapter 15

Dentition Defect and Edentulism

Dentition defect refers to the loss of partial teeth in the maxillary or mandibular dentition. Edentulism refers to the loss of all teeth in the maxillary or mandibular dentition or both the maxillary and mandibular dentitions, also known as edentulous jaws.

Dentition defect and edentulism are common diseases in humans, and the main causes are caries, periodontal diseases, trauma, tumors and congenital malformations, etc. Dentition defect and edentulism can cause dysfunctions in pronunciation, chewing and swallowing, which in turn can affect the temporomandibular joint, digestive system, and the overall health and mental health of the patient.

The restoration of dentition defect and edentulism refers to the use of artificial materials to make prostheses, which can be used to restore the parts of dentition defect and edentulism, and recover the normal morphological and physiological functions of the dentition. Prostheses are generally divided into fixed and removable prostheses.

15.1 Fixed Prosthesis

The fixed prosthesis refers to the treatment method of using fixed restoration for dental defects and dentition defect, also known as fixed denture. It is the preferred treatment for restoration of dental defects and edentulism.

15.1.1 Crown

The crown is a kind of prosthesis that covers the entire crown surface and is used to repair the shape, function and beauty of the missing tooth. It can also be used as a retainer for fixed dentures. It can be divided into full crow and partial crown.

15.1.1.1 Indications

It is used for diseased teeth of various types of dental defects, such as enamel hypoplasia, discolored teeth, dental fluorosis, cone-shaped teeth, etc., which can not be repaired by other methods; patients who need restorative treatment due to excessive dental defect caused by trauma or dental caries; adult's individual malposed tooth and torsion that cannot receive orthodontic treatment; asymptomatic teeth after root canal treatment; fixed bridge repair and retainers fixed with periodontal splints.

Contraindications: severe deep malocclusion or tight occlusion, can not prepare enough space; dental bodies are too small tooth to prepare enough resistance and retention forms; root tips of young permanent teeth root apex have not yet developed well, and the dental pulp cavity is large.

According to different materials, the full crown can be divided into metal full crowns made of metal, non-metal full crowns made of resin and porcelain, and mixed crowns made of metal and porcelain or metal and resin. The full crowns of different materials have their own advantages and disadvantages, and the quantity of tooth preparation is also slightly different.

15.1.1.2   Production methods and procedures

Design: the scheme design is the key to the success or failure of the treatment. The full crown needs to be designed according to the patient's tooth position, oral condition, size of abutment teeth, location, and patient's demands to ensure the beauty and function of the full crown.

Tooth preparation: tooth preparation refers to preparing the material required for the restoration design, and the gap necessary for occlusion and beauty. The anterior tooth full crown is taken as an example. The procedure is listed below: ① prepare the guide groove on the labial side, and prepare three deep positioning grooves parallel to the long axis of the tooth surface on the labial side and the cut end of the dental body. ② Prepare the incisal margin of the tooth, and the cutting amount is based on design requirements. ③ Prepare the labial surface and adjacent surface. ④ Prepare the lingual surface. ⑤ Trim the cervical margin; the cervical margin of lip and cheek is generally placed 0.5 mm below the gingival margin for aesthetic considerations, and the cervical margin of lingual side or adjacent surface is placed at the level of aligning to gingiva or 0.5 mm below the gingiva.

Prepare impressions and models: the accuracy of impression is very important. The procedure is listed below: ① gingival retraction, before and after dental preparation and model taking, the medicinal and/or mechanical methods are taken to expose the gingival sulcus by making gingival margin contracted; so as to make the preparation and impression of the dental neck more accurate and clear. ② Select a tray, the clinician can select based on the size of the dental arch of in the mouth of the patient. When there is no suitable tray, a special tray needs to be made. ③ Select the impression material. At present, clinically applied impression materials mainly include alginate and synthetic rubber. Alginate impression materials are simple to operate and low in cost, but their accuracy and stability are relatively poor. However, the synthetic rubber impression materials are complicated for making models, with long curing time and high cost, but they have good accuracy and stability. The full crown impression is best made of synthetic rubber impression materials. ④ Make a mold, first place the mixed impression material in a tray, apply or inject the impression material on the prepared tooth surface, and immediately place the tray on the dentition, and remove the tray until the impression material is cured and stabilized. Thus the dentition impression is obtained. ⑤ Perfuse the model, the model is perfused with cast with superhard gypsum, prepare a working model, for the preparation of prosthesis. The model should accurately reflect the fine structure of the anatomy of the oral cavity, with stable dimensions, clear models, and without surface defects(Figure 15-1).

Prepare a temporary crown: a temporary crown must be worn during the period after the tooth preparation and before wearing the prosthesis to prevent deformation of the abutment and protect the pulp vitality of the abutment.

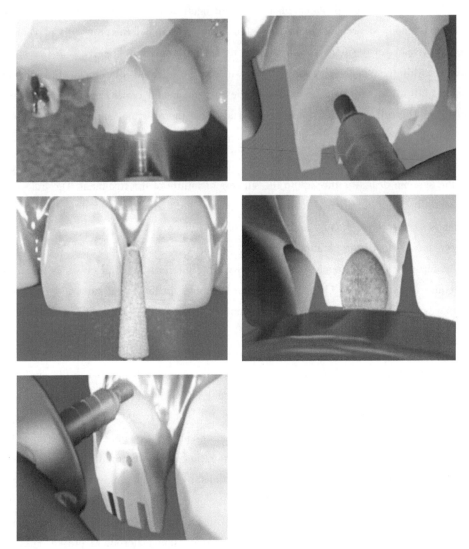

Figure 15-1 **Tooth preparation**

15.1.1.3 Production of the technician

The laboratory processing of the porcelain crowns is divided into two processes: inner crown casting and ceramic layer forming and sintering. Porcelain materials and equipments produced by different manufacturers vary from each other, and there are minor differences in specific operating procedures. Inner crown casting: first, the gypsum pattern is trimmed to make a detachable model, and then the wax molding of the porcelain inner crown is made on this model. Afterwards, the produced inner crown wax molding is cast using the casting process to obtain the inner crown casting parts. Finally, the casting parts are polished, trimmed, and sandblasted to complete the inner crown.

Ceramic layer forming and sintering: the porcelain powder is fused and sintered on the metal inner crown to form the desired crown shape. The order of sintering usually includes: sintering of opaque porcelain, sintering of dental neck porcelain, dental porcelain, sintering of cut-end porcelain and transparent porcelain, trimming and glazing, and other production steps of the laboratory.

15.1.1.4 Try-in and adhesion

When wearing the full crown, remove the temporary crown first, clean the adhesive on the surface of the teeth and in the gingival sulcus, wear the crown to adjust the suitability of the adjoining surface, inner crown and neck margin successively, then adjust the occlusal contact relationship, and try in the porcelain crown. After the satisfactory effect is achieved, then the grinded parts will be glazed and polished, the metal inner crown tissue surface will be sandblasted, and then cemented with suitable cement.

15.1.2　Fixed bridge

The fixed bridge refers to a common prosthesis that uses natural teeth on both side or one side of a missing tooth space as the abutment teeth on which a retainer is made, and the retainer is connected with the artificial tooth into a whole, and then fixes the denture on the abutment teeth.

15.1.2.1　The composition and function of the fixed bridge

Retainer: the retainer connects the abutment with the bridge, forming a functional whole with the fixed bridge and the abutment. The retainer can be a full crown, a partial crown, an inlay, etc.

Bridge: it is a part of the fixed bridge to restore the missing tooth shape and function, and artificial teeth.

Nestor: it is the connecting part between the pontic of fixed bridge and the retainer, and it can be a fixed connector and a movable connector.

15.1.2.2　Indications and contraindications of the fixed bridge

Indications: before the fixed bridge is restored, the patient's oral condition needs to be carefully examined and analyzed in combination with the patient's general condition and individual characteristics. Comprehensive consideration should be given to the following factors: ①number of missing teeth: suitable for the loss of a small number of teeth in the dental arch, or space missing of a few missing teeth, the number is usually 1–2 teeth. ②Missing tooth site: fixed bridge repair can be considered for any missing tooth site in the arch as long as it meets a small number of missing teeth or space missing of a few missing teeth, and the number and condition of abutments can meet the support and retention requirements. ③Abutment conditions: the height of the crown is appropriate, the morphology is normal, the roots are thick, the dental pulps have no lesions, there is enough periodontal potential, and the tooth alignment is basically normal. ④Occlusal relationship: the occlusion is basically normal and there is a proper occlusogingival height. ⑤The alveolar bone in the edentulous area is stable, and it is usually 3 months after tooth extraction.

Contraindication: ①for the young patient: the dental arch has not developed well, leading to the exposure of endodontium in preparation of abutment teeth. ②The number of missing teeth is high: no sufficient support could be provided from the abutment teeth. ③The endodontic or periodontal disease has not been treated. ④The patient with short gingival distance in edentulous area. ⑤The patient could not undergo the removal of dental tissues.

15.1.2.3　Classification of fixed bridge

(1)Classification by structure

1)Rigid fixed bridge: as the most common fixed bridge in clinical settings, there are retainers on both ends of bridge which may be connected via the connector. When the fixed bridge is placed and bonded in abutment tooth, the fixed bridge and the abutment tooth will create together a stationary unit which is stable and may withstand the higher occlusal force.

2)Semi-fixed bridge: this mode is used less clinically, there are retainers on both ends of bridge in which one end is connected via the rigid connector and another end via the origind connector.

3)Free-end fixed bridge: it is also called as cantilever fixed bridge in which only one end of bridge is provided with retainer and is connected via the rigid connector, as another end is the fully-free cantilever without the support supplied by the abutment tooth. The single-end fixed bridge is generally used in the scenario in which the abutment tooth is strong and the edentulous space is limited.

4) Compound fixed bridge: refers to the fixed bridge using the two or more designs from the three basic types above. It is used for the patient with more abutment teeth and edentulous spaces, as well as longer bridge span while the design depends on the truth in the mouth of patient (Figure 15-2).

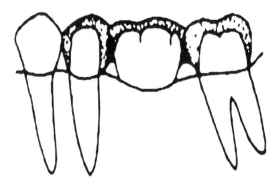

Figure 15-2　Rigid fixed bridge

(2) Classification by materials

1) Metal-ceramic fixed bridge: the retainer of metal-ceramic fixed bridge is made in the form of ceramic crown while its base crown is connected with the metal framework of bridge via the metal connector; the outer part of fixed bridge is covered such with ceramic materials that the whole fixed bridge shows not only the strength of metal materials, but also the esthetics of ceramics. This is an optimal restoring method currently and thus is used widely.

2) Metal-resin fixed bridge: the resin is used to wrap the metal retainer and bridge framework to restore the crown contour of bridge and retainer. With the ceramic materials used in clinical restoration settings, the use of metal-resin fixed bridge is decreased gradually.

3) All ceramic fixed bridge: the all ceramic fixed bridge is the non-metal restoration method, showing the good biosafety and aesthetical and lifelike color. The application of all ceramic fixed bridge is limited mainly by the strength of all ceramic materials. The all ceramic materials represented by zirconia are used in the repairing a variety of all ceramic fixed bridges.

4) Metal fixed bridge: it is commonly the cast metal fixed bridge with the characteristics such as less removed volume of tooth and high strength; however, it is used more for the restoration of posterior teeth due to its poor aesthetical performance.

(3) Classification by bridge design

1) Bridge-contacting fixed bridge: with the gingival surface of bridge contacting the mucosa of alveolar ridge, it is the most popular bridge design showing the aesthetical and comfort features.

2) Bridge-floating fixed bridge: with the gingival surface of bridge not contacting the mucosa of alveolar ridge while minimal 3 mm or more space between them is retained as a result, the design may facilitate the passing of food without the occurrence of retention, leading to the good self-cleaning effect. Thus it is also known as sanitary bridge.

(4) Other types of fixed bridge

1) Implant fixed bridge: the implant is used to support the fixed bridge in place of the abutment tooth.

2) Fixed-removable bridge: literally, it is the removal prosthesis, but its loading mode is similar to that of fixed bridge.

3) Bonding fixed bridge: a fixed bridge for which the major retention is provided by using the etching-

bonding technology to connect the abutment and prosthesis following that no or less abutment is removed.

15.1.2.5 Preparation method and procedure of fixed bridge

Take the ceramic fixed bridge for an example to describe the preparation method and procedure of fixed bridge in brief.

(1)Design of fixed bridge. The excellent design of fixed bridge may maximize restoring the function of missing tooth, protecting the abutment and oral hard and soft tissues, as well as maintaining the oral health in the long run.

1)Select the healthy tooth with the thick root, healthy periodontium and that may form the common path of insertion as the abutment to provide them with sufficient supportive and retentive force, so as to withstand the additional and keep it within the physiological limit over the long term.

2)Based on the factors such as the number and site of missing teeth and the condition of abutment, as well as the age, relationship and health of supportive tissues to comprehensively classify the restoration types, as the retainer should be provided with good retention form and resistance form.

3)The design of bridge should focus on the restoration of integrity for dental arch, meet the demand of oral function and comply with the requirement of oral healthcare.

4) The complicated design of fixed bridge + the analysis model that should be defined prior to treatment, as the analytical research should be carried out outside of mouth.

(2)Preparation of abutment. The tooth preparation should be conducted according to the design of fixed bridge. On the assumption that the health of pulp tissue should be ensured for the tooth, the common path of insertion among the individual abutments must be provided to make the sufficient room for the connector. The preparation volume of retainer should be removed based on the requirement of design as the morphology of gingival margin is required to be considered in such process. The preparation of fixed bridge shows the following features compared with the preparation of full crown.

1)Incisal edge and occlusal surface: for the adjacent tooth is missed regularly, the lack of reference in the preparation is resulted. We thus should emphasize the role of guide groove to control the appropriate preparation volume.

2)Axial surface: consider the common path of insertion in the preparation, and make the research model if necessary. Use the observer to analyze, design the inserting direction, determine the preparation volume and then carry out the clinical preparation.

3)Cervical margin: with the different axial directions of abutment, you may use the design of supragingival margin to be consistent with the requirement of common insertion.

(3)Impression taking and cast pouring, the fabrication of temporary prosthesis follows the procedure similar to that of ceramic full crown. Once the impression is taken, for the large number of teeth involved in the fabrication of fixed bridge, the wax or silicone rubber used for occlusion may be used in the abutment and edentulous area to record the occlusal relationship of patient, facilitating the technician to make correctly the prosthesis.

(4) The fabrication of ceramic fixed bridge by the technician comprises of two major steps including metal base casting and ceramic shaping following the same principle as the fabrication of metal ceramic full crown.

(5)Trial placement and bonding. The operation of trial placement and bonding of fixed bridge is similar to that of full crown, yet some special considerations should be emphasized here.

1)Direction of trial placement: for the large number of abutments on the fixed bridge, the insertion of fixed bridge is more difficult that of single crown. Therefore, you should examine the clinical model and carry out the simulative trial placement before the trial placement is performed inside the mouth of patient.

2) Tissue surface of bridge: the tissue surface of bridge may contact so modestly with the mucosa that there is no gap between them or any pressure on the gingival mucosa to prevent against the significant whitening appearance of gingival caused by pressure and ischemia.

3) Gingival papilla: the crown of abutment on fixed bridge is secured and connected with the bridge via the connector under which there is no gingival papilla, where the embrasure of tooth may be shallow somewhat to avoid the impaction of food.

4) Cleaning of adhesive: the saddle design is most commonly used for the bridge of fixed bridge clinically, causing the adhesive that is prone to remain under the tissue surface of bridge and difficult to be removed. So you should watch out to control the volume and denseness of adhesive during the bonding process. You may pre-place the floss prior to the bonding so as to help the removal of the excessive adhesive.

15.1.3 Inlay

The inlay as one of prostheses may be inserted into the dental tissues to restore the morphology and function of dental defect. As the special alteration of inlay, the inlay can not only be inserted in the dental tissue, but also overtop and cover the occlusal surface of teeth. The inlays may be grouped into single-surface inlay, double-surface inlay and multiple-surface inlay according to the different numbers of dental faces overlaid by such inlay. The inlays may be grouped into metal inlay, resin inlay and ceramic inlay according to the different materials used to make such inlay (Figure 15-3).

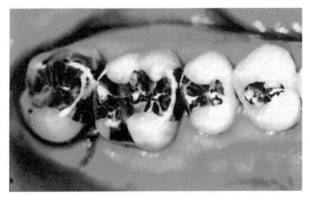

Figure 15-3 **Inlay**

15.1.3.1 Indication and contraindication of inlay

(1) Indication

The various dental defects have involved the dental cusp, incisal angle, marginal ridge and dental face, and can not be repaired with the filling materials; or the dental defects adjoin poorly and cause the severe impaction of food, that require to restore the contact point of approximal surface; it may be used for the tooth in which there is the defect but some larger healthy dental tissues remain yet, and may provide sufficient resistance for the inlay.

(2) Contraindication

Permanent teeth of teenager and deciduous teeth of child; the defect of dental face is small and superficial while the defect of anterior teeth does not affect the incisal angle; the dental defect is extensive with poor retention and resistance.

15. 1. 3. 2   Preparation method and procedure of inlay

(1) Design of inlay

Examine the dental defect, relation with adjacent teeth and opposing teeth, and occlusion of offending tooth; X-ray radiography may be given if necessary to assist the judgment and determine if the inlay option is needed for the restoration, as well as the selection of the contour and materials for the inlay.

(2) Preparation of inlay

The inlay made with the different materials presents the different requirements for the preparation of inlay when the dental preparation is ongoing for the inlay. The common method is to remove totally the infected and necrotic dental tissues to ensure the retention form and resistance form of inlay. If the metal inlay is used for the restoration, the outline form of inlay should be free of undercut with the slant showing at the margin of such outline to prevent against the fracture of tooth at the margin of outline, and to facilitate the control the position of boundary line between the tooth and inlay; furthermore, the resin and ceramic inlay demands to eliminate the infected and necrotic dental tissues while the preparation volume should reach a certain thickness(2-2.5 mm), the line angle should be more rounded and the margin of outline is not provided with slant.

(3) Impression making and taking, and model cast pouring

The oral impression is the female model of teeth and their adjacent oral tissues. The impression related to the oral tissues may be taken by means of impression materials(such as silicone rubber, alginate and agar) placed in the impression tray. Then pour the impression materials(plaster) in the impression to form the male model associated with the oral tissues, i. e. , model, so that the morphological information of oral tissues such as teeth may be replicated on the model. The technician makes the various prostheses on such model.

(4) Inlay made by technician

Most of prostheses including the inlay are completed in the dental laboratory. The technician will complete the fabrication of prosthesis on the plaster model based on the design of clinician. The different making methods may be utilized for the different designs of inlay.

(5) Trial placement and bonding

When the inlay is made, the clinician will try it in the mouth of patient. The process may be divided into two steps: placement and adjustment. The placement refers to the process in which the inlay is inserted to the designed position while the occlusal adjustment refers to adjust and change the inlay and adjacent teeth, as well as align the occlusal teeth until they coordinate with each other. If the patient is satisfied with such trial placement and shows no discomfort, the inlay will undergo the pre-adhesion processing and be bonded finally.

15. 1. 4   Veneer

The veneer is a prosthesis used mainly to cover the side of lip and cheek. When the retention of vital pulp with less or no removal of tooth is necessary, namely, the bonding technology is used to bond and cover the defect, coloration, discoloration and dental deformity of surface with the restorative materials to restore the normal morphology of tooth and improve the color of such surface. The major features of veneer include less removal volume of tooth and good esthetic outcome(Figure 15-4).

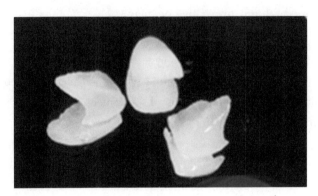

Figure 15-4   **Veneer**

15.1.4.1   Indication and contraindication

(1) Indication

The veneer is used mainly for the poor dental color and the less dental defect of anterior tooth and anterior molar. For example, tetracycline stained teeth with enamel dysplasia, dental fluorosis, distorted tooth, microdontia, cone-shaped tooth, large tooth clearance, proximal caries and incisal defect, are all the indications.

(2) Contraindication

Excessive defect volume of tooth, severe tooth displacement or minor prosthesis clearance for which the veneer can not provide the excellent restoration. ① Severe displacement or translocation of maxillary teeth. ② Mandibular teeth with severe deep overbite occlusion. ③ Severe wear of mandibular labial surface showing no gap between them. ④ Patient with moderate to severe sleep bruxism. ⑤ Excessive defect of tooth and high thickness of prosthesis. ⑥ The bonding effectiveness may be affected by the enamel dysplasia or defect.

15.1.4.2   Classification of veneer

(1) Classification by making method

① Direct-restorative veneer: use the light curing composite resin for bonding, shaping, curing and polishing in the mouth to complete the restoration treatment. ② Indirect-restorative veneer: use mainly the ceramic materials or rigid composite resin to make the veneer on the model, and then carry out the trial placement, bonding and restoration in the mouth. The indirect restoration is not limited by the chair-side operation duration and thus it may implement the thorough trimming, adjustment and polishing, leading to the restoration outcome superior to the direct restoration.

(2) Classification by fabricating materials

① Ceramic veneer: veneer made of the ceramic materials. Based on the type of ceramics, it can be made with casting, slip-casting or CADCAM method. ② Resin veneer: veneer made of resin materials. It may be the light-cured resin veneer formed directly in the mouth or the rigid resin veneer made on the model, and used mostly for the finished resin veneer in the temporary restoration. ③ Ceramic veneer: veneer made by means of ceramic method which is used seldom currently.

15.1.4.3   Making method and procedure of veneer

Take the direct resin veneer restoration and ceramic veneer restoration for an example.

(1) Direct resin veneer restoration

1) Design of veneer: design the veneer restoration plan based on the condition of offending tooth and

the requirement of patient, determine beforehand the preparation volume of tooth, adhesive and bonding method, as well as resin restoration method and so on, and make a preliminary estimate for the effect of restoration; then carry out the veneer restoration.

2) Dental preparation: clean the dental surface and remove a certain volume of enamel surface based on the degree of dental defect or pigmentation, and then the rebasing processing may be conducted as appropriate for the exposed dentine region.

3) Surface processing: the acid etching of bonding surface should be performed for the tooth under the wet insulation condition. There is difference in the acid etching methods according to the etchant.

4) Veneer molding: apply the adhesive at first, then cover the composite resin; for the better esthetic outcome, we should select different type and color of resin to simulate the color of real tooth, such as opaque resin, dentine resin, enamel resin, transparent resin and so on; and shape and polish the prosthesis finally. If necessary, we may coat a layer of polish at last to mimic the color of normal enamel.

(2) Restoration of ceramic veneer

1) Design of veneer: although the ceramic veneer can not be used to complete the treatment at a time, the ceramic veneer is provided with the better mechanical strength and esthetic outcome, and such effect may be persistent and stable. The ceramic veneer should be besigned according to the condition of offending tooth and the requirement of patient as well, select the ceramic materials and determine the preparation volume of tooth. For the fabrication of veneer is completed in the dental laboratory, it is important to select the color of veneer. For the tooth with discoloration, the colorimetric method is used regularly and thus the selection may be done with reference to the normal adjacent tooth or opposing teeth; for the discolored tooth, if only the individual tooth changes the color, the masking should be carried out for the abutment; if most of the teeth change the color, you should consider comprehensively the multiple factors such as tooth staining level, dentition harmony, patient's age and skin color.

2) Preparation of tooth: the preparation of veneered tooth contains in general four parts: labial surface, contiguous zone, cervical margin and incisal margin. The preparation should be conducted orderly according to the requirement of design. It's better that the preparation of labial surface never proceeds beyond the enamel layer; on the one hand, this facilitates the decrease of symptoms such as secondary caries and tooth hypersensitivity, on the other hand, it may lead to the better bonding effect. In general, the contiguous zone stops slightly ahead of adjacent surface of tooth to maintain the adjacent relation of natural tooth; however, the veneer is required to restore the adjacent relationship for the offending tooth with severe discoloration, proximal caries/defect or diastema. The cervical margin is placed usually at the position aligning with gingival margin or slightly above the gingival margin, and may be positioned below the gingival margin for the tooth with the severe discoloration; the preparation of incisal margin should be prepared as window preparation, feathered incisal edge or overlapped incisal edge based on the design.

3) Impression taking and model cast pouring: for the ceramic veneer is more precise prosthesis, the gingival retraction may be performed prior to take the impression, and it's better to take the impression using the individual tray and silicone rubber impression materials.

4) Fabrication by technician: based on the type of ceramics, the ceramic veneer can be made with casting, slip-casting or CAD-CAM method and so on. After the ceramic veneer is made, its tissue surface should be acid etched with hydrofluoric acid to facilitate the bonding.

5) Trial placement and bonding: the ideal veneer should be successful in a trial placement without further adjustment; the offending tooth must be treated for the adhesion at first in the bonding, and then use the adhesive resin cement for the bonding operation.

15.1.5 Implant denture

The implant denture may be implanted in the jaw in place of the implant with natural root to get the prosthesis similar to that fixed and supported by the tooth. Its structure may be divided into three parts: implant, implant abutment and implant superstructure. The implant, implant abutment and implant superstructure may play together the role of retention, support, occlusal force conduction and may restore the chewing function. The indication of implant denture: willingness of patient. If the patients may be followed up on schedule, showing the body in good condition, no severe lesion in the caries soft and hard tissues of missing tooth, no bad occlusal habit, and normal bone quantity and quality in the edentulous area or that such insufficient bone quantity may be addressed via the surgical intervention, these patients could undergo the restoration with implant denture. The implant denture provides the solution essentially for the retention that may be considered for the anodontia on the free end or the complete anodontia for which the traditional denture is used. It may restore preferably the chewing, aesthetical and phonatory function, and save effectively the natural tooth. The restoration with implant denture is a method that best fits the physiological principles when it is used in the scenario following the tooth is missed(Figure 15-5).

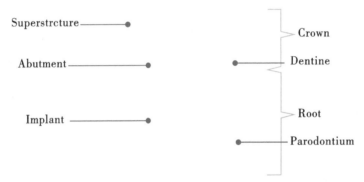

Figure 15-5   Implant and natural teeth

15.2 Removable Prosthesis

15.2.1 Removable partial denture

The removable partial denture(RPD) is the most common restoration method for the dentition defect. When it uses the mucosa and bone tissues covered by natural tooth and denture base as the support, and is retained by the retainer and base of denture, it may restore the morphology and function of missing tooth with the artificial tooth, and restore the morphology of alveolar ridge and soft tissues with the materials of denture base. The patients may remove and wear on their own such prosthesis(Figure 15-6).

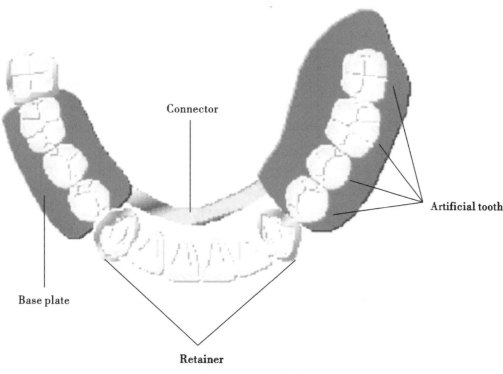

Figure 15-6   **RPD**

15.2.1.1   Indication and contraindication of removable partial denture

(1)Indication

1)Number of missing teeth:from one missed to one remained in a single jaw.

2)Site of missing tooth:any region,especially the missing occurs on the free end.

3)Requirement of abutment:absorption of alveolar bone $\leqslant$ length of root 1/2 mobility $\leqslant$ II, without low clinical crown and low convexity of axial surface.

4)Range of restoration:the missing tooth caused by the various reasons such as caries,periodontal disease and trauma,or accompanied with the defect of alveolar bone,jawbone and soft tissues.

5)Transitional restoration for the unhealed wound by tooth extraction.

6)Restore the vertical distance of lower 1/3 of face.

7)Individual intolerable of the dental removal by fixing the denture or the young permanent teeth unsuitable of the fixation and restoration.

8)Removable splitting fixation for loosen tooth.

9)Special occupation requirement,such as double dentition and chinrest of typecast actor.

(2)Contraindication

1)Tooth that requires no restoration,such as wisdom tooth and small edentulous space.

2)Mental disorder or disability.

3)Diseases of oral mucosa that is not cured for a long time.

4)Foreign body sensation to the denture that can not be overcome or causes the allergic reaction.

15.2.1.2   Components and their roles of removable partial denture

The removable partial denture consists of five components including artificial tooth,base,rest,retainer and connector.

(1)The artificial tooth is used to take the place of missing tooth aiming at restoration of the functions such as chewing and phonation, as well as the prevention against the extension of remaining tooth, the tilting and displacement, as well as the disorder of relations, so as to maintain the vertical distance of jaws and the function of original facial features.

(2) The base plate is the component used to cover the mucosa and integrate the individual parts of denture, which may play a role in conducting and dispersing the occlusal force, restoring the appearance of soft and hard tissues of defect and enhancing the functions of denture retention and stability. They may be classified as plastic base, metal base and plastic–metal base on the basis of the materials used for the fabrication

(3) The occlusal rest which is placed on the natural tooth may pass the occlusal force in the vertical direction, prevent against the dislocation of denture in gingival direction and act as the supportive part, which is generally located at mesial–distal margin of abutment.

(4) The retainer is the device that may be used to fix the removable partial denture on the dental arch. The clasp retainer is the most common retainer among them. The clasp consists of occlusal rest, clasp arm, clasp body and minor connector. The clasp arm may be divided into two parts; the flexible tip of clasp arm which is located in undercut area will bring about the retention; the rigid starting part of clasp arm plays a role of stability and support in the undercut area. The clasp body, the rigid part which is used to connect the clasp arm, rest and minor connector, plays a role of stability and support in the undercut area. The minor connector, as the part which is the clasp embedded in base plate or connected with major connector, plays a role of stability and support in the undercut area.

(5) The connector (nestor) is the component used to integrate the individual parts of denture, which may play a role in conducting and dispersing the occlusal force, facilitating the protection of abutment, health of soft and hard tissues and increase of denture strength(Figure 15-7).

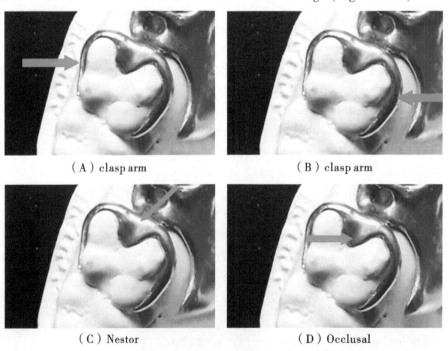

(A) clasp arm   (B) clasp arm

(C) Nestor   (D) Occlusal

Figure 15-7   **The components of clasp**

A: The flexible clasp arm located in undercut area brings about the retention; B: The rigid clasp arm
plays a role of stability and support; C: The nestor is used to integrate the individual parts of denture;
D: The occlusal rest passes the occlusal force and prevent against the dislocation of denture.

15.2.1.3   Design of removable partial denture

(1)The Kennedy classification is the most common method for classification of dentition defect

Class 1: both ends of dental arch miss while the distal end is the free end without the presence of natural tooth.

Class 2: the unilateral posterior tooth of dental arch misses while the distal end is the free end without the presence of natural tooth.

Class 3: the unilateral posterior tooth of dental arch misses while the natural tooth is seen in mesial-distal defect.

Class 4: the anterior teeth miss consecutively and run across the midline while the natural tooth is seen in the defect.

There are subclasses in Class 1,2 and 3 of Kennedy classification, and no subclass in Class 4. In the subclass, there are additional defects other than the major defect, while the number of former defects is represented as subclasses.

(2)Design of removable partial denture

To restore the appearance and function of missing tooth and the surrounding soft & hard tissues, the reasonable denture design is crucial.

1)Basic requirement of removable partial denture: with the capacity to protect the health of soft & hard tissues in the mouth; with good retention, support and stability; may restore the function, comply with the esthetic requirement; sturdy and durable, and is convenient in removal and wear.

2)Retention of denture: the retention force refers to the force which may prevent against the denture off in the direction opposing to the path of insertion. The retention force contains mainly the friction force, adsorption force, atmospheric pressure and gravity as the friction force is the major part among them. The retention force of retainer may be adjusted appropriately to make the denture in consistent with the physiological requirement and functional demands, and avoid the higher or lower retention force.

3)Stability of denture: the good stability may facilitate the application of retention and chewing function of denture. The main factor which may influence the stability of denture is rotational instability of which the major clinical signs mainly include tilting, swinging, rotation and sinking. The main solution is that you should make sure the complaint and associated medical history of patient, and administrate the required clinical examinations and the preparation prior to restoration, before try to restore the dentition defect using the pivot point removal method and counterbalance method.

15.2.1.4   Making and initial wear of denture

(1)Making of Denture

1)Preparation of tooth: use the appropriate bur to prepare the guide-plane, rest recess, gap-clasp groove and so on, and to adjust the occlusion.

2)Impression and model making and taking: select the suitable stock impression tray or make the individual tray to take the impression if necessary. The commonly used impression materials.

The alginate and silicone rubber impression materials, the latter is ideal but its cost is higher. To establish the proper maxillo-mandibular relationship, it is necessary to record the maxillomandibular relation.

3)Design and preparation of model: draw the surveying line on the model of working region and record the position of clasp arm tip. Draw the edge line of rest, connector, proximal plate and base and the soft and hard tissues which require the buffering, and then fill the undercut and close the margin and the padding in saddle area.

4)Making of technician: the commonly used casting rest materials include high fusing chrome cobalt alloy, pure titanium and titanium alloy, etc.

(2)The initial wear of dentures

Check and remove the excessive small tubercles on the tissue surface of denture prior to the placement. Following the placement, check if the base is coupled closely with the soft tissues, the clasp arm, rest and abutment is tightly sealed, the depth that the tip of clasp arm enters the undercut, extension range of base and if the appearance of artificial teeth is suitable, etc. The grinding, modification and adjustment, as well as the necessary oral education may be carried out in the light of the circumstances.

15.2.2　Complete denture

The complete denture is made for the patient with edentulism. The complete denture consists of denture base and artificial teeth, which may adsorb to alveolar bones of upper and lower jaws to restore the facial morphology and function of patient by means of the intention caused by the adsorption force and atmospheric pressure from the tight seal and margin closing between base and mucosa. The traditional complete denture is the mucosa support type while the complete overdenture or implant complete denture may be the mixing support type or even the tooth – support denture. This section introduces mainly the traditional complete denture

15.2.2.1　Change of tissues following the edentulism

After the edentulism, alveolar process will be absorbed gradually to form the alveolar ridge. The alveolar ridge in the upper jaw is absorbed upwards and inwards as the more bone plate internally to the lateral plate will be absorbed, causing the contour of upper jaw reduces gradually; the alveolar ridge in the lower jaw is absorbed inferoanterior and outwards, causing the low dental arch increases gradually. For the lack of support of soft and hard tissues, the lip and cheek will become depress inwards, leading to poor fullness of upper lip, increase of facial wrinkles, deepening of nasolabial fold, sinking of angulus oris and shortening of lower 1/3 distance of face, so that the facial features show the significant aging sign. The alveolar ridge will be absorbed rapidly 3 months following the missing of teeth, and the absorption rate decreases significantly after approx. 6 months. The absorption rate becomes more stable 2 years following the tooth extraction, i. e. ,0. 5 mm/year. Therefore, the restoration with complete denture should be performed as soon as possible, generally 3 – 6 months after the teeth of patient with edentulism are extracted.

15.2.2.2　Retention and stability of complete denture

The retention of complete denture refers to the ability that the denture withstands the vertical dislodgment from the oral position. The denture may dislodge easily when the patient opens his/her mouth if the retention of complete denture is poor. The complete denture may adsorb to the upper and lower jaw due to the physical effect by adsorption force, surface tension and atmospheric pressure. The factors such as patient's oral anatomic form, quality and quantity of saliva, area of denture base and extension of margin may be associated with the retention of denture(Figure 15–8).

The stability of complete denture refers to the resistance level and rotational power of denture, so as to prevent the denture against the lateral and anterior – posterior dislodgement. When the complete denture functions the chewing, talking or the like, even there is good retention of denture, if the position of denture or artificial tooth and the contour of polished surface can not coordinate with the muscular function of lip, cheek and tongue, the denture will be exposed to the horizontal or lateral force, causing the displacement or tilting, damage of margin sealing, so that the denture will dislodge and generate the traumatic force against the alveolar ridge. Therefore, you should notice the tooth – arrangement, occlusal relationship and contour of polished surface.

The good retention and stability is the basis for the success of complete denture.

15.2.2.3   Complete denture fabrication

Recording jaws relation and preparing impression are two critical steps to complete denture success.

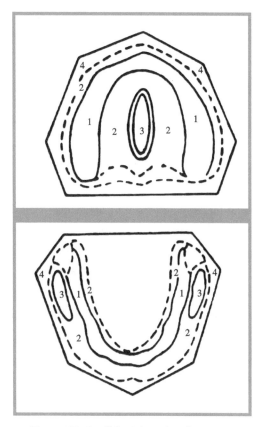

Figure 15-8   **Edentulous jaw fowrareas**

1. Primary stress-bearing area; 2. Secondary stress-bearing
area; 3. Periphery border seal area; 4. Relief area.

Impression preparation is the first step of full dental prosthesis. Edentulous jaw has a series of significant anatomical landmarks. Maxilla includes labial and buccal frenum, incisive papilla, maxillary tuberosity, palatine rugae, foveola, pterygomaxillary notch and vibrating line; underjaw includes frenum linguae, buccal flange area, distobuccal angles area, lingual flange area and retromolar pad. Standard impression precisely reflects anatomic form which including these critical landmarks and the activity of physiological function of surrounding tissue which including breadth and height of migration groove and the motion trail of labial, buccal and lingual muscles. Complete denture model is the male die of edentulous jaw which formed by perfusion model material in edentulous jaw impression. It should fully reflect the fine lines of tissue surface of edentulous jaw. And there should be repair trace of muscle function manifested on the edge of the impression.

According to the relation between the organizational structure of edentulous jaw and the complete denture, edentulous jaw can be divided into four areas: primary stress-bearing area, secondary stress-bearing area, periphery border seal area and relief area. The model can not show the thickness or elasticity of the mucosa as it's made of die stone, so do an intraoral checking to make sure the condition of the four areas and record it on the model. And then make a plan and do relevant process which includes the following: ①marking baseplate edge line; ②processing postdam area; ③filling undercut.

Recording maxillomandibular relation is the record of maxillomandibular position relation between the suitable height of lower 1/3 part of patient's face determined and recorded by bite plate and the condyle on both sides at the physiological position of temporomandibular joint concave, which transferred on articulator by plaster model. Recording maxillomandibular relation includes vertical relation record and horizontal relation record. Vertical distance determination method includes freeway space measuring, facial observing and articulating, etc. ; horizontal jaw position determination method includes Gothic arch measuring and direct occluding, etc.

Complete denture is an occlusal reconstruction for edentulous patients. After maxillomandibular relation recording is done, it must be fixed to articulator. And the articulator should be the one that imitates patient's mandibular movement the most for further tooth arrangement. The common articulators for complete denture are plainline articulator, average articulator and half–adaptable articulator. The plainline articulator can only achieve centric occlusion; average articulator can conduct moderate sideway and protrusive movement of the mandible; half–adaptable articulator can establish more accurate and personalized sideway and protrusive movement of the mandible as well as centric occlusion. Artificial teeth arrangement is a crucial part of complete denture functional restoration and cosmetology. As for complete denture making, the basic goal of teeth arrangement is to meet the requirement of masticating and articulating functions while aesthetics, function and tissue health protection are all considered. When edentulism happens, the space that dentition originally takes up forms into a potential space which in the neutral area of internal and external force of lip muscle, buccinator and lingualis. If the artificial teeth are placed in neutral area, it can still take the basically balanced force while buccinator exerting it inwardly and lingual muscle exerting it outwardly; and this is good for the retention of complete denture. Therefore, complete denture should be arranged in neutral area. Anterior teeth requires the dental arch degree being consistent with bite block size; shallow covering, shallow covered occlusion; keeping lip fullness; showing patient's personality. Posterior teeth requires the central fossa or apex linguae of maxillary posterior teeth and the frequency point or central fossa of mandibular posterior teeth to be arranged on respective alveolar ridge crest: upper and lower artificial posterior teeth should be arranged on alveolar ridge, and the ligature of lower alveolar ridge crest. Balanced occlusion is the main difference between the occlusal form of complete denture and natural dentition. It means that relevant upper and lower teeth are able to touch during noncentral occlusion movement such as protrusive and sideway movements(Figure 15–9).

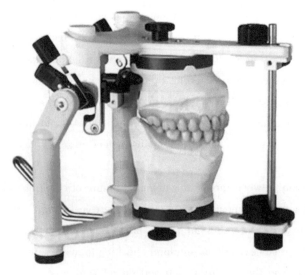

Figure 15–9　**Articulator**

15.2.2.4 Initial wear of complete denture

Before patients wearing the denture, clinicians should check the tissue surface, polished surface and occlusal surface of the denture carefully and then proceed to intraoral checking of the denture. The checking usually has three steps: maxillary denture checking, mandibular denture checking, occlusal checking. Checking contents mainly include denture stability, extension range of baseplate, stress condition of stress−bearing area, occlusal balance condition, etc. Appropriate adjustment of complete denture can then be done according to the actual situation. After properly wearing the complete denture, clinicians should help patients so that they can adjust to it and denture can begin to function. When initially wearing complete denture, patients should be guided as per following aspects: application method of new denture, time of rechecking, protection method of the denture, future maintenance of the denture, etc.

15.2.2.5 Rechecking and maintenance

Usually rechecking should be arranged after 1 week of wearing the complete denture and every detail of the rechecking should be proceeded carefully. Possible problems that might be encountered during rechecking can be divided into the following aspects: appearance, function, comfort, voice and mentality, etc. Problems during rechecking should be solved individually. As for complete denture maintenance, the first step is educating and supervising patients about oral hygiene, and checking oral cavity and mastication organ; meanwhile assessing the impact caused by continuous alveolar ridge absorption during denture wearing; adjusting occlusion and handling tissue surface of the denture to ensure its stability. Necessary methods of cleaning and preserving the denture should be taught to patients.

15.2.3 Overdenture

Overdenture is a removable partial denture or a complete denture whose baseplate covering natural teeth, treated tooth root or the implant while gaining support from them. The covered natural teeth or tooth root is called overdenture abutment. It can reduce alveolar ridge absorption, retain parodontium proprioceptor, and fortify denture support, retention and stabilization. Overdenture abutment can be divided into three categories according to different production time: immediate overdenture, transitional overdenture, definitive overdenture which also called as remote overdenture.

15.2.3.1 Advantage and disadvantage of overdenture

(1) Advantage of overdenture

①The existence of overdenture abutment, to a great extent, reduces alveolar ridge absorption and fortifies denture support, retention and stabilization. ②Because the retention of tooth root retains parodontium proprioceptor and reactively adjusts occlusal force, overdenture can prevent or delay alveolar bone absorption. ③Overdenture changes crown−to−root ratio by crown removal and this decreases force generation and is helpful to periodontal tissue health. ④Overdenture abutment without the far−end can effectively decrease denture sinking. ⑤Keeping the tooth or tooth root which need to be extracted during traditional denture repair alleviates the pain of tooth extraction from the patients, decreases the baseplate area of the denture, and enhances the comfort degree of the denture. ⑥Denture is easy to repair and adjust. After the extraction of overdenture abutment, just padding the tooth extraction area and it can be modified into traditional denture.

(2) Disadvantage of overdenture

①Overdenture abutment can cause dental caries or gingivitis easily. ②Upheaval and undercut are often seen at labial and buccal side of the retained tooth and it sometimes affects esthetics. ③Long treatment session, difficult fabrication, high treatment price.

15.2.3.2　Indications and contraindications of overdenture

(1) Indications of overdenture

①For patients who have congenital mouth defect/deform or malocclusion, it is not suitable for using surgical operation or orthodontic treatment. ②Most of dental crown is missing, wearing or too short, who is not suitable for doing conventional fixed denture restoration. ③Teeth with periodontal disease and partial alveolar resorption but it still can support. ④For free-end edentulous patients, whose paired jaw teeth are natural teeth, try best to keep the remaining root and crown as overdenture. ⑤Because patients have some systemic diseases, they are not suitable for teeth removal. ⑥Overdenture can be used as gap retainers and transitional restoration for adult and adolescent patients.

(2) Contraindication of overdenture

①Tooth, dental pulp, tooth with unhealed periodontal disease. ②Patients who can not maintain oral hygiene. ③Repair contraindication of dentition defect or deficiency.

15.2.3.3　Overdenture abutment

(1) Abutment choosing

1) Abutment quantity: preserve ideally 2 – 4 mono-maxillary abutments. If there's only 1 abutment left, best endeavors should be used to preserve it.

2) Abutment position: ideally there should be abutment at both front and back of dental arch and it should be at the area with maximum occlusal force and be helpful to the health of soft and hard tissues of the baseplate.

3) Endodontics condition of abutment: if there is no inflammation in periapical periodontal, the overdenture abutment should receive complete endodontic therapy.

4) The condition of abutment periodontium condition: the loose level of abutment is no less than degree I. The gum of abutment is normal and there is no inflammation. There is no periodontal pocket or alveolar bone resorption.

(2) The preparation and treatment of overdenture abutment.

1) Preparation for surgical surgery: extract teeth that can not be remained and the remaining teeth that are not ideal. Cut hyperplastic soft tissue that affects dental prosthesis. Trim the bone that is obviously sticking out, which may affect the placement of the denture.

2) The treatment of disease of tooth, dental pulp and periapical tissue: do root canal therapy to most of the abutments. Keep alive pulp for minority of long crown abutment.

(3) Periodontal treatment: do thorough periodontal treatment for overdenture abutments. Improve periodontal status of abutments. It is good for the tolerance for artificial tooth.

15.2.3.4　Adhesion

Adhesion of overdenture abutment is usually made by two parts: negative adhesion and positive adhesion. One part combined with abutment and the other part combined with the removable part of the denture so denture can be provided with good retention, stability and esthetics.

(1) The category of adhesion

1) According to the relationship between prosthesis and retention post: it can be classified as rigid attachment, non-rigid attachment and resilient attachment.

2) According to the position and structure of adhesion: above root attachment, in root attachment, bar clip attachment, magnetic retainer.

(2)The advantage of magnetic attachment

1)Strengthen retention of denture.

2)Denture is stable and has high mastication efficiency.

3)Denture can move horizontally to decrease sideway force generation.

4)Esthetic and comfortable, no sensation of foreign body.

15.2.3.5   The making of overdenture abutment

The manufacturing process includes make treatment plan of overdenture abutment. Prepare overdenture abutment and make the top part. Take impression and perfusion model. Record jaw relationship and transfer it to frame. Design dental base plate, arrange the teeth, try-in, finish making denture. Place the attachment.

15.2.3.6   The maintenance of overdenture

(1)Strengthen awareness of oral health. Change your diet.

(2)The cleaning of abutment tooth.

(3)The maintenance of overdenture: use toothbrush to do mechanical cleaning, assisted by denture detergent.

(4)Check overdenture regularly.

15.2.4   Immediate denture

Immediate denture: your dentist makes a model of your teeth by taking impressions before removal of your teeth. It is fabricated for placement immediately following the removal of natural teeth. Immediate denture includes removable partial denture, complete dentures and overdenture. Among them, partial denture is commonly used in clinical use. It is one type of temporal removable partial denture.

Temporary restoration: it offers esthetics and improves the chewing function while you wait for your final restoration to be made and placed. Features: you only wear it for a short term. The cost of repair material is low. The production procedure is simple. Manufacture periodicity is short. It is also easy to adjust.

15.2.4.1   The aims of making temporal removable partial denture

(1)Offer aesthetics. Usually the wound will heal well 3 months after the removal of your teeth. The alveolar ridge absorption tends to be stable. At this point, you can have dentist to do formal restoration. When having missing anterior teeth, especially for those who have missing anterior teeth, the lip-cheek soft tissues lose their supporting surface so they sink in, which has a huge impact on aesthetics. Before formal restoration, wearing removable partial denture can offer aesthetics.

(2)Keep gaps. The gap caused by extraction of teeth-maintain it well throughout the healing process of soft tissues. For adult patients, keeping teeth gap can effectively prevent adjacent teeth drifting and elongation of antagonistic tooth before the formal restoration treatment. For adolescent patients, they should keep the gap until adjacent teeth are mature and when it can work as abutment for fixed restoration or it is good time to do implant restoration.

(3)Occlusal reconstruction. For patients whose vertical distance is too short, which causes that there is no space for dental prosthesis or even temporomandibular joint disorders because of severe natural teeth wear, also for patients who have too many missing teeth or whose stomatognathic system disorders, they all need to reconstruct occlusal. As occlusal reconstruction is complicated to operate, cost is expensive, plus it is difficult to predict the how it will react to the change of occlusal reconstruction, it is better to do temporary removable denture to do restoration, so it is convenient to change the design according to patients' condition.

(4) Adjusting butment and residual ridge before distal-extension prosthesis restoration or using temporary removable denture can adjust alveolar crest where is missing teeth, which can make it strengthen function exercise, providing stronger support for formal restoration. It can make butment become relatively stable through wearing temporary removable denture.

(5) Adjust patients' psychology. Provisional restoration both provides patients with chances to get adapted and also heightens their confidence for treatment after they see prosthetic effect, so they will actively cooperate with treatment.

15.2.4.2　The category of temporary removable partial denture

According to production structure, it can be divided into simple and complicated temporary removable denture.

(1) Simple temporary removable partial denture is usually used in the case that anterior teeth would be removed. Do immediate restoration due to need of aesthetics. The production method is as follows.

1) Make a by taking an impression of your upper and lower jaws. Design a simple clasp or use base plate to do retention according to the need of retention.

2) Cut and scrape the teeth that will be removed to 2 mm below gum. Please be cautious not to damage adjacent teeth.

3) They production way of professional operation is the same as normal removable partial denture.

4) Wear the disinfected provisional restoration 12 hours after removal of teeth. The tissue surface of base plate should not compress wound. For the first 24 hours, it is better not to get rid of it.

5) This type of restoration usually lasts for 3 months or so. If it needs last longer, the tissue surface of prosthesis needs to rebased.

(2) Complicated temporary removable partial denture is mainly used in complicated case of stomatognathic system related disease, especially in case of occlusal reconstruction. The production method is as follows.

1) Do primary diagnosis by asking past medical history and doing all kinds of inspection. Take impression to make models when needed and determine the restoration design.

2) For patients who have posterior free-end edentulism or whose occlusion needs to lift up, do wax base or wax rim.

3) After baking wax rim soft, ask patients to do centricocclusion to certain vertical distance. For patients whose natural teeth are severely wearing, but they don't have temporomandibular joint disorder, they only need manufactured dental restoration-lift up by 2 mm for occlusion. For patients who have temporomandibular joint disorder, lift up by 4 mm for occlusion. Do continuous adjustment to proper level during rechecking.

4) As normal put articulator, carve the form of tooth arrangement and occlusal pad with wax. Have a good contact relationship with occlusion. Then box it, fill compound, boil box, open box and polish it.

5) When initial wearing prosthesis, dental base and occlusal pad should be compatible with the soft and hard tissues in oral cavity. Also adjust occlusion to make natural teeth and artificial tooth have uniform contact.

6) To do recheck regularly. Adjust to proper occlusal position and vertical dimension. Then consider doing formal restoration.

He Liming, Liu Bin

Chapter 16

Malocclusion

Malocclusion is commonly known as irregular dentition, which can cause the disorder of oral function and facial beauty. Orthodontics is a branch of dentistry concerned with the supervision, guidance and correction of the growing and mature dentofacial structures, including those conditions that require movement of teeth or correction of malrelationships and malformations of related structures. Orthodontic treatment focuses on adjustment of relationships between and among teeth and facial bones by the application of forces and/or the stimulation and redirection of the functional forces within the craniofacial complex. Major responsibilities of orthodontics practice include the diagnosis, prevention and treatment of all forms of malocclusion of the teeth and associated alterations in their surrounding structures; the design, application, and control of functional and corrective appliances; and the guidance of the dentition and its supporting structures to attain and maintain optimum relations in physiologic and esthetic harmony among facial and cranial structures.

16.1 The Etiology of Malocclusion

It is difficult to know the precise cause of most malocclusions, but we do know in general what the possibilities are, and these must be considered before treatment is conducted. Malocclusion can occur as a result of genetically determined factors, which are inherited, or environmental factors, or more commonly a combination of both. Inherited conditions include congenitally missing teeth, malformed and supernumerary teeth. abnormal formations of the jaws and face, such as a cleft lip and palate. Environmental factors include bad oral habits(such as digital sucking and tongue thrusting), premature loss of teeth as a result of either trauma or caries, and some medical conditions(such as enlarged tonsils and adenoids that lead to mouth breathing). This section concludes these factors with a perspective that the interaction between hereditary and environmental has great influences on the development of the major types of malocclusion.

16.1.1 Hereditary influences

16.1.1.1 Race evolution

Although malocclusion now occurs in a majority of the population, this does not mean it is normal. Skeletal remains indicate that the present prevalence is several times greater than it was only a few hundred years ago. Crowding and malalignment of teeth were unusual until relatively recently. The fossil record documents evolutionary trends over many thousands of years that affect the present dentition, including a decrease in the number of the teeth, and a decrease in the size of the jaws.

Compared with primitive peoples, modem human beings have quite underdeveloped jaws. It is easy to find that the progressive reduction in jaw size, if not well matched to a decrease in tooth size and number, could lead to crowding and malalignment. It is easier to see why dental crowding should have increased quite recently, but this seems to have paralleled the transition from primitive agricultural to modern urbanized societies. Because of escalating conditions of modern life, the worsening malocclusions perhaps result partly from less use of the masticatory apparatus with softer and more delicate diet. Under primitive conditions, of course, excellent function of the jaws and teeth was important for surviving and reproducing.

In fact, both dental caries and periodontal disease are rare on the primitive diet and appear rapidly when the diet changes, it is complicated to determine whether changes in jaw function have increased the prevalence of malocclusion. The resulting dental pathology can make it difficult to establish what the occlusion might have been in the absence of early loss of teeth, gingivitis and periodontal breakdown. The increase in malocclusion in modern times certainly parallels the development of modem civilization, but a reduction in jaw size related to disuse atrophy is hard to document.

16.1.1.2 Generic influences

A strong influence of inheritance on facial features is obvious at a glance. It is easy to recognize familial features in the tilt of the nose, the shape of the jaw, and the look of the smile. It is apparent that certain types of malocclusion run in families. Dentists see repeated instances of similar malocclusions in parents and their offspring(Figure 16-1). The pertinent question for the etiologic process of malocclusion is not whether there are inherited influences on the jaws and teeth, because apparently there are, but whether malocclusion is often caused by inherited characteristics.

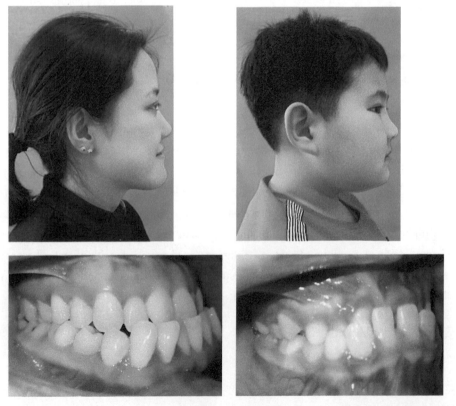

Figure 16-1 The mother and her son showing a strong inheritance of prognathic mandible and teeth

Evidence for the role of inherited factors in the etiology of malocclusion has come from studies of families and twins. Malocclusion could be produced by inherited characteristics in two major ways. The first would be an inherited disproportion between the size of the teeth and the size of the jaws, which would produce crowding or spacing. The second would be an inherited disproportion between size or shape of the upper and lower jaws, which would cause improper occlusal relationships. The more independently these characteristics are determined, the more likely that disproportions could be inherited. However, more direct testimony is provided in studies of twins and triplets, which indicate that skeletal pattern and tooth size and number are largely genetically determined.

16.1.2   Environmental Influences

Environmental Influences include systemic disorders and localized disturbances.

16.1.2.1   Systemic disorders

Systemic disorders are in the fetal period, because the mother, fetus or both at the same time be affected and lead to malocclusion, and because some systemic diseases caused by cranial and maxillofacial dysplasia after birth. During the embryo period, maternal malnutrition, exposure to radiation, and early pregnancy, such as rubella and syphilis, can result in fetal maxillofacial deformity. When the baby is born, from birth to stop development, vitamin D deficiency caused by rickets can lead to abnormal bone development, showing upper dental arch stenosis, high arch of the palate, anterior teeth crowding, protrusion, openbite, etc.

16.1.2.2   Localized disturbances

Localized disturbances refer to the abnormal growth of the teeth during the growth and development of children.

(1) Supernumerary teeth

This type resembles a tooth and occurs at the end of a tooth series, for example an additional lateral incisor, second premolar. Supernumerary teeth can occur within the arch, but when they develop between the central incisors they are often described as a mesiodens.

(2) Conical teeth

The conical supernumerary most often occurs between the upper central incisors. It is said to be more commonly associated with displacement of the adjacent teeth, which can also cause failure of eruption or have no effect at all.

(3) Impacted first permanent molars

Impaction of a first permanent molar tooth against the second deciduous molar occurs in approximately 2% – 6% of children and is indicative of crowding. It most commonly occurs in the upper arch. Spontaneous disimpaction may occur, but this is rare after 8 years of age. In more severe cases the impaction can be kept under observation although extraction of the deciduous tooth may be indicated if it becomes abscessed or the permanent tooth becomes carious and restoration precluded by poor access. The resultant space loss can be dealt with in the permanent dentition.

(4) Congenitally missing teeth

Congenital absence of teeth results from disturbances during the initial stages of formation of a tooth—initiation and proliferation. Anodontia, the total absence of teeth, is the extreme form. Anodontia and oligodontia are rare to be seen, but hypodontia is relatively common. As a general rule, if only one or a few teeth are missing, the absent tooth will be the most distal tooth of any given type. If a molar tooth is congenitally missing, it is almost always the third molar. If an incisor is missing, it is nearly always the lateral. If a premolar is missing, it almost always is the second rather than the first. Rarely is a canine the only missing tooth.

(5) Retained deciduous teeth

A difference of more than 6 months between the shedding of contralateral teeth should be regarded with suspicion, provided that the permanent successor is present, retained primary teeth should be extracted, particularly if they are causing deflection of the permanent tooth.

16.1.3　Oral bad habits

The effect of a habit will depend upon the frequency and intensity of indulgence.

16.1.3.1　Sucking habit

Although almost all normal children engage in non–nutritive sucking, prolonged sucking habits can lead to malocclusion. As a general rule, sucking habits during the primary dentition years have little effect. If these habits persist beyond the time that the permanent teeth begin to erupt, however, malocclusion characterized by flared and spaced maxillary incisors, lingually positioned lower incisors, anterior openbite and a narrow upper arch is the likely result(Figure 16–2). The characteristic malocclusion associated with sucking arises from a combination of direct pressure on the teeth and an alteration in the pattern of resting cheek and lip pressures.

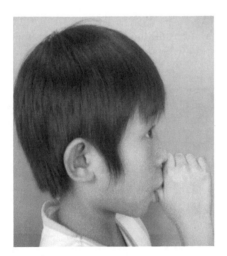
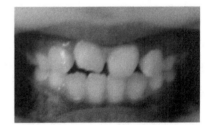

Figure 16–2　**Sucking habit**

The effects of sucking habit will be superimposed upon the child's existing skeletal pattern and incisor relationship, and thus can lead to an increased overjet in a child with a Class Ⅰ or Class Ⅲ Skeletal pattern can worsen a pre–existing Class Ⅱ malocclusion. The effects may be asymmetric if a single finger sucked.

16.1.3.2　Tongue thrusting

Much attention has been paid at various times to the tongue and tongue habits as possible etiologic factors in malocclusion. The tongue thrust swallowing is defined as placement of the tongue tip forward between the incisors during swallowing.

Swallowing is not a learned behavior but is integrated and controlled physiologically at subconscious levels. So the pattern of swallow, it can not be considered a habit in the usual sense. It is true, however, that individuals with an anterior openbite malocclusion place the tongue between the anterior teeth when they swallow while those who have a normal incisor relationship usually do not, and it is tempting to blame the openbite or crossbite on this pattern of tongue activity(Figure 16–3).

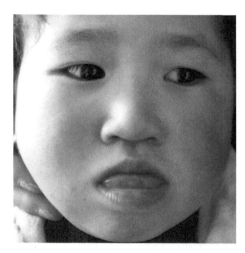
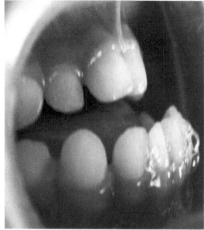

Figure 16-3   **Tongue thrusting**

Nowadays, orthodontists tend to believe that tongue thrust swallowing is normally seen in two kinds of patients. One is younger children with reasonably normal occlusion with normal displaced incisors. in whom this activity represents only a transitional stage during normal physiologic maturation. The other is individuals of any age with displaced incisors. In whom tongue thrust swallowing is an adaptation to the space between the teeth. The presence of overjet and anterior openbite conditions a child or adult thrust swallowing therefore should be considered the result of displaced incisors, not the cause. It follows, of course that correcting the tooth position should cause a change in swallow pattern, and this usually happens. It is neither necessary nor desirable to try to teach the patient to swallow differently before beginning orthodontic treatment.

16.1.3.3   Respiratory pattern

Respiratory needs are the primary determinant of the posture of the jaws and tongue. Therefore, it seems entirely reasonable that an altered respiratory pattern, such as breathing through the mouth rather than the nose, could change the posture of the head, jaw, and tongue. In order to breathe through the mouth, it is necessary to lower the mandible and tongue, and extend the head if these postural changes were maintained, face height would increase, and posterior teeth would super-erupt; unless there was unusual vertical growth of the ramus, the mandible would rotate down and back, opening the bite anteriorly and increasing overjet; and increased pressure from the stretched cheeks might cause a narrower maxillary dental arch.

In addition, the occlusion habit, sleep habit and so on can lead to obstructing normal facial growth and development.

16.2   The Harmfulness of Malocclusion

15.2.1   Affecting the development of the maxillofacial region and the teeth

In the process of growth and development of children, malocclusion will seriously affect the normal development of the soft and hard tissue of the maxillofacial and mandibular region. Anterior teeth crossbite, for example, the teeth, because of the dental arch is located in the dental arch on the front, limit the growth of the maxillary anterior forward, causing shortages of maxillary development and excessive mandibular forward growth, eventually forming concave maxillary and mandible deformity, crescent shaped face. Unilateral reverse bite can lead to lateral deviation of the lower jaw, which can lead to condyle dysplasia, resulting in facial asymmetry.

16.2.2　Affecting oral health

Malocclusion due to dislocation, torsion, elongation of the teeth or inadequate of place, can cause abnormal teeth contact zones, which is easy to cause plaque accumulation, food embedded plug, and not easy to self-cleaning. It is prone to tooth decay and gingivitis. There are also some severely misaligned teeth that stimulate the mucosa and the tongue to cause ulcers. In addition, some malocclusion, such as the anterior protrusion of the jaw and the opening of the lip, significantly increased the incidence of tooth trauma.

16.2.3　Affecting the oral function

16.2.3.1　Affect chewing function

Anterior teeth openbite or posterior teeth crossbite due to the upper and lower teeth can't normal to splint, function cusps can not fully play a role, not cut properly, biting and chewing food and makes the masticatory efficiency lower. Oral cavity is an important part of digestive system, and the decrease of chewing efficiency can cause gastrointestinal diseases such as dyspepsia(Figure 16-4).

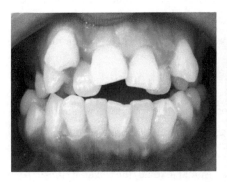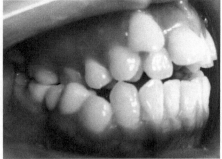

Figure 16-4　Anterior teeth openbite, Posterior teeth crossbite

16.2.3.2　Affect swallowing function

Most malocclusion of the swallowing function can result in abnormal position of the tongue, and the movement of swallowing is accomplished by the perfect coordination of the tongue, teeth and muscles of the oral cavity. When a patient with malformed teeth is engaged in swallowing exercise, the swallowing activity can not be completed well due to the abnormal position of the tongue and teeth.

16.2.3.3　Affect pronunciation function

It also requires perfect coordination of the various parts of the mouth. Some malformations such as anterior teeth openbite and mandibular protrusion can affect normal pronunciation.

16.2.3.4　Affect breathing function

The deformity of the lower jaw that affects the respiratory function can affect the normal breathing movement. Malocclusion can affect temporomandibular joint movement too.

16.2.4　Affecting the appearance

The eyes are the window of the soul, the nose is the backbone of the face, and the mouth occupies the majority of the 1/3 of the surface, which plays a crucial role in the appearance. The malocclusion can greatly affect the appearance of a person, and can be seen the mandibular protrusion, the opening of the lips, and the deformity of the beak.

16.2.5　Affecting mental health

No matter what kind of malformation, it can cause psychological and mental stress and even trauma to children and adults, which can have a great impact on patients. Especially in adolescent patients with severe or wrong tooth deformity, with their own appearance not confident even timid, creates a huge psychological burden and inferiority complex, most introverted, caused great impact on the physical and mental health of teenager growth.

16.3　The Diagnosis of Malocclusion

15.3.1　Classifications

The categorization of a malocclusion by its significant features is helpful for describing and documenting a patient's occlusion. In addition, classifications and indices could be used to record the prevalence of a malocclusion within a population and also aid in the assessment of need, difficulty, and success of orthodontic treatment.

Malocclusion can be recorded qualitatively and quantitatively. However, various indices and classifications were introduced and then devised, all of them have their limitations, and these should be borne in mind when they are applied.

Angle's and Mao's classification are two important classifications of malocclusion. The Angle's classification was proposed by E. H Angle in 1889. The Mao's classification was proposed by Chinese orthodontist Mao Xie-jun in 1959. These two classifications have their own advantages and disadvantages respectively. In this section, we will only introduce the Angle's classification.

Angle's classification was based upon the premise that the first permanent molars erupted into a constant position within the facial skeleton, which could be used to assess the anteroposterior relationship of the arches. In addition to the fact that Angle's classification was based upon an incorrect assumption, the problems experienced in categorizing cases with forward drift or loss of the first permanent molars have resulted in this particular approach being substituted by other classifications. However, Angle's classification is still used to describe molar relationship, and the terms used to describe incisor relationship have been adapted into incisor classification.

Class I or neutrocclusion: the mesiobuccal cusp of the upper first molar occludes with the mesiobuccal groove of the lower first molar in practice, discrepancies of up to half a cusp width either way are also included in this category(Figure 16-5).

Class II or distocclusion: the mesiobuccal cusp of the lower first molar occludes distal to the Class I position. This is also known as a postnormal relationship. Two subtypes of Class II malocclusion exist. Both have Class II molar relationship, but the difference lies in the position of the upper incisors.

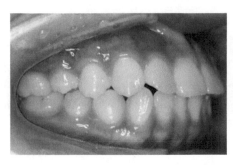
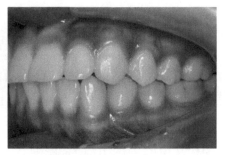

Figure 16-5　Angle's class Ⅰ malocclusion

Class Ⅱ division 1：the upper incisors are labially tilted，creating significant overjet（Figure 16-6）.

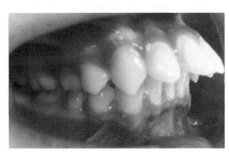
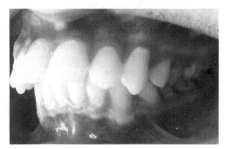

Figure 16-6　Angle's class Ⅱ division 1 malocclusion

Class Ⅱ division 2：the upper incisors are lingually inclined，the first incisors overjet is within normal limits（Figure 16-7）.

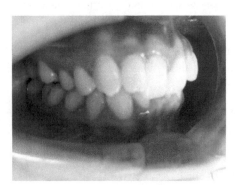
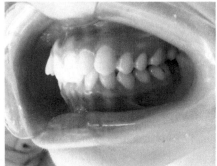

Figure 16-7　Angle's class Ⅱ division 2 malocclusion

Class Ⅲ or mesiocclusion：the mesiobuccal cusp of the lower first molar occludes mesial to the Class Ⅰ position. This is also known as a prenormal relationship（Figure 16-8）.

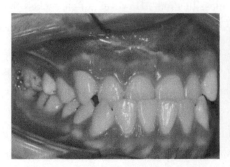
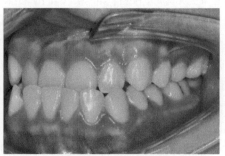

Figure 16-8　Angle's class Ⅲ malocclusion

Normal occlusion and Class Ⅰ malocclusion share the same molar relationship but differ in the arrangement of the teeth relative to the line of occlusion. The line of occlusion may or may not be correct in Class Ⅱ and Class Ⅲ.

16.3.2　Diagnostic methods

16.3.2.1　General examination

General examination is the basis for the implementation of diagnostic procedures. First, the basic information of the patient is collected: name, gender, date of birth, occupation, address and telephone number.

(1) Chief complaint

The main purpose and requirement of the patient. If the problem is not clear, it is likely to cause a medical dispute after treatment.

(2) Systemic history

Whether or not children have epilepsy, rheumatism, diabetes, hemophilia, rickets and endocrine system diseases. What's the situation now?

(3) Oral history

The parents dental health is a good indicator of the patient's susceptibility to periodontal disease or caries. Another important question to ask whether the patient has atraumatic injury to the teeth. Orthodontic treatment can exacerbate periapical symptoms that are already present because of trauma. Usually tooth movement is blamed if problems arise.

(4) Congenital factors and genetic history

Inquiring about material health and drug use during pregnancy and childbirth, and whether there are innate factors or not. There is no similar malformation in the parents of three generations of immediate family members, so as to determine whether there are genetic factors.

(5) Psychology

Many facial deformities have psychological barriers, deformity itself the function of the damage caused by far less psychological damage, the deformation of different age and different nature, different psychological characteristics of the patients. The orthodontist should have the psychological knowledge and keen observation ability, and be good at detecting the inner activities of the patient's words and deeds, so as to take different counter measures. The patient's psychological adaptability and cooperation are important for the success of orthodontic treatment.

16.3.2.2　Clinical examination

(1) Soft tissue examination

First of all, it is necessary to check the shape of the frenum and the position of the accessory. If the upper lip frenum is tight, the attachment is between the maxillary central incisor, so when the upper lip is attached, the maxillary incisor is white. This can be diagnosed as the interdental space is caused by the upper lip frenum with a large or low attachment.

Gingivitis is a common disease of orthodontic children. Long-term antiepileptic drugs such as phenytoin sodium can cause gingival hyperplasia or fibroid change, requiring surgical excision to do orthodontic treatment. Adult cases must be treated before orthodontic treatment.

The change of tongue position and movement is usually related to the lingual frenum. The relationship between the size of the tongue and the size of the mouth can be roughly estimated by analyzing the cephalometric measurement.

Palatal pharynx has cleft palate, pharyngitis, tonsillitis, adenoid hyperplasia and mucosal disease or not.

(2) Dentition and dental arch examination

In general, the tooth begins to sprout after the crown is formed. When the root of the tooth is more than 1/2, the crown of the tooth is worn through the alveolar ridge. When the root canal is basically formed and the apical hole is not completely closed, the tooth can sprout to the occlusal surface. The girl's tooth developed earlier than the boys, and the lower jaw developed earlier than the upper jaw. The timing of tooth development is related to heredity.

The order in which permanent dentition is normal: the maxillary is generally 6,1,2,4,5,3,7 or 6, 1,2,4,3,5,7. The mandibular is usually 6,1,2,3,4,5,7 or 6,1,2,4,3,5,7. The maxillary second premolar and the cuspid teeth are often present in the same time. Abnormal order of teeth often results in malocclusion.

When examining the number of teeth, it is important not only to understand the teeth that have been erupted, but also to the teeth that are developing or developing in the jawbone. It is generally necessary to take a panoramic film, especially to pay attention to the congenital absence of the teeth. In addition, multiple teeth should also be noticed.

The shape of the dental arch is based on the position of the cutting edge of the maxillary incisor to the distant transposition. The arch can be divided into a circumference, an ellipse and a pointed circle. Most people are elliptic. The variation of dental arch shape is large, and the adaptability is small. It should be paid attention to maintaining the shape of the dental arch in the treatment, otherwise the treatment will fail.

Dental arch symmetry includes to dental arch width of left and right sides of the symmetry, the center line of the dental arch teeth with osseous midline are consistent, and dental arch left and right sides of the corresponding teeth nearly far in symmetrical positioning.

(3) Occlusion examination

Overjet: the upper and lower anterior teeth cutting edge are more than 3 mm in sagittal direction, which is called deep overjet. Deep overjet divided into three degrees. I degree deep overjet: covered 3-5 mm; II degree deep overjet: covered for 5-8 mm; III degree deep overjet: covered over 8 mm.

Reverse overjet: the lower anterior teeth are located on the labial surface of the upper anterior teeth and often present in a severe mandible protrusion.

Overbite: the upper anterior teeth cutting edge cover more than 1/3 of the anterior lower teeth cutting edge in the vertical direction. Deep overbite divided into three degrees. I degree deep overbite: the anterior crown covers more than 1/3 of the anterior crown and less than 1/2; II degree deep overjet: the anterior crown covers more than 1/2 of the anterior crown and less than 2/3; III degree deep overjet: the anterior crown covers more than 2/3 of the anterior crown.

Openbite: there was no covering between the upper and lower anterior teeth, and there is space in the vertical direction.

(4) Facial examination

Positive view: check whether the facial proportion is coordinated, whether the facial development is symmetrical, facial type and other facial deformities, the closure degree and lip shape of the lips, tooth exposure of the gums, etc.

Profile view: check the profile convexity, depth and angle of the lower jaw, the degree of the chin, the shape of the lips, the depth of the inferior sulcus, the extension of the lower jaw and the degree of retraction.

16.3.2.3　Model analysis

The analysis of tooth size and arch length is usually performed on the dental cast, which is one of the patients' special examination items—dental cast analysis. Dental cast analysis can give orthodontist more detailed understanding of the number, size, shape, width and symmetry of the patient's teeth to make up for the lack of information obtained from clinical examination. Dental cast analysis can be carried out directly on the model, or it can be digitized and measured on a computer. Laser—scanned dental cast could convert to the STL files which can be read by most 3D software. Tooth size, arch length, space analysis, overjet, overbite, and the Bolton ratio can be obtained with digital models.

(1) Space analysis

Space available: the first step of space analysis is calculation of space available which is accomplished by measuring arch perimeter from the mesial of one first molar to the other (Figure 16-9).

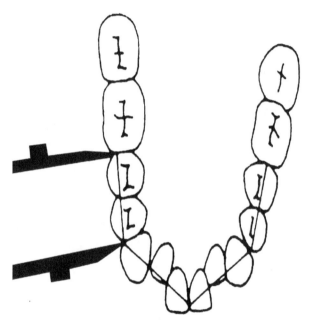

Figure 16-9   Space available

The second step of space analysis is to measure the amount of space required (or alignment of the teeth). This can be done by measuring the mesiodistal width of each erupted tooth from contact point to contact point (Figure 16-10). If the space analysis is done in the mixed dentition the size of unerupted permanent teeth can be estimated on individual periapical radiographs of panoramic radiographs image. However, there is an image enlargement existing in these types of radiographic images and it needs to compensate for. With the popularity of CBCT applications, the size of unerupted permanent teeth can be measured directly in CBCT image or in 3D—reconstruction model.

(2) Crowding

If the space required is greater than space available, crowding would occur. If available space is larger than the space required, excess space will lead to gaps between the teeth.

(3) Arch symmetry

The arch symmetry analysis can be done directly by using a transparent ruled grid placed over the upper dental arch in the software. Firstly, the transparent ruled grid should orient to the midpalatal raphe, and then the distortion of arch form could be measured from the ruled grid.

(4) Curve of Spee

The curve of Spee can be measured directly in the model or software. Steps to measure SP include the following: ① drawing a line from the tip of the lower cuspid to the terminal molar. ② Measuring the distance from the lowest point of the Spee curve to the line(Figure 16-11).

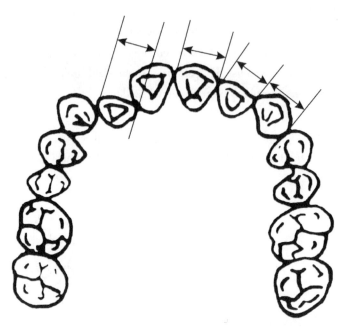

Figure 16-10 **Space required**

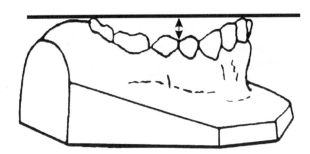

Figure 16-11 **Curve of Spee**

(5)Bolton analysis

Bolton analysis is carried out by measuring the mesiodistal(MD) width of each permanent tooth. For digital model analysis,the Bolton ratio can be calculated directly after measuring the mesiodistal width of each permanent tooth. The formulas are as follows.

Overall ratio= [Sum of MD widths of mandibular 12 teeth(first molar to first molar)/(sum of MD widths of maxillary 12 teeth(first molar to first molar)]×100.

Anterior ratio=(sum of mandibular 6 teeth)/(sum of mandibular 6 teeth)×100.

16.3.2.4 Cephalometric analysis

Cephalometric analysis was first introduced to the profession by Hofrath in Germany and Broadbent in the United States in 1934. Cephalometric radiography is a helpful diagnostic guide through measuring the head in the living individual. Nowadays,cephalometric radiographs provided both a research and a clinical tool for the study of malocclusion and underlying skeletal disproportions and are routinely used in orthodontic and orthognathic practices.

There are amounts of cephalometric analysis. Which involves measuring,comparing,and relating various linear and angular measurements of the hard and soft tissue structures of the face. The following analysis is a complication of measurements found to be useful in making a diagnosis and developing a treatment plan. It is divided into cephalometric analysis of hard tissue. dental relations and soft tissue.

（1）Hard tissue landmarks（Figure 16-12）

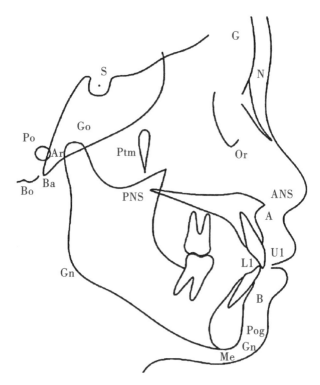

Figure 16-12   **Hard tissue landmarks**

Cranial base landmarks include the following：

Glabella（G）：the most anterior point of the frontal bone.

Nasion（N）：the most arterior point on the fronto-nasal suture.

Sella（S）：the mid-point of sellaturcica.

Basion（Ba）：the point where the median sagittal plane of the skull intersects the lowest point in the anterior margin of the foramen magnum.

Bolton：the most concave point in the posterior margin of the foramen magnum.

Porion（Po）：the most superior point on the bone external auditory meatus.

Maxilla landmarks include the following：

Orbitale（Or）：the most inferior anterior point on the bony margin of the orbit.

Pterygomaxillary fissure（Ptm）：the most inferior point of pterygomaxillary fissure.

Anterior Nasal Spine（ANS）：the most anterior point on the maxilla at the level floor of the nose.

Posterior Nasal Spine（PNS）：the most posterior point on the maxilla at the level floor of the nose.

Point（A）：the deepest point on the anterior contour of the maxilla between ANS and alveolar crest usually it is approximately 2 mm anterior to the apices of maxillary central incisor.

Mandible landmarks include the following：

Condylion（Co）：the superior point of the condyle.

Articulare（Ar）：the intersection of the inferior margin of cranial base and the posterior margin of condyle. It is always considered stable when Co can not be identified.

Point B (B): the deepest point on the anterior contour of the mandible between the chin and alveolar crest.

Pogonion(Pog):the most anterior point on the mandibular of bony chin.

Menton(Me):the most inferior point on the mandibular symphysis.

Gnathion(Gn):the median point between pogonion and menton.

Gonion(Go):the most inferior posterior point on the angle of the mandible.

(2)Hard tissue planes(Figure 16-13)

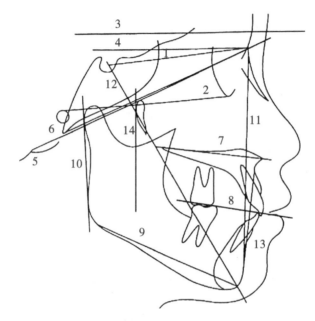

Figure 16-13　Hard tissue planes

1. SN;2. FH;3. HP;4. cHP;5. Bolton;6. Ba-N;7. ANS-PNS;8. OP;9. MP;
10. RP;11. N-Po;12. Y axis;13. dental plane;14. Ptv.

SN line:this line,connecting the mid-point of sellaturcica with nasion,is taken to represent the cranial base.

Frankfort plane:this is the line joining porion and orbitale.

"True horizontal" plane(HP):a line perpendicular to a plumb line on the radiograph will be the HP for a specific patient.

Constructed horizontal plane(cHP):this is a horizontal plane constructed by drawing a line through nasion at an angle of 7 degrees to S-N. This plane tends to be close to true horizon.

Bolton-nasion plane(bolton):the line joining Bolton and nasion.

Basion-nasion plane(Ba-N):extends between basion and nasion and dividesthe face and the cranium.

Maxillary plane(ANS-PNS):the line joining anterior nasal spine with posterior nasal spine.

Mandibular plane(MP):the line joining gonion and menton.

Y axis:the line joining sella and gnathion.

(3)Skeletal relationships

Skeletal anteroposterior relationships(Figure 16-14)include the following:

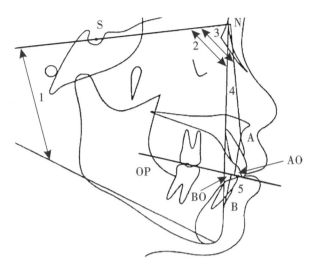

Figure 16-14 Skeletal anteroposterior relationships
1. SN/GoGn;2. SNA;3. SNB;4. ANB;5. wits appraisal.

SNA:measured at the junction of SN line and NA line. It evaluates the anteroposterior position of the maxilla in relation to the anterior cranial base. The normal average is $82°\pm 2°$. When this angle is above the normal range, it would be interpreted as protruded or prognathic maxilla, and when it is below the norm al range, retruded or retrognathic maxilla.

SNB:measured at the junction of SN line and NB line. It evaluates the anteroposterior position of the mandible in relation to the anterior cranial base. The normal average is $80°\pm 2°$. When this angle is a-bove the normal range, it would be interpreted as protruded or prognathic mandible, and when it is below the normal range, retruded or retrognathic mandible.

ANB:this angle is the difference between SNA and SNB angle and indicates the amount of skeletal dis-crepancy between maxilla and mandible in anteroposterior position. The normal average is $2°$. Larger than $5°$ would indicate a skeletal class Ⅱ malocclusion, and smaller than $0°$ a skeletal class Ⅲ malocclusion.

Wits appraisal:a linear measurement between the maxilla and mandible. Points AO and BO are estab-lished by dropping perpendicular lines from the A-point and B-point. Respectively, onto the occlusal plane (OP). The mean in males is BO-1 mm ahead of AO. In females, BO and AO coincide.

NP-FH:measured at the junction of NP line and FH line. it evaluates the anteroposterior position of the maxilla in relation to the anterior cranial base. The normal average range is $82°-95°$.

NA-PA:angle between N-A and P-A. It evaluates the anteroposterior position of the maxilla in rela-tion to the lower 1/3 facial height. The normal average is $6°$.

N-S-Ar(saddle angle):angle formed by joining N,S and Ar provides a parameter for assessment of relationship between anterior and posterolateral cranial bases. The average number is $127.3°\pm3.8°$.

S-Ar-Go(articular angle):the angle is constructed angle between the upper and lower parts of the posterior contours of the facial skeleton. The average number is $149.6°\pm5.6°$.

Ar-Go-Me(gonial angle):the angle formed by tangents to the body of the mandible and posterior bor-der of the ramus is of special interest, because it not only expresses the form of the mandible but also gives information on mandibular growth direction. The average number is $119.8°\pm5.6°$.

Skeletal vertical relationships include the following:

MP-FH:angle between FH plane and mandibular plane. This angle expresses slope of mandibular body, degree of gonial angle and lower 1/3 facial height. The average number is $32°$.

N-Me: anterior facial height, distance from nasion to menton.

S-Go: posterior facial height, distance from sella togonion.

(4) Analysis of dental relationship(Figure 16-15)

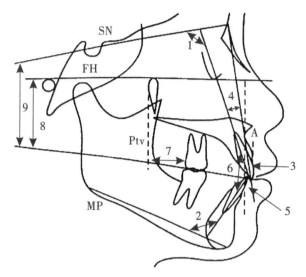

Figure 16-15   **Dental relationship**

1. U1-SN;2. L1-MP;3. Protrusion of upper incisors;4. U1-NA(°);5. U1-NA(mm);6. U1-L1;7. U6-Ptv;8. OP-LFH;9. OP-SN.

U1-NA(°): angle formed by the longaxis of the upper central incisor and NA line. It averages 22°.

U1-NA(mm): this is a linear distance measured in millimeter from the most prominent incisal edge of the upper incisor perpendicular to NA line. It averages 4 mm.

L1-NB(°): this is an angle formed by the long axis of the lower central incisor and NB line. It averages 25°.

L1-NB(mm): this is a linear distance measured in millimeter from the most prominent incisal edge of the lower incisor perpendicular to NB line. It averages 4 mm.

Protrusion of lower incisors: this is measured by the distance between labial surface of lower central incisor and parallel line dropping from B. The average number is 4 mm.

U1-L1(°): the interincisal angle measure at the junction of the long axis of upper central incisor with the lower central incisor. It averages 130± 6°.

U6-Ptv(mm): the distance between posterior margin of upper first molars and a line dropping from posterior margin of pteryomaxillary fissure. For adolescent patients, it averages his age plus 3 mm.

U1-SN: measured at the intersection of the long axis of the upper central incisor with the anterior cranial base. It evaluates the anteroposterior inclination of the most prominent maxillary central incisor. This angle averages 105.7°±6.3°.

L1-MP: measured at the intersection of the long axis of the lower central incisor with mandibular plane. It evaluates the anteroposterior inclination of the most prominent mandibular central incisor. This angle averages 90°±7°.

Protrusion of upper incisors: this is measured by the distance between labial surface of upper central incisor and parallel line dropping from A. The average number is 4-6 mm.

(5) Analysis of soft tissue relationships

Soft tissue landmarks(Figure 16-16) include the following:

Soft tissue glabella(G'): the most anterior point of the forehead.

Soft tissue nasion(N') : the deepest point of concavity in the midline between the forehead and the nose.

Pronasale(Pn) : the most anterior point of the nose.

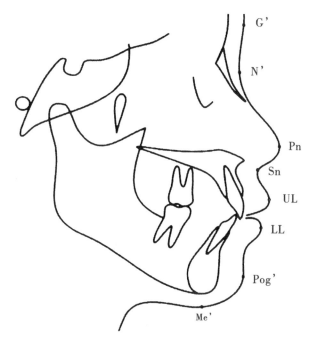

Figure 16-16   Soft tissue landmarks

Subnasale(Sn) : the point at which the columella of the nose merges with the upper lip in the midsaggittal plane.

Upper lip point(UL) : the most anterior point of upper lip profile.

Lower lip point(LL) : the most anterior point of lower lip profile.

Soft tissue pogonion(pog') : the most anterior point on the profile of soft tissue chin.

Soft tissue menton(Me') : the lowest point on the contour of the soft tissue chin.

Soft tissue planes(Figure 16-17) include the following :

Facial plane(N'-Pog') : extends from nasion to pogonion.

Upper facial plane(G'-Sn) : extends from soft tissue to subnasale.

Lower facial plane(Sn-Pog') : extends from subnasale to soft tissue pogonion.

S-line : formed by connecting soft tissue pogonion to a point midway between pronasale and subnasale.

Esthetic plane(E-line) : extends from the tip of nose to soft tissue pogonion.

Analysis of soft tissue include the following :

UU-EL : this is a linear distance measured from the most anterior point on the upper lip perpendicular to esthetic plane. It averages 1.4 mm ±1.9 mm. A larger angle indicates the protrusion of the upper lip and a smaller angle indicates the retrusion of the upper lip.

LL-EL : This is a linear measurement from the most anterior point on the lower lip perpendicular to esthetic plane. It averages 0 mm ±1 mm. A larger angle indicates the protrusion of the lower lip and a smaller angle indicates the retrusion of the lower lip.

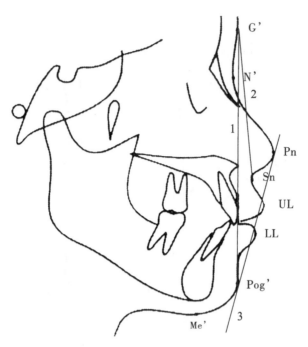

Figure 16-17　Soft tissue planes

16.3.2.5　X-ray examination

(1) The apical radiograph shows the development of the teeth, the order of the teeth, the multiple teeth, missing teeth, abnormal teeth, etc.

(2) The occlusal radiograph shows the position of the multiple teeth, the location of the impacted teeth, and the root lesions.

(3) The temporomandibular joint radiograph shows the position of the condylar process relative to the joint, the width of the joint space, the shape and structure of the joint head and socket.

(4) Panoramic radiograph shows the development of the whole mouth, the condition of the upper and lower jaw, the temporomandibular joint, and whether there was pathological damage.

(5) Wrist X-ray: The most commonly used method of wrist X-ray is the degree of calcification of the left wrist skeleton. Grave's wrist film is one of the more widely used indicators. According to the calcification of the wrist bone, domestic professor Shicai Zhang found that girls aged from 9-10 years old and boys from 12-13 years old entered the rapid period, and boys reached the peak period from 14-15 years of age, while females were 14 and males were 16 years old.

(6) Cervical vertebra X-ray is another method of estimating bone age, which can show the six stages of cervical development. S1 is the initial stage, S2 is the acceleration stage, S3 is the transition stage, S4 is the deceleration stage), S5 is the maturation stage, and S6 is the completion period.

(7) A posteroanterior(PA) cephalometric film should be taken if an asymmetry is noted in the clinical examination, or if skeletal transverse problems exist.

(8) CBCT is a medical image acquisition technique and is specifically designed for dental, oral and maxillofacial surgery and orthodontic indication. In the maxillofacial region, CBCT is used for the evaluation of impacted teeth, implant treatment planning, diagnostics of the TMJ, simulations tor orthodontic and surgical planning, etc.

16.3.2.6　Orthodontic treatment planning

Orthodontic treatment planning is the very difficult important element. The knowledge of dental development, facial growth, psychology, and appliance mechanics are all prerequisites for success. Whilst much can be learnt from textbooks there is no substitute for clinical experience gained over time. In the vast majority of cases definitive orthodontic treatment is best carried out in the early permanent dentition, however, due to the complexity of orthodontic treatment, the timing of treatment for different malformations is different.

(1) Deciduous dentition

The general tooth malposition does not need to be corrected, but when the tooth malposition caused by the oral harmful habit, should be treated actively. There is still some controversy about the treatment of the deciduous teeth class Ⅲ malocclusion. A mild form of deciduous teeth class Ⅲ malocclusion is only to observe, and then to decide whether to correct when the teeth are replaced. If the teeth class Ⅲ malocclusion is serious, which is related to the jaw bone, should be actively treated to facilitate the development of the maxillofacial region of the child.

(2) Mixed dentition

It is not necessary to treat mild dental malocclusion and functional development, but it should be treated actively if it is expected to affect the occlusion of permanent teeth. In general, a simpler applianced is used for the localized correction of the dislocation teeth. The course of treatment is usually about half a year, and the series teeth extraction method can be used to treat severe crowded cause.

It should be treated actively for the skeletal malformation. Orthodontic treatment is also called growth modified therapy. In order to achieve significant growth modified, orthodontist must implement growth modified treatment before or after the growth spurt of youth, for most children, it is in the later stage of mixed dentition. However, the optimal timing for the initiation of modified treatment is not the same for the different types of orthodontic teeth, and the optimal treatment time is 8-10 years for the protrusive mandible and the deficient maxilla. For patients with lower mandibular retraction, the best treatment time is about 11 years. For regions, therefore, in the children's treatment plan and treatment opportunity, to comprehensively the patient's malocclusion type, severity and multiple factors such as the growth of whole body, form a scientific treatment.

(3) permanent dentition

In permanent dentition, a fixed appliance is installed as the main means, to each kind of teeth dislocation, abnormal occlusion with a comprehensive, treatments of the system, so as to establish the best tooth arrangement and relations. Treatment for the best time of puberty, the teeth have been fully established, the development of the jaw and the soft tissue are nearing completion, all kinds of malocclusion deformity extent and complexity has been largely, is beneficial to diagnosis and treatment. At the same time, the jaw bone still has certain growth potential, the orthodontic treatment has a good reaction, the alveolar bone reconstruction is also relatively quick.

16.4　The Treatment of Malocclusion

16.4.1　Early orthodontics treatment

Crowded, irregular, and protruding teeth have been a problem for some individuals since antiquity, and attempts to correct this disorder go back at least to 1000 B. C. As dentistry developed in the 18th and 19th centuries, a number of devices for the "regulation" of the teeth were described by various authors and apparently used sporadically by the dentists of that era.

However, their emphasis in orthodontics remained the alignment of the teeth and the correction of facial proportions. Little attention was paid to bite relationships.

Angle's classification of malocclusion in the 1890s was an important step in the orthodontics because it not only subdivided major types of malocclusion but also included the fires clear and simple definition of normal occlusion in the natural dentition. With the establishing of a concept of normal occlusion and a classification scheme that incorporated the line of occlusion, by the early 1900s orthodontics was no longer just the alignment of irregular teeth. Instead, it had evolved into the treatment of malocclusion, defined as any deviation from the ideal occlusal scheme described by Angle. With the emphasis on dental occlusion that followed, however, less attention came to be paid to facial proportions and esthetics. He solved the problem of dental and facial appearance by simply postulating that the best esthetics always were achieved when the patient had ideal occlusion.

As time passed, it became clear that even an excellent occlusion was unsatisfactory if it was achieved at the expense of proper facial proportions.

Cephalometric radiography, which enabled orthodontists to measure the changes in tooth and jaw position produced by growth and treatment came into widespread use after World War Ⅱ. These radiographs made it clear that many Class Ⅱ and Class Ⅲ malocclusions resulted from faulty jaw relationships, not just malposed teeth. By use of cephalometrics, it also was possible to see that jaw growth could be altered by orthodontic treatment. At present, both functional and extraoral appliances are used internationally to control and modify growth and form. Obtaining correct or at least improved jaw relationships became a goal of treatment by the mid-twentieth century.

The changes in the goals of orthodontic treatment, which are to focus on facial proportions and the impact of the dentition on facial appearance, have been codified now in the form of the soft tissue paradigm.

16.4.2 Modern treatment goals: the soft tissue paradigm

A paradigm can be defined as "a set of shared beliefs and assumptions that represent the conceptual foundation of an area of science or clinical practice". The soft tissue paradigm states that both the goals and limitations of modern orthodontic and orthognathic treatment are determined by the soft tissues of the face, not by the teeth and bones. This reorientation of orthodontics away from the Angle paradigm that dominated the 20th century is most easily understood by comparing treatment goals, diagnostic emphasis, and treatment approach in the two paradigms.

More specifically, what difference does the soft tissue paradigm make in planning treatment? There are several major effects: the primary goal of treatment became soft tissue relationships and adaptations, not Angle's ideal occlusion. This goal is not incompatible with Angle's ideal occlusion, but it acknowledges that to provide maximum benefit for the patient, ideal occlusion can not always be the major focus of a treatment plan. Soft tissue relationships, both the proportions of the soft tissue integument of the face and the relationship of the dentition to the lips and face, are the major determinants of facial appearance. Soft tissue adaptations to the position of the teeth determine whether the orthodontic result will be stable. Keeping this in mind while planning treatment is critically important.

The secondary goals of treatment become functional occlusion. Temporomandibular(TM)dysfunction, to the extent that it relates to the dental occlusion, is best thought of as the rest of injury to the soft tissues around the TM joint caused by clenching and grinding the teeth. Given that, an important goal of treatment is to arrange the occlusion to minimize the chance of injury. In this also, Angle's ideal occlusion is not incompatible with the broader goal, but deviations from the Angle ideal may provide greater benefit for some patients. It should be considered when treatment is planned.

The thought process that goes into "solving the patient's problems" is reversed. In the past, the clinician's focus was on dental and skeletal relationships, with the tacit assumption that if these were correct, soft tissue relationships would take care of themselves. With the broader focus on facial and oral soft tissues, the thought process is to establish what these soft tissue goals. Why is this important in establishing the goals of treatment? It relates very much to why patients/parents seek orthodontic treatment and what they expect to gain from it.

16.4.3   Aims of orthodontic treatment

The treatment provided should not only satisfy the patient's esthetic desires but also satisfy certain functional and physiologic requirements.

16.4.3.1   Functional efficiency

The teeth along with their surrounding structures are required to perform certain important functions. The orthodontic treatment should increase the efficiency of the functions performed by the stomatognathic system.

16.4.3.2   Structural balance

The structures affected by the orthodontic treatment include, not only the teeth but also the surrounding soft tissue envelop and the associated skeletal structures. The treatment should maintain a balance between these structures, and the correction of one should not be detrimental to the health of another.

16.4.3.3   Esthetic harmony

The orthodontic treatment should increase the overall esthetic appear of the individual. This might just require the alignment of certain teeth or the forward movement of the complete jaw including its basal bone. The aim is to get results which gear with the patient's personality and make him/her to look more esthetic.

16.4.4   Contemporary orthodontic appliances

Orthodontics has come far since the days when finger pressure was being advocated to move teeth. With the development of this branch of dentistry is associated an inseparable quest of researchers to create appliances which can move teeth "ideally".

This endeavor to achieve "ideal" tooth movement has led clinicians to create numerous appliances, which move teeth. Orthodontic appliances can be defined as devices, which create and/or transmit forces to individual teeth/a group of teeth and/or maxillo – facial skeletal units so as to bring about changes within the bone with or/without tooth movement which will help to achieve the treatment goals of functional efficiency, structural balance and esthetic harmony.

Most of the orthodontic appliances are restricted to bringing about tooth movement. But as our knowledge of growth and development of the maxillofacial unit has increased, so has our endeavor to modify the growth of underlying skeletal structures.

16.4.4.1   Removable appliances

As the name suggests, these are appliances that can be removed by the patient without any supervision by the orthodontist. Removable orthodontic appliances are useful in a variety of situations but present the inherent disadvantage of the treatment being in control of the patient. Also, movement of teeth in all the three planes of space can not be carried out simultaneously.

Removable appliances are capable of the following types of tooth movement: tipping movements, movement of blocks of teeth, influencing the eruption of opposing teeth.

The removable orthodontic appliances are made up of three components:

Force or active components—comprises of springs(Figure 16-18, Figure 16-19), screws(Figure 16-20) or elastics.

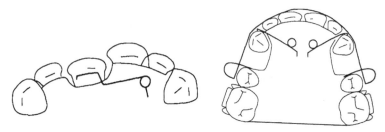

Figure 16-18　Finger spring

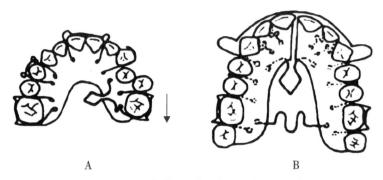

A   B

Figure 16-19　Coffin spring: for arch expansion

A: The split spling pushes the molars away; B: The expansion spring enlarges the maxillary arch.

Base plate or framework—can be made of cold cure or heat cure acrylic.

Commonly used removable appliances include the following:

(1) To correct anterior crossbite in mixed dentition

Movement labially of upper incisors in the mixed dentition can be accomplished either using a spring or screw design depending upon the number of incisors to be moved. To move a single incisor buccally a Z-spring is commonly used. This design is also known as a double-cantilever spring(Figure 16-21) when it is used for moving more than one tooth. A Z-spring for a single tooth should be fabricated in 0.5 mm wire, but for longer spans 0.6 or 0.7 mm is advisable. Good anterior retention is required to resist the displacing effect of this spring.

Activation is by pulling the spring about 1-2 mm away from the baseplate at an angle of approximately 45° in the direction of desired movement[so that the spring is not caught on the incisal edge(s) as the appliace is inserted].

A screw design is often used where three or all of the upper incisors need to be moved labially as then the teeth to be moved can be used for retention of the appliance. However, the disadvantage is that this results in a much bulkier appliance anteriorly.

Buccal capping is usually incorporated into this appliance to free the occlusion with the lower arch.

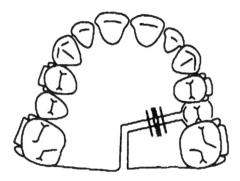

Figure 16-20 Screw for distal movement of maxillary 1st molar

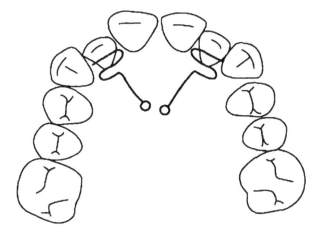

Figure 16-21 Double cantilever/Z-Spring

Fixation orretentive components—usually include clasps(Figure 16-22).

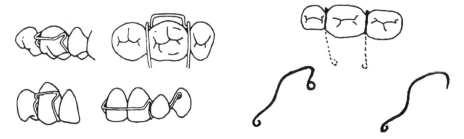

Figure 16-22 Adams clasp and Ball-ended clasp

(2)Screw appliance to expand upper arch

A design incorporating a screw(Figure 16-23)is useful for moving blocks of teeth and has the additional advantage that the teeth being moved can also be clasped for retention. Buccal capping is also used to free occlusion with the lower arch.

Activation is by means of turning the screw a one-quarter turn. One quarter-turnopens the two sections of the appliance by 0.25 mm. For active movement the patient should turn the screw twice a week(for example on a Wednesday and a Saturday). If opened too far, the screw will come apart; therefore patients should be warned that if the screw portion becomes loose they should turn it back one turn and not advance the screw again.

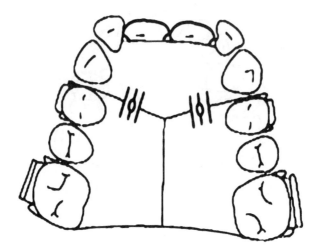

Figure 16-23 **Screw for arch expansion**

(3) Anterior bite-plane

Increasing the thickness of acrylic behind the upper incisors forms a bite-plane onto which the lower incisors occlude. A bite-plane is prescribed when either the overbite needs to be reduced by eruption of the lower buccal segment teeth or elimination of possible occlusal interferences is necessary to allow tooth movement to occur. The thickness should be sufficient to open the bite in the premolar region by 4-5 mm. As the overbite reduces, additional acrylic can be added to raise the platform and continue overbite reduction. Grooves can be provided in the anterior bite plate (Figure 16-24) to support the incisal tips of the mandibular incisors. Also, the maxillary incisors may be capped to prevent their supra-eruption or flaring. It also aids in retention and increases the anchorage potential of the appliance. An inclined guide plane (Figure 16-25) can also be provided as a modification of the anterior bite plane. This will cause the patient to bite more forward as compared to normal and may cause the mandible to grow forward. It can also procline the mandibular incisors.

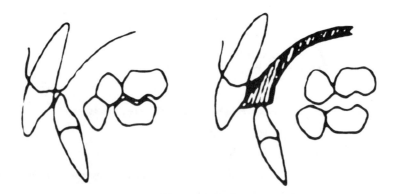

Figure 16-24 **Anterior bite-plane**

(4) Posterior bite-plane

Posterior bite-plane is used mainly when teeth have to be pushed over the bite. The height of the platform should be sufficient enough to free the teeth, that are to be moved, from occlusal interference with the opposing teeth. It is better to adjust the posterior bite planes to obliterate the freeway space to aid compliance.

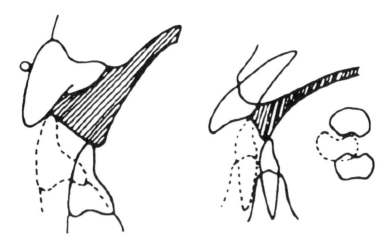

Figure 16-25   An inclined guide plane anterior bite plane

(5) Hawley retainer

This passive appliance is used for retention following active orthodontic treatment. It is a simple and robust appliance made from an acrylic baseplate with a metal labial bow. It has the advantages of being simple to construct, reasonably robust, rigid enough to maintain transverse corrections and it is easy to add a prosthetic tooth. When replacing missing teeth it is important to put rigid stops on the retainer mesial and distal to any prosthetic tooth, to prevent relapse. Hawley retainers(Figure 16-26) also allow more rapid vertical settling of teeth than vacuum-formed retainer, due to the lack of complete occlusal coverage.

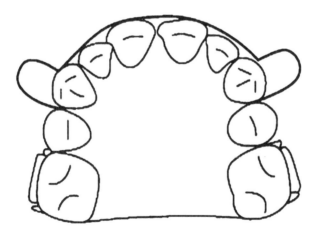

Figure 16-26   Hawley retainer

(6) Clear aligner therapy(CAT)

The use of clear aligners in orthodontic treatment for adults became possible as vacuum-formed clear thermoplastic sheets to fit tightly over the teeth were introduced into orthodontics in the 1980s.

In the late 1990s, a new company with no ties to previous suppliers of dental and orthodontic materials, obtained venture capital to computerize the process of producing a sequence of casts with incremental changes, on which aligners could be fabricated. The approach was to scan dental casts to create a digital model, make small changes in the position of the teeth on the digital model, produce a stereolithographic cast from the digital model on which an aligner could be made, then make a series of additional incremental changes on the digital model and produce a matching series of modified casts for aligner fabrication. With careful planning, this would result in a sequence of aligners that could correct more complex problem. From the beginning, it was recognized that since growth changes could not be predicted, the method would be useful only for treatment of adults or adolescents in whom growth modification was not needed, but these are the patients most interested in making an orthodontic appliance invisible or minimally visible.

Currently, these appliances have been shown to perform well, particularly in adults, in the following circumstances: mild-to-moderate crowing in conjunction with interproximal stripping or expansion; lower incisor extraction for severe crowing; closure of mild-moderate spacing; posterior dental expansion; intrusion of one or two teeth. Severely rotated teeth, high canines, overbite reduction by relative intrusion, molar uprighting do not lend themselves easily to correction by these appliance. In conjunction with fixed attachments, however, it is possible to extend their use to closure of premolar extraction spaces, extrusion of incisors and molar translation.

16.4.4.2　Functional appliances

Functional appliances correct malocclusion by using, removing or modifying the forces generated by the orofacial musculature, tooth eruption and dento-facial growth.

(1) Mechanism of action

How functional appliances work is not completely understood. They are generally devoid of active components, such as springs, and are incapable of moving teeth individually. Instead, they operate by applying or eliminating forces that are generated through the facial and masticatory musculature and by harnessing those that occur through natural growth processes. They are, therefore, only effective in growing children, preferably just prior to their pubertal growth spurt. The specific force system set up by any appliance will depend on its particular design. Essentially, forces are developed by posturing the mandible—either downward and forward in class Ⅱ or downward and backward in class Ⅲ. This applies intermaxillary traction between the arches, as can be produced by elastics with fixed appliances. As the scope for posturing the mandible backward is far less than for posturing it forward, functional appliances are more successful in, and are indicated almost exclusively for, class Ⅱ malocclusion. For this reason, the possible mechanisms of action will only be considered for class Ⅱ malocclusion. In these cases, the result is a forward tipping of the lower incisors and the entire mandibular dentition, with acceleration of mandibular growth, as well as a backward tipping of the upper incisors and restraint of maxillary growth. Overall mandibular growth is modified—the total amount is unaffected but the expression of growth is altered.

(2) Indications

Where the appliance is the sole means of correcting the malocclusion in a growing child, the following features should be present:

1) Mildskeletal class Ⅱ owing to mandibular retrusion or mild skeletal class Ⅲ owing to mandibular protrusion.

2) Average or reduced FMPA.

3) Uncrowded arches.

4) Lower incisors upright or slightly retroclined in class Ⅱ, and proclined in class Ⅲ; proclined lower incisors in class Ⅱ usually contraindicates functional appliance therapy.

5) In severe class Ⅱ malocclusion, a preliminary phase of functional appliance therapy in the mixed dentition may be useful to aid overbite reduction and occlusal correction prior to proceeding to further treatment with fixed appliances and possible extractions.

6) One of the important criteria in case selection for the functional appliance therapy is eliciting a posi-

tive VTO. VTO is said to be positive if the profile of the patient improves noticeably when the patient advances the mandible voluntarily to correct the overjet. A negative VTO, i. e. , patient whose profile does not improve/worsens on voluntary forward posturing of the mandible, are not good candidates for the functional appliance therapy.

(3) Types of functional appliance

The following account describes some standard functional appliances. However, current thinking regarding design is to "pick and mix" the components that necessary for the specific correction of a particular malocclusion. Such a "components approach" to design requires considerable insight into the working of these appliances which necessitates specialist knowledge and expertise.

1) Twin-block appliance

The twin-block appliance (Figure 16-27) was developed by Clark in 1977. It is the most popular functional appliance in the UK. The reason for its popularity is that it is well tolerated by patients as it is constructed in two parts. The upper and lower parts fit together using posterior bite blocks with interlocking bite-planes, which posture the mandible forward. The blocks need to be at least 5 mm high, which prevents the patient from biting one block on top of the other. Instead the patient is encouraged to posture the mandible forwards, so that the lower block occludes in front of the upper block. The appliance can be worn full time, including during eating in some cases, which means that rapid correction is possible. It is also possible to modify the appliance to allow expansion of the upper arch during the functional appliance phase. A modification to allow correction of class Ⅱ division 2 malocclusions is also used.

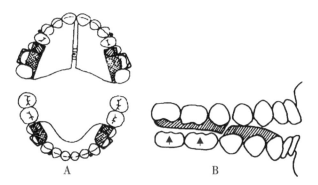

Figure 16-27 **Twin-block appliance**
A: Occlusal view; B: lateral view.

It is also easy to reactivate the twin-block appliance. This means that during treatment if further advancement of the mandible is required, it is possible to modify the existing appliance rather than having to construct a new appliance.

One of the side-effects of the twin-block appliance is the residual posterior lateral open bites at the end of the functional phase. This is seen particularly in cases initially presenting with a deep overbite. The posterior teeth are prevented from erupting by the occlusal coverage of the bite blocks. Some clinicians will trim the acrylic away from the occlusal surfaces of the upper block to allow the lower molars to erupt. Any remaining lateral open bites are closed down in the fixed appliance phase of treatment.

2) Activator

Activator (Figure 16-28) is a loose fitting appliance which was designed by Andreasen and Haupl to correct retrognathic mandible. The present form of the appliance came through various stages of development starting with the concept of "bite jumping" introduced by Norman Kingsley. He used a vulcanite palatal plate consisting of an anterior inclined plane, which guided the mandible into a forward position when the patient closed on it.

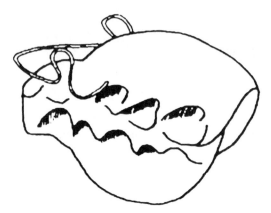

Figure 16−28 Andresen activator

This was followed by Hotz's Vorbissplatte which was a modification of Kingsley's plate and was used to correct retrognathic mandible with deep bite.

Monobloc which was made up of a single block of vulcanite, was used by Pierre Robin to correct the airway obstruction in patients with micrognathia.

Later in 1908 Viggo Andreasen, modified the Hawley's type of retainer, on the maxillary arch, to which he added a lower lingual horse shoe shaped flange which helped to position the mandible forward. He called it the biomechanical working retainer. Later he teamed with Karl Haupl, and developed an appliance which they called as Norwefian appliance and later came to be known as the activator.

The Andresen activator is constructed to a bite giving 2 − 3 mm of incisal opening, usually with an edge−to−edge incisor relationship. A second advancement may be necessary with a large overjet. Specific design aspects include no clasps, a passive labial bow and upper and lower acrylic base plates fused together. Acrylic capping extends over the lower incisors to allow overbite reduction while the buccal interocclusal acrylic is trimmed to direct mesial movement of the lower teeth and distal and buccal movement of the upper teeth.

Various views have been put forward to explain the mode of action of the activator. Some implicate the reflex myotactic activity and isometric contractions while others attribute the results to the viscoelastic properties and stretching of the muscles and soft tissues.

However, the basic fact remains that most of the changes are induced by holding the mandible forward and the ensuing reaction of the stretched muscles and soft tissues, transmitted to the periosteum, bones and the teeth.

A restraining effect on the growth of the maxilla and the maxillary dentoalveolar complex is also seen along with the stimulation of mandibular growth and mandibular alveolar adaptation. Research has also shown favorable changes in the TMJ region.

3) Bionator

The bulkiness of the activator and its limitation to night−time wear was a major deterrent in its greater use by clinicians to obtain maximum potential of functional growth guidance. The appliance was too bulky for day−time wear. Moreover, during sleep, the function is minimized or virtually nonexistent. This led to the development of the bionator.

The bionator (Figure 16−29) is a less bulky (therefore more popular) derivative of the Andresen activator. In addition, the construction bite is taken edge to edge. The labial bow is extended back to hold the cheeks out of contact with the buccal segment teeth and allow arch expansion, while a thick palatal loop takes the place of acrylic. The palate is free for proprioceptive contact with the tongue and the buccinator wire loops hold away the potentially deforming muscles. The appliance developed by Balters in 1960. Full-time wear is advisable except for meals.

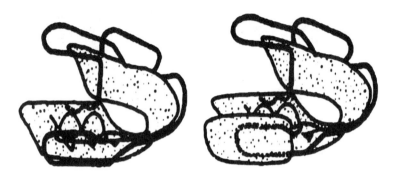

Figure 16-29   **Bionator**

According to Balters, the equilibrium between the tongue and the circumoral muscles is responsible for the shape of the dental arches and that the functional space for the tongue is essential for the normal development of the orofacial system, e. g. , posterior displacement of the tongue could cause Class Ⅱ malocclusion. Taking into consideration the dominant role of the tongue, Balters designed an appliance, which could take advantage of tongue posture. Thus he constructed anteriorly, with the incisors in an edge to edge position. This forward positioning brought the dorsum of the tongue in contact with the soft palate and helped accomplish lip closure.

Thus the principle of bionator is not to activate the muscles but to modulate muscle activity, thereby enhancing the normal development of the inherent growth pattern and eliminate abnormal and potentially deforming environmental factors.

4) Frankel appliance

The Frankel appliance was originally termed a "function regulator". These were developed by Rolf Frankel(Germany). Frankel believed that the active muscle and tissuc mass, i. e. , the buccinator mechanism and the orbicularis oris complex have a major role in the development of skeletal and dentofacial deformities.

Hence he developed function regulators as orthopedic exercise devices, to aid in the maturation, training and reprogramming of the orofacial neuro-muscular system.

It has particular use in the management of abnormal soft tissue pattern, for example hyperactive mentails muscle, which is often associated with partial or complete lip trapping and retroclination of the lower labial segment. Buccal shields hold the cheeks away from the teeth and stretch the mucoperiosteum at the sulcus depth, intending to expand the arches and widen the alveolar processes. Stability of such changes are doubtful over the long term.

There are four subtypes:

Fr Ⅰ is used to correct class Ⅰ and class Ⅱ division 1 malocclusion.

Fr Ⅱ (Figure 16-30)is used for correction of class Ⅱ division 2 malocclusion.

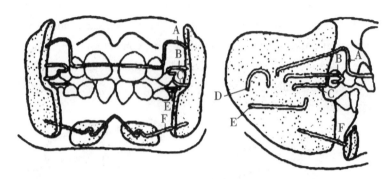

Figure 16-30　Frankel Ⅱ appliance

FrⅢ (Figure 16-31) is used for correction of class Ⅲ malocclusion.

FrⅣ is used for correction of anterior open bite.

Fr V is Fr with headgear.

Fr Ⅰ is the most popular and includes acrylic pads labial of the lower incisors to encourage development of the mandibular alveolar process. Although lower incisor capping is not traditionally prescribed, it may be incorporated to aid overbite correction. The construction bite is usually as in the medium opening activator. Wear is gradually built up from 2-3 hours per day in the first few weeks, to night-time and then full-time apart from sports and while eating.

FrⅢ has labial pads in the upper labial sulcus, and heavy wires palatal to the upper and labial to the lower incisors. For the construction bite, the mandible is postured down and slightly backward to achieve an edge-to-edge incisor relationship. Instructions regarding wear are as for the Fr Ⅰ .

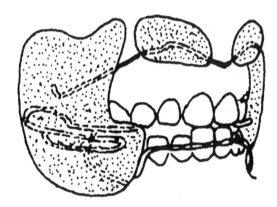

Figure 16-31　Frankel Ⅲ appliance

Frankel appliances are complex in design, expensive to make and repair and easy to damage and distort. They can, however, be reactivated by sectioning the buccal shields and repositioning them forward.

5) Headgear addition to functional appliances

In cases where maximal anteroposterior and vertical maxillary restraint is desirable, occipital – pull headgear may be added to tubes incorporated in the acrylic or soldered to the clasp bridges. Forces of about 500 g should be used for 14 - 16 hours per day and usual headgear safety precautions and instructions should be followed. If the FMPA is increased, molar capping is essential to promote a closing rotation of the mandible and prevent molar eruption, thereby facilitating an increase in overbite. The addition of high-pull headgear to the appliance will facilitate this process(Figure 16-32).

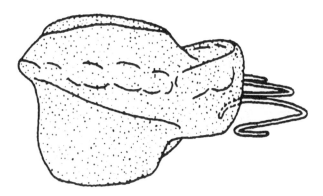

Figure 16-32   Van Beek appliance

6) Fixed functional appliances

Successful orthodontic treatment often relies heavily on patient's cooperation in the wearing of removable functional appliances, elastics or headgears. It is eliminating the need to use these places the treatment result more under the control of the orthodontist. This led to the development of "non-compliant appliances". The appliances in "noncompliance" treatment have a couple of features in common.

Forces are applied using auxiliaries between the arches. Most often multi-banded fixed appliances are used with lingual arched and palatal bars. Most of them use superelastics nickel titanium and Titan-molydenum alloy springs.

The commonly used fixed functional appliances are Herbst appliance (Figure 16-33), Jasper jumper (Figure 16-34), Adjustable bite corrector, Eureka spring, Saif springs, Mandibular anterior repositioning appliance (MARA), Klapper super spring, Forsus fatigue resistant device (Figure 16-35), Sabbagh universal spring (SUS).

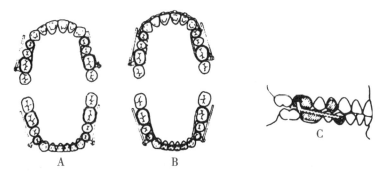

Figure 16-33   Herbst appliance

A, B: Occlusal view; C: Lateral view.

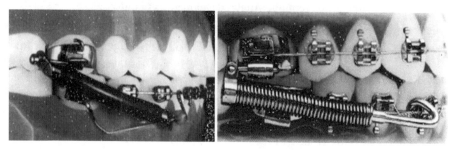

Figure 16-34   Jasper jumper

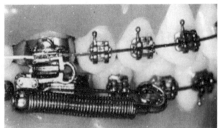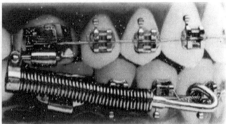

Figure 16-35 **Forsus appliance**

The Herbst appliance is a fixed functional appliance and is the most popular functional appliance in the US. There is a section attached to the upper buccal segment teeth and a section attached to the lower buccal segment teeth. These sections are joined by a rigid arm that postures the mandible forwards. As it is a fixed appliance, it removes some (but not all) compliance factors. It is however slightly better tolerated than the bulkier twin-block appliance, with patients finding it easier to eat and talk with it in place. The principal disadvantages are the increased breakages and higher cost of the Herbst appliance.

16.4.4.3　Fixed appliance

Fixed appliances are attached to the teeth and are thus capable of a greater range of tooth movements than is possible with a removable appliance. Not only does the attachment on the tooth surface (called a bracket) allow the tooth to be moved vertically or tilted, but also a force couple can be generated by the interaction between the bracket and an archwire running through the bracket. Thus rotational and apical movements are also possible. The interplay between the archwire and the bracket slot determines the type and direction of movement achieved.

With fixed orthodontic appliances the control over treatment mechanics shifts more directly into the clinicians hands and the patient is restricted to simply maintaining the appliance and oral hygiene and may be changing certain force applying devices, e. g. , elastics. Patient compliance is rarely a problem. The control achieved with fixed orthodontic appliance is far greater as compared to removable appliances and the teeth can be moved virtually in all the three planes of space.

(1) The development of contemporary fixed appliances

1) Angle's progression to the edgewise appliance

Edward Angle's (Figure 16 - 36) position as the "father of modern orthodontics" is based not only on his contributions to classification and diagnosis but also on his creativity in developing new orthodontic appliances. With few exceptions, the fixed appliances used in contemporary orthodontics are based on Angle's designs from the early 20th century. Angle developed four major appliance systems.

* E-arch

In the late 1800s, a typical orthodontic appliance depended on some sort of rigid framework to which the teeth were tied so that they could be expended to the arch form dictated by the appliance. Angle's first appliance, the E-arch (Figure 16-37), was

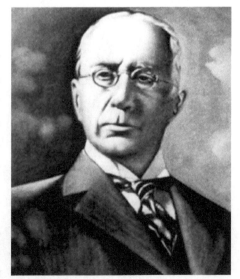

Figure 16-36 **Edward H. Angle**

an improvement on this basic design. Bands were placed only on molar teeth, and a heavy labial archwire extended around the arch. The end of the wire was threaded, and a small nut placed on the threaded portion

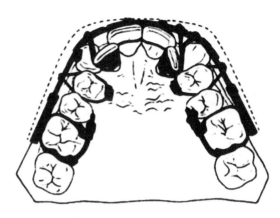

Figure 16-37   **E-arch**

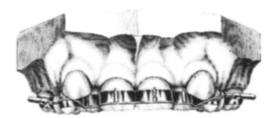

Figure 16-38   **Pin and tube**

of the arch allowed the archwire to be advanced so that the arch perimeter increased. Individual teeth were simply ligated to this expansion arch. This appliance still could be found in the catalogs of some mail-order orthodontic laboratories as late as the 1980s, perhaps because of its simplicity, and despite the fact that it can deliver only heavy interrupted force.

• Pin and tube

The E-arch was capable only of tipping teeth to a new position. It was not able to precisely position any individual tooth. To overcome this difficulty, Angle began placing bands on other teeth and used a vertical tube on each tooth into which a soldered pin from a smaller archwire was placed. With this appliance, tooth movement was accomplished by repositioning the individual pins at each appointment. An incredible degree of craftsmanship was involved in constructing and adjusting this pin and tube appliance (Figure 16-38), and although it was theoretically capable of great precision in tooth movement, it proved impractical in clinical use. It is said that only Angle himself and one of his students ever mastered the appliance. The relatively heavy base arch meant that spring qualities were poor, and the problem therefore was compounded because many small adjustments were needed.

• Ribbon arch

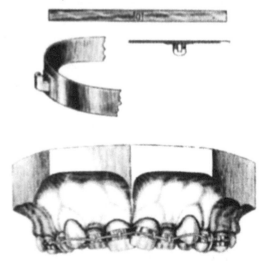

Figure 16-39   **Ribbon arch**

Angle's next appliance modified the tube on each tooth to provide a vertically positioned rectangular slot behind the tube. A ribbon arch of 10×20 gold wire was placed into the slot and held with pins. The ribbon arch (Figure 16-39) was an immediate success, primarily because the archwire, unlike any of its predecessors, was small enough to have good spring qualities and was quite efficient in aligning malposed teeth. Although the ribbon arch could be twisted as it was inserted into its slot, the major weakness of the appliance was that it provided relatively poor control of root position. The resiliency of the ribbon archwire simply did not allow generation of the moments necessary to torque roots to a new position.

• Edgewise

To overcome the deficiencies of the ribbon arch, angle reoriented the slot from vertical to horizontal and inserted a rectangular wire rotated 90 degrees to the orientation it had with the ribbon arch—thus the name "edgewise" (Figure 16-40). The dimensions of the slot were altered to 22×28 precious metal wire was used. These dimensions, arrived at after extensive experimentation, did allow excellent control of crown and root position in all three planes of space. After its introduction in 1928, this appliance became the mainstay of multibanded fixed appliance therapy, although the ribbon arch continued in common use for another decade.

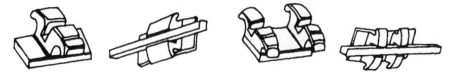

Figure 16-40 **Edgewise bracket**

2) Other early fixed appliance systems

● Tweed technique

Given Angle's insistence on expansion of the arches rather than extraction to deal with crowding problems, it is ironic that the edgewise appliance finally provided the control of root position necessary for successful extraction treatment. The appliance was being used for this purpose within a few years of its introduction. Charles Tweed, one of Angle's last students, was the leader in the United States in adapting the edgewise appliance for exreaction treatment. In fact, little adaptation of the appliance was needed. Tweed used the diagnostic facial trangle for diagnosis and treatment planning. He also advocated the concept of "anchorage preparation". Anchorage preparation was done to prevent the mandibular and maxillary molars from drifting anteriorly in response to the intermaxillary elastics used for retracting the anterior teeth. Tweed moved the teeth bodily and used the subdivision approach for anchorage control, first sliding the canines distally along the archwire, then retracting the incisors.

The technique though far advanced than any previously known was complex and required the clinician to be extremely dedicated and meticulous in his/her wire bending. Patient cooperation in wearing headgears was a must. Since the forces used were heavy the incidence of patient discomfort and root resorption were high.

● Begg appliance

Raymond Begg had been taught use of the ribbon arch appliance at the Angle school before his return to Australia in the 1920s. Working independently in Adelaide, Begg also concluded that extraction of teeth was often necessary, and set out to adapt the ribbon arch appliance so that it could be used for better control of root position. Dr Begg's studies on the normal occlusion of man made him realize that the teeth continuously migrate mesially and vertically to compensate for attritions of their proximal and occluso-incisal surfaces. Based on this premise, he devised the light wire differential force technique.

The technique is designed such that it permits teeth to move towards their anatomically correct positions in the jaws under the influence of very light forces, as would occur naturally in the presence of attrition.

Begg's adaptation took three forms: ① he replaced the precious metal ribbon arch with high-strength 16 mil stainless steel wire as this became available in the late 1930s; ② he retained the original ribbon arch bracket, but turned it upside down so that the bracket slot pointed gingivally rather than occlusally; ③ he added auxiliary springs to the appliance for control of root position.

In the resulting Begg appliance(Figure 16-41), friction was minimized because the area of archwire was also small and the force of the wire against the bracket was also small. Begg's strategy for anchorage control was tipping/uprighting. In other words, Begg advocated the tipping of teeth crowns instead of bodily movement, which were later uprighted, roots paralleled and repositioning achieved.

Although the progress records with his approach looked vastly different, it is not surpring that Begg' overall result in anchorage control was similar to Tweed's, since both used two steps to overcome some frictional problems. The Begg appliance is still seen in contemporary use though it has declined in popularity and often appears now in a hybrid form, with brackets that allow the use of rectangular wires in finishing. It is a complete appliance in the sense that it allows good control of crown and root position in all three planes of space.

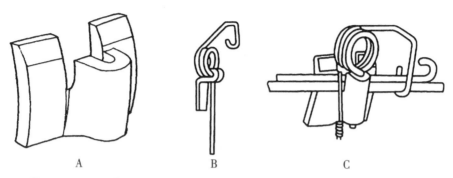

Figure 16-41   **First-,second-,and third-order bends in the edgewise wires**

A. First-order bends in a maxillary(left) and mandibular(right) archwire. Note the lateral inset required in the maxillary archwire, and the canine and molar offset bends that are required in both. B. Second-order bends in the maxillary incisor segment to compensate for the inclination of the incisal edge of these teeth relative to the long axis of the tooth. C. Third-order bends for the maxillary central incisors and maxillary first molars showing the twist in the archwire to provide a passive fit in a bracket or tube on these teeth. Twist in an archwire provides torque in a bracket; the torque is positive for the incisor, negative for the molar.

3) Contemporary edgewise

The Begg appliance became widely popular in the 1960s because it was more efficient than the edgewise appliance of that era, in the sense that equivalent results could be produced with less investment of the clinician's time. Developments since then have reversed the balance: the contemporary edgewise appliance has evolved far beyond the original design while retaining the basic principle of a rectangular wire in a rectangular slot, and now is more efficient than the Begg appliance—which is the reason for its almost universal use now. Major steps in the evolution of the edgewise appliance are as below:

Automatic retational control. In the original appliance, Angle soldered eyelets to the corners of the bands, so a separate ligature tie could be used as needed to correct rotations or control the tendency for a tooth to rotate as it was moved. Now rotation control is achieved without the necessary for an additional ligature by using either twin brackets or single brackets with extension wings that contact the underside of the archwire(Lewis or Lang brackets) to obtain the necessary moment in the rotational plane of space.

Alteration in bracket slot dimensions. Reducing Angle's original slot size from 22-18 mils. There are now two modern edgewise appliances, because the 18 and 22 slot appliances are used rather differently (Figure 16-42).

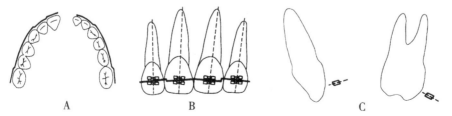

Figure 16-42   **Begg bracket auxiliary springs for control of root position**

A: First order bend; B: Second order bend; C: Third order bend.

4）The pre-adjusted edgewise appliance

Because of their advantages these systems are now universally accepted. The need for first -, second-, and third-order bends in the archwire during treatment is considerably reduced because the brackets are manufactured with the slot positioned to the bracket base in such a way that these movements are built in. Therefore plain preformed archwires can be used so that the teeth are moved progressively from the very start of treatment to their ideal position. Hence they are also known as the straight wire appliance. However, a pre-adjusted bracket system will not eliminate the need for wire bending as only average values are built into the appliance, and often additional individual bends need to be placed in the archwire.

Not surprisingly, there are many different opinions as to the correct position of each tooth, and many manufacturers keen to join a lucrative market. The result is an almost bewildering array of pre-adjusted systems, all with slightly differing degrees of torque and tip. Of these perhaps the best known are the Andrews' prescription, developed by Andrews, the father of the straight wire appliance; the Roth system and the MBT prescription.

• Andrews' prescription

In 1972 Lawrence Andrews listed the ingredients of occlusion which he considered essential to accomplish the anatomical goal and achieve harmony of occlusion are the six keys to optimal occlusion.

Key Ⅰ ; interarch relationships

Key I is the first of the six significant characteristics that were consistently present in the sample of 120 dental casts with optimal occlusion. Key I pertains to the occlusion and the interarch relationships of the teeth. This key consists of seven parts.

The mesiobuccal cusp of the permanent maxillary first molar occludes in the groove between the mesial and middle buccal cusps of the permanent mandibular first molar, as explained by Angle.

The distal marginal ridge of the maxillary first molar occludes with the mesial marginal ridge of the mandibular second molar.

The mesiolingual cusp of the maxillary first molar occludes in the central fossa of the mandibular first molar.

The buccal cusps of the maxillary premolars have a cusp-embrasure relationship with the mandibular premolars.

The lingual cusps of the maxillary premolars have a cusp-fossa relationship with the mandibular premolars.

The maxillary canine has a cusp-embrasure relationship with the mandibular canine and first premolar. The tip of its cusp is slightly mesial to the embrasure.

The maxillary incisors overlap the mandibular incisors, and the midlines of the arches match.

Key Ⅱ ; crown angulation(Figure 16-43)

The angle formed by the facial axis of the clinical crown(FACC)and a line perpendicular to the occlusal plane.

Crown angulation is considered positive when the occlusal portion of the FACC is mesial to the gingival portion, negative when distal.

Essentially all crowns in the sample have a positive angulation. All crowns of each tooth type are similar in the amount of angulation.

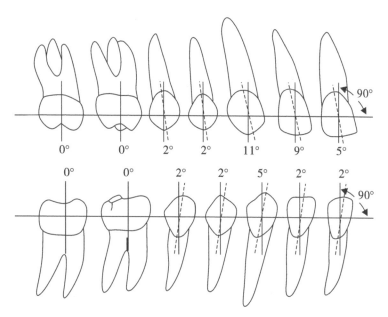

Figure 16-43 **Crown angulation**

Key Ⅲ: crown inclination(Figure 16-44)

Crown inclination which the angle between a line perpendicular to the occlusal plane and a line that is parallel and tangent to the FACC at its midpoint (the FA point) is determined from the mesial or distal perspective. It is sometimes incorrectly called torque, which means a twisting force. Crown inclination is considered positive if the occlusal portion of the crown, tangent line, or FACC is facial to its gingival portion, negative if lingual.

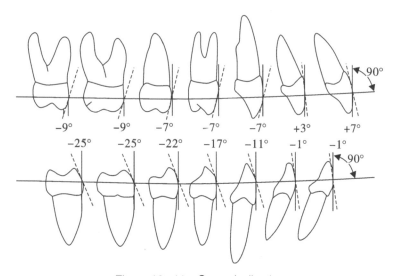

Figure 16-44 **Crown inclination**

As they do in angulation, consistent patterns also prevail in crown inclination, with the following characteristics for individual teeth.

Most maxillary incisors(81.5%)have a positive inclination; mandibular incisors have a slightly negative inclination. In most of the optimal sample, the interincisal crown angle is less than 180. The crowns of maxillary incisors are more positively inclined, relative to a line 90° to the occlusal plane, than the mandibular incisors are negatively inclined to the same line.

The inclinations of the maxillary incisor crowns are generally positive—the centrals more positive than the laterals. Canines and premolars are negative and quite similar. The inclinations of the maxillary first and second molars are also similar and negative, but slightly more negative than those of the canines and premolars. The molars are more negative because they are measured from the groove instead of from the promonent facial ridge, from which the canines and premolars are measured.

The inclinations of the mandibular crowns are progressively more negative from the incisors through the second molars.

Key IV : rotations

The fourth key to optimal occlusion is an absence of tooth rotations.

Key V : tight Contacts

Contact points should abound unless a discrepancy exists in mesiodostal crownd diameter.

Key VI : curve of spee

The depth of the curve of Spee ranges from a plane to a slightly concave surface.

Andrews developed bracket modifications for specific teeth, to eliminate the many repetitive bends in archwires that were necessary to compensate for differences in tooth anatomy. The result was the "straight wire" appliance. This was the key step in improving the efficiency of the edgewise appliance. In Angle's terminology for his appliance, first – order bends were used to compensate for differences in tooth thickness, second – order bends to position roots correctly in a mesio – distal direction, and third – order (torque) bends to position roots in a facio–lingual direction. All the bends have to be built into the archwire by the clinician. But as the name suggests, in the pre–adjusted edgewise appliance (PAE) all these are built into the brackets or the appliance.

Compensations for first–order bends (Figure 16 – 45). For anterior teeth and premolars, varying the bracket thickness eliminates in–out bends in the anterior portions of each archwire, but an offset position of molar tubes is necessary to prevent molar rotation. For good occlusion, the buccal surface must sit at an angle to the line of occlusion, with the mesio–buccal cusp more prominent than the disto–buccal cusp. For this reason, the tube or bracket specified for the upper molar should have at least a 10 – degree offset, as should the tube for the upper second molar. The offset for the lower first molar should be 5–7 degrees, about half as much as for the upper molar. The offset for the lower second molar should be at least as large as for the first molar.

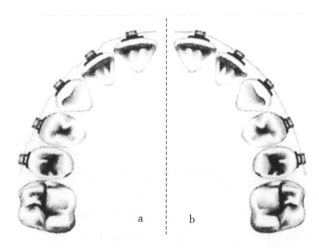

Figure 16–45   **First-order bends**
a : Edgewise ; b : Straight wire.

Compensations for second−order bends(Figure 16−46). In the original edgewise appliance, second−order bends, sometimes called artistic positioning bends, were an important part of the finishing phase of treatment. These bends were necessary because the long axis of each tooth is inclined relative to the plane of a continuous archwire. Contemporary edgewise brackets have a built−in tip for maxillary incisor teeth, which varies among the appliances that are now available. A distal tip of the upper first molar is also needed to obtain good interdigition of the posterior teeth. If the upper molar is too vertically upright, even though a proper Class Ⅰ relationship apparently exists, good interdigition can not be achieved. Tipping the molar distally brings its distal cusps into occlusion and creates the space needed for proper relationships of the premolars.

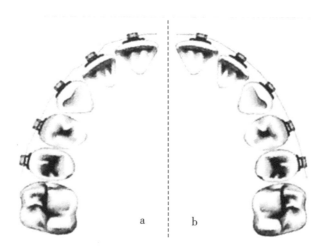

a   b

Figure 16−46   **Second−order bends**

Compensation for third−order bends (Figure 16−47). If the bracket for a rectangular archwire is placed flat against the labial or buccal surface of any tooth, the plane of the bracket slot will twist away from the horizontal, often to a considerable extent. With the original edgewise appliance, it was necessary to place a twist in each rectangular archwire to compensate for this. Failure to place third−order bends meant that in the anterior region, the teeth would become too upright, while posteriorly the buccal cusps of molars would be depressed and the lingual cusps elevated. Cutting the bracket slot into the bracket at an angle, which is called placing torque in the bracket, allows a horizontally flat rectangular archwire to be placed into the bracket slots without incorporating twist bends.

Based on the "prescription", i. e., the in out, tip and torque values—various clinicians have brought out various PAE systems. Andrew proposed the first prescription for the PEA and called it the straight wire appliance. In fact, Andrew created various prescription based on the malocclusion, extractions and the underlying skeletal structure of the patient. He advocated the placement of brackets on the Andrew's plane, which is the plane or surface on which the mid−transverse plane of every crown in an arch will fall when the teeth are ideally positioned.

Figure 16−45 Compensations for first−order bends. Varying the pre−adjusted edgewise appliance bracket thickness eliminates in−out bends in the original edgewise wires.

Figure 16−46 Compensations for second−order bends. Pre−adjusted edgewise brackets have a built−in tip for each teeth, which varies among the appliances that are now available.

Figure 16−47 Compensation for third−order bends. Pre−adjusted edgewise cutting the bracket slot into the bracket at an angle, which is called placing torque in the bracket, allows a horizontally flat rectangular archwire to be placed into the bracket slots without incorporating twist bends.

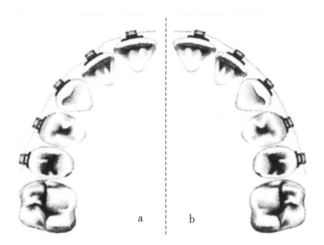

Figure 16-47　**Third-order bends**

● Roth system

Roth modified the tip and torque values of his prescription making a series which was common for extraction and non-extraction cases.

● MBT system

In the early 1990s, Drs. Richard McLaughlin, John Bennett and Hugo Trevisi collaborated with 3M to develop the MBT Versatile+Appliance System. Combining the doctors' decades of clinical experience with 3M's legacy of quality and innovation, the result was a set of integrated tools and methods based on a set of fundamental concepts:

Improving the values of pre-adjusted appliances. Over the previous two decades, pre-adjusted appliances had become widely accepted globally over standard edgewise brackets, yet all systems were based on the research and techniques available at the time that Andrews published *The Six Keys to Normal Occlusion* in 1972. The MBT system updates the tip and torque values based on further research.

Customizing archwire selection to patient need. The shape of the arch form, the material type and archform size can be selected based on the treatment need for the patient. The MBT system equips doctors with tools and information on how to choose archwires that best meet the patient's situation at each stage of movement.

Assisting the accurate vertical placement of brackets. The visual cues traditionally used to properly orient brackets are frequently deceptive. The MBT system (Figure 16 – 48) provides a quantitative means to consistently arrive at a more effective vertical placement.

Using light-force, sliding mechanics. Anchorage control can be achieved early in treatment, and does not have to be sacrificed to achieve other movement goals. The MBT system offers a number of techniques to achieve treatment goals effectively (Table 16-1).

①Improving the values of pre-adjusted appliances, and updates the tip, torque, offset values based on further research. ②Laceback. ③Cinch back. ④Using light-force, sliding mechanics.

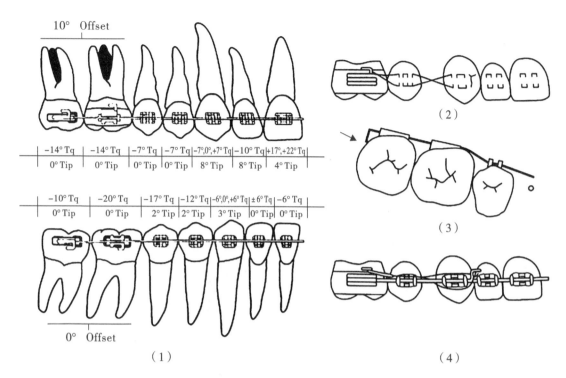

Figure 16-48 **The MBT system**

(1) Pre-adjusted appliances; (2) Laceback; (3) Cinch bock; (4) Sliding mechanic.

Table 16-1 **Three systems' summary of values**

	Maxillary									
	Central		Lateral		Canine		1st Premolar		2nd Premola	
	Torque	Tip	Torque	Tip	Torque	Tip	Torque	Tip	Torque	Tip
Andrews	7	5	3	9	−7	11	−7	2	−7	2
Roth	12	5	8	9	−2	9	−7	0	−7	0
MBT	17	4	10	8	−7	8	−7	0	−7	0
	Mandibular									
	Central		Lateral		Canine		1st Premolar		2nd Premola	
	Torque	Tip	Torque	Tip	Torque	Tip	Torque	Tip	Torque	Tip
Andrews	−1	2	−1	2	−11	5	−17	2	−22	2
Roth	0	0	0	0	−11	7	−17	0	−22	0
MBT	−6	0	−6	0	−6	3	−12	2	−17	2
	Maxillary									
	1st Molar			2nd Molar						
	Torque	Tip	Rotation	Torque	Tip	Rotation				
Andrews	−9	5	10	−9	0	10				
Roth	−14	0	14	−14	0	14				
MBT	−14	0	10	−14	0	10				

Continue to Table 16-1

	Mandibular					
	1st Molar			2nd Molar		
	Torque	Tip	Rotation	Torque	Tip	Rotation
Andrews	-25	2	0	-30	0	0
Roth	-30	1	4	-30	0	4
MBT	-20	0	0	-10	0	0

5) Tip-edge appliance

The Tip-edge appliance (Figure 16-49) was developed from the Begg appliance with the aim of combining the advantages of both the straight wire and the Begg systems. Named after its originator, the Begg appliance was based on the use of round wire which fitted fairly loosely into a channel at the top of the bracket. Light forces were used and tipping movements, with apical and rotational movement achieved by means of auxiliary springs or by loops placed in the archwire. However, the main drawback to the Begg system was difficult to position the teeth precisely at the end of treatment. There was also a height-

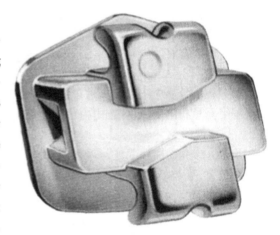

Figure 16-49　**Tip-edge plus bracket**

ened awareness of the advantages of the rectangular wire finish which provided the three-dimensional control of each individual tooth.

The advent of the tip edge bracket by Peter C Kesling, was a step in this direction. The Tip-edge bracket, allows tipping of the tooth in the initial stages of treatment when round archwires are employed, as in the Begg technique, but when full-sized rectangular archwires are used in the latter stages, the built-in pre-adjustments help to give a better degree of control of final tooth positioning.

The Tip-edge appliance may not be the most popular appliance today but it has certainly provided an opportunity to both Begg and edgewise practitioners to come closer, to a common more versatile appliance system.

6) Ceramic brackets

These were first made available commercially in the late 1980s, largely overcome the esthetic limitations of plastic brackets in that they are quite durable and resist staining. In addition, they can be custom-molded for individual teeth and are dimensionally stable, so that the precise bracket angulations and slots of the straight-wire appliance can be incorporated. Several different types of ceramic brackets currently are available.

Ceramic brackets were received enthusiastically and immediately achieved widespread use, but problems with fractures of brackets, friction within bracket slots, wear on teeth contacting a bracket, and enamel damage from brackets removal soon became apparent. Fractures of ceramic brackets occur in two ways: loss of part of the brackets (e. g. , tie wings) during archwire changes or eating, and cracking of the bracket when torque forces are applied. Ceramics are a form of glass, and like glass, ceramic brackets tend to be brittle. Because the fracture toughness of steel is much greater, ceramic brackets must be bulkier than stainless steel brackets, and the ceramic design is much closer to a single wide bracket than is usual in steel.

Most currently—available ceramic brackets are produced from alumina, either as single—crystal or poly-crystalline units. In theory, single—crystal brackets should offer greater strength, which is true until the bracket surface is scratched. At that point, the small surface crack tends to spread, and fracture resistance is reduced to or below the level of the polycrystalline materials. Scratches, of course, are likely to occur during the course of treatment.

7) Self—ligating brackets

Placing wire ligatures around tie wings on brackets to hold archwires in the bracket slot is a time—consuming procedure. The elastomeric modules introduced in the 1970s largely replaced wire ligatures for two reasons: they are quicker and easier to place, and they can be used in chains to close small spaces within the arch or prevent spaces from opening.

It also is possible to use a cap or clip, attached over the bracket or built into the bracker itself, to hold wires in position. Three types of self—ligating mechanisms (Figure 16-50) built into the bracket are available at present (with more probably on the way) : a springy latching cap, springy retaining bracket walls, and rigid latching caps. The principal advantage is a reduction of friction between the wire and bracket because the archwire is not pressed against the base of the bracket, as it is by a wire ligature or elastomeric module. This makes it easier to slide teeth along the archwire as spaces are opened or closed. Easier placement and removal of archwires may or may not be a secondary benefit, depending on how user—friendly the design is. However, what is an advantage for sliding is a disadvantage for frictionless space closure. The springy clips of both types may not hold a wire in place well enough to deliver adequate moments to prevent tipping when closing loops are used, and with rigid clips, it can be quite difficult to completely engage full—dimension wires in the finishing stage of treatment.

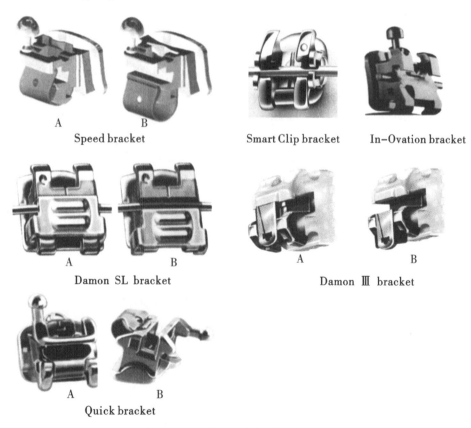

A   B
Speed bracket

Smart Clip bracket

In—Ovation bracket

A   B
Damon SL bracket

A   B
Damon Ⅲ bracket

A   B
Quick bracket

Figure 16-50   Self—ligating bracket

8) Individually customized brackets

Because of the marked individual variations in the contour of the teeth, no appliance prescription can be optimal for all patients, and compensatory bends in finishing archwires often are necessary. Custom brackets for the facial surface of teeth offer the prospect of eliminating almost all archwire bending, i. e. , they could provide the perfect straight wire appliance.

Whether custom brackets are to be made for the facial or lingual surfaces, the technology is much the same. The first step is a 3 - dimensional digital scan of casts of the patient's teeth on a laboratory bench, using a laser beam with a resolution at least as good as 50 microns. The current approach to custom labial brackets is to precisely cut each bracket using CAD-CAM technology, so that the base of each bracket is contoured for a particular place on the surface of a particular tooth, and the slot for each bracket has the appropriate thickness, inclination and torque needed for ideal positioning of that tooth. Using such brackets, it would be possible to place a sequence of a minimal number of archwires, each selected for optimal performance, so that treatment time would be minimized for the doctor and treatment duration minimized for the patient. The technology now exists to produce such brackets from laboratory or intraoral laser scans, with a 2-3 week turnaround time.

Individual custom brackets must be attached to the teeth with precision equal to that used in making them—so an indirect bonding system with an accurate placement template is required. What happens when one of the custom brackets is lost and requires replacement and rebonding, or is loose and requires rebonding? Because the specifications for each bracket can be maintained in computer memory, it is possible to obtain a replacement bracket within 2-3 weeks (but of course not instantaneously), and a secondary template can be provided with it. Rebonding a loose bracket is done most efficiently by using the original bonding template, which should be kept with the patient's records for this possible re-use.

9) Lingual appliances

A major objection to fixed orthodontic appliances always has their visible placement on the facial surface of the teeth. This is one reason for using removable appliances, and then is the major reason for the current popularity of clear aligners in treatment of adults. The introduction of bonding in the 1970s made it possible to place fixed attachments on the lingual surface of teeth to provide an invisible fixed appliance. Brackets designed for the lingual surface were first offered soon after bonding was introduced. Although it is possible to obtain the same 3-dimension control of crown and root position from the lingual surface as the labial, the difficulty, duration and cost of treatment are all significantly increased. In the United States, most orthodontists who experimented with the lingual appliances available in the 1980s abandoned this appliance as more trouble than it was worth, lingual appliance (Figure 16-51) treatment all but disappeared until quite recently.

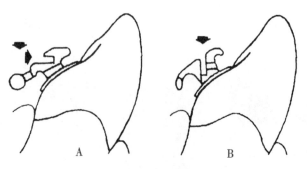

Figure 16-51　Lingual bracket

A : Horizontal slot ; B : Vertical slot.

Recent progress in Europe has made lingual orthodontics much more widely used there. One successful European approach is to fabricate a custom precious metal pad that covers as much as possible of the lingual surface of each tooth, and then attach low-profile brackets to the custom pads. These brackets, designed so the archwire can be inserted from the tops, are the same for each tooth, so eliminating wire bending is not a major goal with this approach. Computer-controlled wire bending devices are particulaly applicable to the fabrication of the lingual archwires and are a part of the more advanced applications of lingual techniques.

(2) Practical procedures

Accurate bracket placement is crucial to achieving success with fixed appliances. The "correct" position of the bracket on the facial surface will depend upon the bracket system used. Most pre-adjusted systems require the bracket to be placed in the middle of the tooth along the long axis of the clinical crown. Bracket placement is particularly important with the pre-adjusted technique, as the values for tip and torque are calculated for the midpoint of the facial surface of the tooth. Incorrect bracket positioning will lead to incorrect tooth position and ultimately affect the functional and aesthetic result; therefore errors in bracket placement should be corrected as early as possible in the treatment. Alternatively, adjustments can be made to each archwire to compensate, but over the course of a treatment this can be time-consuming.

When a fixed appliance is first placed a flexible archwire is advisable to avoid applying excessive forces to displaced teeth, which can be painful for the patient and result in bond failure. Usually, a round, pre-formed nickel titanium archwire is used to achieve initial alignment.

It is important to move on form these initial aligning archwire as soon as alignment is achieved, as by virtue of their flexibility they do not afford much control of tooth position. However, it is equally important to ensure that full bracket engagement has been achieved before proceeding to a more rigid archwire. Correction of inter-arch relationships and space closure is usually best carried out using rectangular wires for apical control. The exact archwire sequence will depend upon the dimensions of the archwire slot and operator preference.

Adjustments to the appliance need to be made on a regular basis, usually every 6-10 weeks. Once space closure is complete and incisor position corrected, some operators will place a more flexible full-sized archwire, often in conjunction with vertical elastic traction, to help "sock-in" the buccal occlusion.

Following the attainment of the goals of treatment it is important to retain the finished result.

When treating cases with the pre-adjusted edgewise appliance, the management can be divided into six distinct yet overlapping stages:

1) Anchorage control: Anchorage control can be achieved using intraoral means like transpalatal arches or Nance palatal button, etc., or extraoral means, e. g., head gears.

2) Leveling and aligning: Leveling and aligning is done with light continuous force wires like, nickel titanium alloy wires sequentially increasing in stiffness and diameter.

3) Overbite control: Overbite control is achieved using utility arches or wires with a reverse curve of Spee. Molar extrusion might even be achieved using headgears.

4) Overjet reduction.

5) Space closures: Overjet reduction and space closures are accomplished with the help of elastics, closed coil springs or elastic modules, or elastic chains or loops incorporated into the arch wire.

6) Finishing and detailing: Finishing and detailing involves the use of stiff rectangular stainless steel wires with or without the use of artistic bends.

The stages are sequential in their order, with the effective management of one stage being a prerequisite for the successful completion of the next stage.

A retention sequence follows, once all corrections have been achieved to satisfaction. Retention appliances are a must whatever the appliance chosen for treatment.

16.4.4.4 Orthopedic appliance

A disproportion in the size or position of the jaws result in a skeletal discrepancy in either the sagittal, coronal or transverse plane. The three approaches to management of a skeletal problem are-growth modification, camouflage treatment, and surgical correction. Growth modification is, by far, the best option if possible. Growth modification helps in altering the expression, direction and magnitude of growth, thus bringing about favorable jaw growth.

"Orthopedic therapy" is aimed at the correction of skeletal imbalance with the correction of any dentoalveolar malocclusion being of less importance, in which little or no tooth movement is desired. Therefore, orthopedic forces are heavier(=400 g) when compared to orthodontic forces(50–100 g).

Orthopedic appliances make use of the teeth as a "handle" to tramit forces to the underlying skeletal structures. Forces in excess of 400 gm should be applied to bring about favorable skeletal change. Orthopedic appliances are most effective during the mixed dentition period as it takes advantage of the prepubertal growth spurt. However, treatment should be maintained till growth is complete as these appliances change only the expression of growth and not the underlying growth pattern, which may later reassert.

Orthopedic appliances included headgear, facemask and chin cup.

(1) Headgear

Headgears(Figure 16–52) are the most common among all the orthopedic appliances. They are ideally indicated in patients with excessive horizontal growth of the maxilla with or without vertical changes along with some protrusion of the maxillary teeth, reasonably good mandibular dental and skeletal morphology. They are most effective in the prepubertal period. Headgears can also be used to distalize the maxillary dentition along with the maxilla. They are an important adjunct to gain or maintain anchorage.

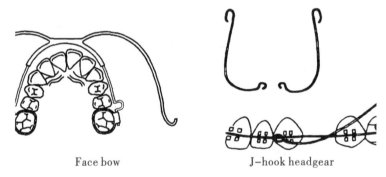

Face bow   J–hook headgear

Figure 16–52 **Headgear**

1) Cervical headgear: the anchor unit in this headgear is the nape of the neck. It causes extrusion and distalization of the molars along with distal movement of the maxilla(Figure 16–53).

2) Occipital headgear: derives anchorage from the occipital region, i. e. , back of the head. It produces distal translation of the molar. Sometimes a slight superior component of force may also be seen (Figure 16–54).

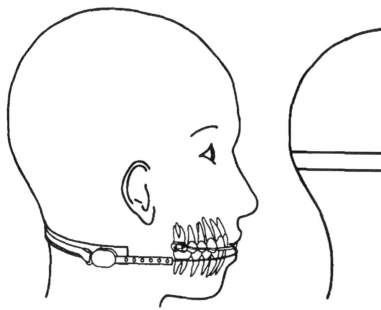

Figure 16-35 **Cervical headgear**

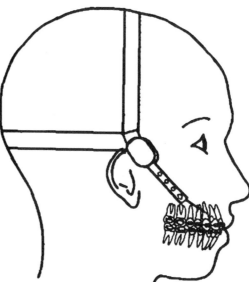

Figure 16-54 **Occipital headgear**

3) High pull headgear: deriving anchorage from the parietal region, i. e., front of the head it produces intrusion and distalization of teeth.

4) Combination pull headgear: derives anchorage from at least two regions, i. e., the neck and occiput. It causes a distal and slightly superior force on the maxilla and dentition(Figure 16-55).

(1)Treatment effects

1) Skeletal effect: the maxillary sutures namely the frontomaxillary, zygomaticotemporal, zygomaticomaxillary and pterygopalatine sutures are the most important growth sites for development of maxilla. Therefore, to alter the maxillary growth, the headgears act by compressing the sutures thus restricting the normal downward and forward growth of the maxilla, while at the same time the mandible is allowed to grow normally.

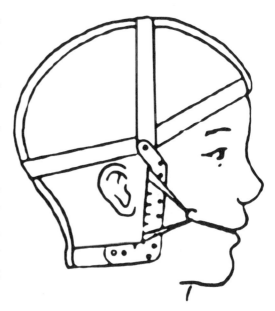

Figure 16-55 **Combination pull headgear**

2)Dental effect: headgear being a tooth-borne appliance, produces certain dental effects along with a skeletal change. Headgears usually cause distalization of the maxillary molars. Along with this, extrusion or intrusion of the molar may also be seen if the extroral attachment is cervical or occipital respectively. In most skeletal Class II problems a cervical headgear is not desired as the extrusion of the maxillary molar caused by the inferiorly directed force which causes downward and backward mandibular rotation, thus worsening the problem.

(2)Uses of Headgear

1)To restrain the forward and downward growth of the maxilla and redirectioning maxillary growth.

2)Molar distalization: headgear may be used to distalize the maxillary molar to correct the Class II molar relationship or to gain space for relief of crowding.

3）Headgears can be used to reinforce molar anchorage in high anchorage a minimum force of 300 gm per side.

4）Headgear is an effective means of maintaining arch length by preventing mesial migration of molars.

5）Molar rotation can also be brought about with the inner bow of the headgear.

3.2.4.2　Facemask

Class Ⅲ malocclusion is usually a result of a combination of maxillary deficiency and mandibular excess. Growth modification for Class Ⅲ problems is the reverse of Class Ⅱ, i. e. , treatment involves restriction of mandibular growth along with downward and forward maxillary growth. When headgear applies a distal force to the maxilla, compression of the maxillary sutures can inhibit forward maxillary growth. Likewise, pulling the maxilla forward and separating the sutures should stimulate forward growth of the maxilla. Headgears which cause a forward pull on the maxilla are, therefore, called reverse pull headgear. Facemask, popularized by Delaire in 1970 s is one of the most common reverse pull headgears in use today. A facemask works on the principle of pulling the maxillary structures forward with the help of anchorage from the chin or forehead or usually both. A forward maxillary pull is applied with the help of heavy elastics that are attached to hooks on the rigid framework.

（1）Indications

1）Mild to moderate Class Ⅲ skeletal malocclusion due to maxillary retrusion, reverse pull headgear works best in young, growing children(around 8 years).

2）Ideal patients for facemask should have normal or retrusive but not protrusive maxillary teeth as facemask causes forward movement of the maxillary teeth relative to the maxilla. Short or normal, but not long, anterior vertical facial dimensions, i. e. , a hypodivergent growth pattern.

3）Correction of postsurgical relapse after osteotomies.

4）Selective rearrangement of palatal shelves in cleft patients.

（2）Parts of a facemask

Usually, a facemask is made up of the following components(Figure 16-56):

1）Metal framework.

2）Chin cup/pad.

3）Forehead cap.

4）Intraoral appliance.

5）Heavy elastics.

The reverse pull headgear is made up of a rigid extraoral framework connecting two pads that contact the soft tissues in the forehead and chin regions. The pads are usually adjustable through the use of screws. The elastics are attached to an adjustable anterior wire with hooks which is connected to the framework. Anchorage is usually derived from both chin and forehead, however, some forms of reverse pull headgears derive anchorage from only chin or forehead. Two sites of anchorage have the advantage that anchorage is spread over a larger area thus reducing the amount of force exerted. Along with the facemask, banded or bonded palatal expansion appliance may also be used to correct cross bites. To resist tooth movement, it is better to splint the maxillary teeth together as a single unit. Whatever the maxillary appliance, it should have hooks in the canine-primary molar region above the occlusal level for attachment of elastics. This places the force vector closer to the center of resistance of the maxilla and helps in pure forward translation.

The heavy elastics apply a forward traction on the upper arch. Elastics attached from the vertical posts of the chin cup to the molar tubes or soldered hooks can bring about tooth movement.

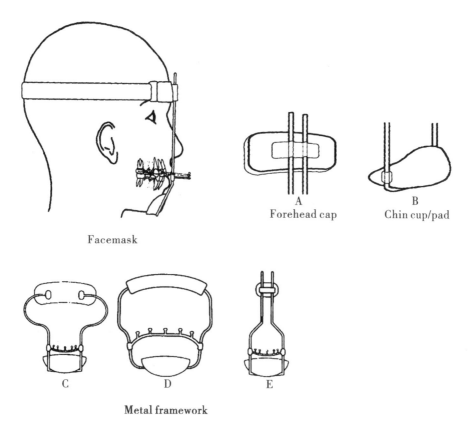

Facemask

A
Forehead cap

B
Chin cup/pad

C   D   E

Metal framework

Figure 16-56   Components of framework

16.4.4.5   Chin cup

It is an extraoral orthopedic device, which is useful in the treatment of Class Ⅲ malocclusions that occurs due to a protrusive mandible but a relatively normal maxilla. Chin cup therapy attempts to retard or redirect the growth of the mandible in order to obtain a better anteroposterior relation between the two jaws.

Mandible grows by apposition of bone at the condyle and along its free posterior border. Condyle is not a growth center and condylar growth is largely a response to translation of surrounding tissues. This contemporary view offers a more optimistic view of the possibilities for growth restraint of the mandible, as with chin cup therapy.

The chin cup(Figure 16-57) is an extraoral appliance that utilizes a head cap, which is firmly fitted/ seated on the posterosuperior aspects of the cranium as anchorage and has attachments for the placement and activation of the chin cup. It consists of the following:

Force module: elastic/metal spring that provides the desired tension levels on the chin cup.

Chin cup: custom made or preformed, hard or soft. A hard chin cup can be custom made from plastic using a chin impression. A soft cup can be made from a football helmet chinstrap. A commercial metal or plastic cup can be used if it fits well enough. Soft cups produce more tooth movement than hard ones.

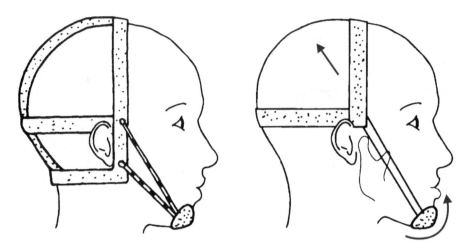

Figure 16-57 Chin cup

Wang Gaofang , Huang Min

Chapter 17

Dentomaxillofacial Deformities and Orthognathic Surgery

17.1 Introduction

Dentomaxillofacial deformity is a term that refers to the significant deviations from normal morphologies and sizes of the jaws, the discrepancy in positions of the jaws as they relate to each other and to the upper facial skeleton, the accompanied malocclusion and compromise in oral and maxillofacial functions and facial ethics. The relative functions include breathing, swallowing, talking and chewing.

Orthognathic surgery is a branch of oral and maxillofacial surgery that focused on the diagnosis and surgical treatment of dentomaxllofacial deformities to restore the proper anatomic and functional relationship of the jaws. The term "orthognathic" comes from the Greek words "orthos" meaning straighten and "gnathic" meaning of or related to the jaw. Hence the term orthognathic, meaning "straighten the jaw."

Although the first anterior mandibular dento-alveolar segmental osteotomy was performed in 1849, until 1970's, William H. Bell carried out a series of experimental studies, which confirmed the biologic basis for standard orthognathic procedures and promoted the development of orthognathic surgery. With the rapid development of orthodontic treatment, combined orthodontic and orthognathic surgical approach has been a standard treatment strategy for severe dentomaxillofacial deformities.

17.2 Etiology

17.2.1 Congenital factors

17.2.1.1 Hereditary factors

The craniofacial morphology is controlled by genetics and characterized by ethnic and familial features. Dentomaxillofacial deformities could be caused by genetic factors, such as maxillary protrusion, mandibular retraction, can be expressed as parental inheritance or intergenerational inheritance. Congenital anomalies, from syndromic conditions such as Apert and Crouzon syndromes to facial clefts, affect normal growth and development.

17.2.1.2 Abnormal embryonic development

Certain teratogenic factors could cause the abnormal embryonic development of the craniofacial region, such as malnutrition, endocrine disorders, infection, and drug effects. For example, the 6–7th week of embryonic development phase, cleft palate can occur, usually accompanied with maxillary malformation, and orthognathic surgery is often needed to correct the skeletal deformity.

17.2.2 Acquired factors

17.2.2.1 Systemic diseases

Some metabolic and endocrine diseases in childhood can lead to developmental abnormalities in the maxillofacial region, such as rickets and pituitary diseases.

Rickets is a dystrophic disease caused by insufficient vitamin D resulting in abnormal calcium and phosphorus metabolism. Calcium and phosphorus can not be deposited properly in the bone growth site and then bone deformation occured. In the maxillofacial region, narrowed maxillary dental arch, crowded anterior teeth, open bite, insufficient height of the mandibular ramus are often expressed.

Pituitary disease could lead to excessive or insufficient production of growth hormone, the jaws could appear as excess or deficiency deformities relevantly.

17.2.2.2 Abnormal habits

Abnormal habit during the childhood might affect the growth and development of jaws and result in dentomaxillofacial deformities and other dysfunctions. For example, thumb sucking persisting over 6 years old is strongly associated with the development of open bite malocclusion in mixed dentition or permanent dentition. But it is not every child who has such a habit will develop open bite. When the thumb is put between the upper and lower dentions, the teeth might be forced to show a circular gap, the cheeks might be contracted to press and narrow the dental arches. The upper anterior teeth might protrude and an inadequate lip seal might present. If the habit is not released in time, it will lead to maxillary protrusion and mandibular retraction.

17.2.2.3 Oral and maxillofacialtrauma and infection

In infants, children and adolescents, trauma to the craniofacial skeleton might disturb the growth potential of the jaws. Proliferating cartilage at the base of the fibrocartilage layer that covers the articular surface results in mandibular growth. Damage to one or both of the temporomandibular joints might lead to ankylosis of the temporomandibular joints and in consequence induce severe mandibular deficiency. Infant osteomyelitis of jaws can damage the bone, which could lead to facial deformities.

17.2.2.4 Tumors

The common tumor causing jaw deformity is osteoma of condyle. Condylar osteoma may cause a progressive change in the patient's occlusion with a deviation of the midline of the chin towards the opposite side. The most common clinical manifestations are malocclusion, facial asymmetry and temporomandibular joint dysfunction.

17.3   Clinical Classification

17.3.1   Congenital deformities

Congenital dentomaxillofacial deformities can be grouped into following categories according to the abnormal positions of the maxilla and/or the mandible.

17.3.1.1   Deformities in relation to anteroposterior direction

Maxillary prognathism.

Maxillary retrognathism.

Mandibular prognathism.

Mandibular retrognathism.

Maxillary prognathism and mandibular retrognathism.

Maxillary retrognathism and mandibular prognathism.

Bimaxillary prognathism.

Chin retrognathism.

17.3.1.2   Deformities in relation to vertical direction

Long face symdrome with/without open bite.

Short face syndrome with long ramus/with short ramus.

17.3.1.3   Deformities in relation to transverse direction

Mandibular deviation.

Hemifacial microsomia.

Hemifacial hyperplasia.

Hemifacial atrophy.

Unilateral condylar hyperplasia.

Unilateral condylar osteochondroma.

17.3.1.4   Occlusal deformities

Anterior open bite.

Anterior crossbite.

Posterior open bite.

Posterior closed bite.

17.3.2   Secondary dentomaxillofacial deformities

Deformities secondary to:

Temporomandibular joint ankylosis.

Oral and maxillofacial bone fractures.

Oral and maxillofacial neoplasia.

17.3.3   Craniofacial syndrome

Apert syndrome.

Crouzon syndrome.

Treacher—collins syndrome.

17.4 Clinical Examination and Diagnosis

17.4.1 Clinical examination

17.4.1.1 Frontal examination

Facial symmetry, horizontal and vertical proportions of the face, morphologies of the lip and nose, and the relationship between the teeth, gingiva and lip(the incisor exposure) should be assessed from the frontal view.

17.4.1.2 Lateral examination

The protrusion of the jaws, the canting of the mandible, the protrusion of the chin, the morphology and soft tissue thickness of the lip, the chin depth, the nasolabial angle, the morphology of the paranasal areas, etc. , should be assessed from the lateral view. Normally, the nasolabial angle is from 90°to 110°.

17.4.1.3 TMJ examination

The movement, tenderness, clicking and noise of the condyle could be assessed by palpation in front of the bilateral tragi simultaneously with two index fingers, while the patient keeps opening and closing the mouth. The extent of maximum opening should also be recorded.

17.4.1.4 Intraoral examination

The shape, size and number of teeth, whether or not periodontal lesions exist, the form of dental arch, the coordination between upper and lower arches, whether the midline is aligned, the alignment of teeth, the sagittal and vertical relationship and whether the sagittal and transverse curve of occlusion is normal or not should be examined.

17.4.2 Cephalometric analysis

Cephalometric analysis is an important part for the orthognathic treatment planning. It enables the surgeon to classify and quantify the dentofacial deformities, creating a treatment plan via a visual treatment objective(VTO) , study specific changes after the surgery and during the follow—up.

The cephalometric radiograph must be taken with the patient's head in a reproducible position with the aid of a craniostat, so that the radiographs are standardized and each radiograph of the same person at different time could be compared.

Cephalometric analysis involves various linear, angular and proportion measurements of the hard and soft tissue structures of the face.

Cephalometric landmarks: these landmarks should be easy to locate and stable. The commonly used landmarks are as follows(Table 17-1, Figure 17-1).

Table 17-1　The commonly used landmarks in orthognathic surgery

Classification	Abbreviation	Full name	Definition
Cranial landmarks	S.	Sella	The geometric center of the pituitary fossa
	N.	Nasion	The most anterior point on the frontonasal suture in the midsagittal plane
Bony landmarks of the jaws	P.	Porion	The most superiorly positioned point of the external auditory meatus
	Or.	Orbitale	The lowest point on the inferior rim of the orbit
	ANS.	Anterior nasalspine	The anterior tip of the sharp bony process of the maxilla at the lower margin of the anterior nasal opening
	PNS.	Posterior nasalspine	The posterior spine of the palatine bone constituting the hard palate
	A.	Subspinale	The most posterior midline point in the concavity between the ANS and the prosthion(the most inferior point on the alveolar bone overlying in the maxillary incisors)
	Go.	Gonion	A point on the curvature of the angle of the mandible located by bisecting the angle formed by lines tangent to the posterior ramus and the inferior border of the mandible
	B.	Supramental	The most posterior midline point in the concavity between the most superior point on the alveolar bone overlying the mandibular incisors(infradentale) and Pog
Soft tissue landmarks	Gs.	Glabella of soft tissue	The most prominent anterior point in the mid sagittal plane of the forehead
	Ns.	Nasion of soft tissue	The point of the greatest concavity in the midline between the forehead and the nose
	Prn.	Pronasale	The most prominent or anterior point of the nose(tip of the nose)
	Sn.	Subnasale	The point at which the columella(nasal septum)merges with the upper lip in the midsagittal plane
	UL.	Upper lip (labrale superius)	The point indicating the most anterior point of the upper lip
	LL.	Lower lip (labrale inferius)	The point indicating the most anterior point of the lower lip
	Pgs.	Pogonion of soft tissue	The most protruding point of the soft tissue chin contour
	Gns.	Gnathion of soft tissue	A point located by taking the midpoint between the anterior(pogonion of soft tissue)and inferior(menton of soft tissue)points of the chin
	Mes.	Menton of soft tissue	Lowest point on the contour of the soft issue chin. Found by dropping a perpendicular from horizontal plane through skeletal menton

Planes: some landmarks could indicate planes. The planes could be divided into two kind: the reference planes and the measurement planes. The planes commonly used in the cephalometry are as follows(Table 17-2, Figure 17-2).

Table 17-2   The commonly used planes

Classification	Abbreviation	Full name	Composition points
Reference planes	FH plane	Frankfort horizontal plane	Or. and P.
	SN plane	SN plane	S. and N.
Measurement planes	PP.	Patatal plane	ANS. and PNS.
	OP.	Occlusal plane	The midpoint of U6 and L6, and the midpoint of UI. and LI.
	MP.	Mandibular plane	Go. and Gn.

Measurement items: the most commonly used measurement items in orthognathic surgery are as follows (Table 17-3, Figure 17-2).

Table 17-3   Clinical classification

Classification	Items	Implication
Hard tissue angles	SNA(S-N-A)	The relationship between maxilla and skull base
	SNB(S-N-B)	The relationship between mandible and skull base
	ANB(A-N-B)	The relationship between maxilla and mandible
Soft tissue distances	Gs-Mes	The whole face height
	Gs-Sn	The upper face height
	Sn-Mes	The lower face height
	Sn-Stoms	The upper lip height
	Stoms-Mes	The height of lower lip and chin

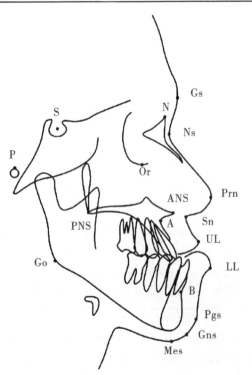

Figure 17-1   Commonly used landmarks

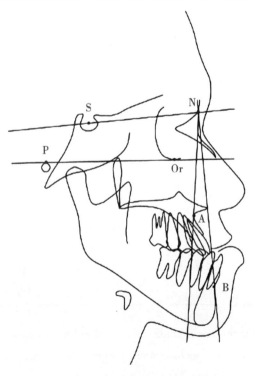

Figure 17-2   Commonly used plans and angels(FH, SN, ∠SNA, ∠SNB, ∠ANB)

17.4.3 Diagnosis

Diagnosis is based on a comprehensive assessment that includes clinical examination, skeletal evaluation with standardized radiographs, and dental evaluation. Only by collecting the appropriate data, can the accurate diagnosis be obtained and then can the patient be treated appropriately(Table 17-3).

17.5 Treatment Design

Correct diagnosis is the basic of corrective treatment design. Once a patient has been determined to be a candidate for orthognathic surgery, the treatment plan should be appropriately established according to the classification and severity of deformities. The aim of a logistic treatment plan is to achieve satisfying facial and dental aesthetics, functional and stable occlusion. Good communication should be carried out to ensure the plan suits the patient's need.

The treatment plan for dentomaxillofacial deformity should include three key phases: presurgical orthodontics, orthognathic surgery, postsurgical orthodontics.

17.5.1 Presurgical and postsurgical veorthodontic treatment

Usually, the presurgical orthodontic treatment is planned to maximum the deformities by removing dental compensations and is the opposite of normal orthodontic treatment. The purpose of pre-and postsurgical orthodontic treatment is listed below.

(1) Reduce the surgery time and the chance of segmental surgery.

(2) Achieve a good occlusion and aesthetic outcome.

(3) Control the relapse tendencies.

Therefore, preoperative and postoperative orthodontic objectives include the following.

(1) Align the teeth with inclination and angulation correction.

(2) Remove the dental compensations and correct the incisor torque.

(3) Flatten the occlusal plane.

(4) Close the spaces in the dentitions.

(5) Coordinate the relation of the upper and lower dental arches.

(6) Eliminate gross dental interferences.

17.5.2 Virtual treatment objective(VTO)

After demonstrating the mechanism of the dentomaxillofacial deformity, VTO should be carried out to further determine the direction and distance to move the jaws and to ensure the orthognathic surgery could be performed quantitatively. In addition, VTO can predict the post-operative facial profile and obtain a visualized prognostic outcome. VTO is a basic training for young surgeon to make the definitive surgical plan.

17.5.2.1 Contents of VTO

(1) Determine the types of surgery.

(2) Predict the direction and distance of movement of the bone segment.

(3) Predict the postoperative occlusal relationship. To achieve good occlusion is one of the key aims of orthognathic surgery. The movement of the bony segment must coordinate with the movement of the teeth, so as to obtain good relationship between the upper and lower jaws with good occlusion.

(4) Predict the postoperative facial profile. After the bony segments are moved to new positions, it will lead to changes of the patient's soft tissue profile of the face. Based on the proportional relation of soft and hard tissue movement, VTO could illustrate the visualized postoperative lateral appearance and evaluate the rationality of the surgical plan.

17.5.2.2 Procedure of VTO

(1) Perform cephalometric analysis, label the marks of soft and hard tissues, and measure a variety of parameters of the jaws, teeth, and dental arch (Figure 17-3A). Compare the results with normal values to determine the mechanism and severity of dentomaxillofacial deformity. Thus the surgical type, the distance and direction of jaw movement could be decided.

(2) Trace the lateral profiles of soft and hard tissue.

(3) Make the templates of the upper and lower jaws (Figure 17-3B).

(4) Put the templates on the original cephalometric tracing. Move them to the desired position until their positions is close to or consistent with the normal values (Figure 17-3C).

(5) According to the proportional relation of soft tissue and hard tissue movement, trace the soft tissue profile.

(6) Make a template for the chin, and predict the movement of the chin according to the aesthetic plane.

(7) Trace the final postoperative profile (Figure 17-3D). If necessary, repeat the above steps to correct the prediction. Communicate with the patient on the VTO result to obtain his/her consent.

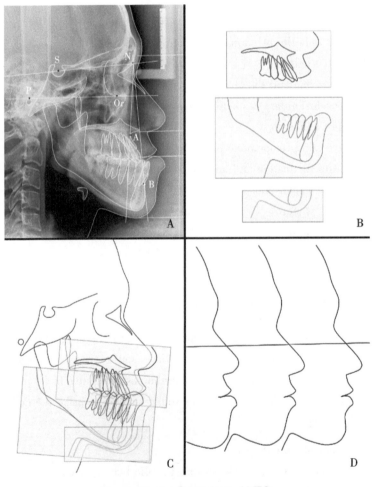

Figure 17-3 **Procedure of VTO**

A: Cephalometric analysis; B: Make the template; C: Moved to the desired position; D: Changes in profile.

17.5.3 Model surgery

According to the clinical examination, X-ray cephalometric analysis and VTO results, the plaster models transferred to the articular will be cut and moved to the desired position to simulate the position of the osteotomy, the direction and distance of the movement of the bony segments, in order to achieve good jaws position and occlusion.

17.5.3.1 Significance of model surgery

Model surgery is an important part of the preoperative design of orthognathic surgery. Model surgery must be performed before call orthognathic surgeries. It needs to change the occlusal relationship to ensure the bony segments could be adjusted to the designed position and the occlusion to the designed relationship.

(1) The 3-dimensional relationship of the jaws could be observed, making up for the limitation of the X-ray cephalometric analysis which is 2-dimensional analysis.

(2) To evaluate the coordination of upper and lower dental arches and explore ways to adjust the occlusal relationship.

(3) To simulate the movement of the bony segment.

(4) To fabricate surgical splints on the finished model plaster casts in order to guide the surgery.

17.5.3.2 Procedure of model surgery

(1) Generate dental casts using alginate impressions of the patient's dentitions.

(2) Record the relationship between the upper jaw and the skull with facebow transfer system then record the relationship between the upper and lower jaws with wax-occlusion records(Figure 17-4A).

(3) Mount the plaster casts to the articular by the aiding of the facebow transfer system and the wax-occlusion records(Figure 17-4B).

(4) Draw horizontal and vertical reference line and measure the height of the occlusal plane(Figure 17-4C).

(5) Cut the plaster casts and move them to the desired position according the surgical plan. Fix the casts at the new position with wax(Figure 17-4D, Figure 17-4E).

(6) The intermediate splint and final splint are respectively made on the plaster model after the movement(Figure 17-4F).

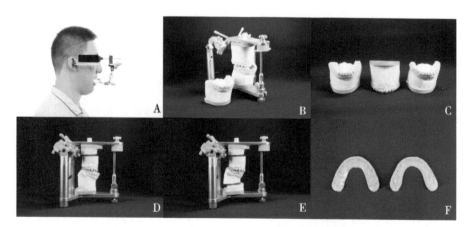

Figure 17-4   **Procedure of model surgery**

A: Occlusion records; B: Mount the plaster casts; C: Draw the reference line; D、E: Model surgery;
F: Intermediate and final splint.

17.5.4 Computer aided surgical simulation(CASS)

More recently, 3 – dimensional surgical planning has been used in the field of oral and maxillofacial surgery, and CASS has been employed in various orthognathic surgical processes, including diagnosis, tridimensional analysis(Figure 17 – 5a, Figure 17 – 5b), tridimensional surgical planning(Figure 17 – 5c), virtual design (Figure 17 – 6A) and 3D printing of the splints(Figure 17 – 6B), 3D printed plates, and predicting clinical outcomes.

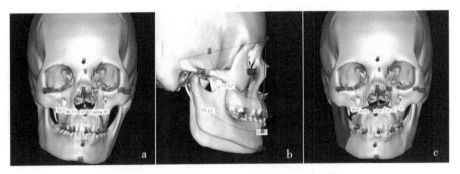

Figure 17 – 5   Computer aided surgical simulation
a、b:Tridimensional analysis;c:Tridimensional surgical planning.

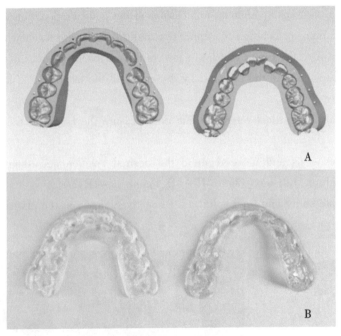

Figure 17 – 6   Virtual design and 3D printing of the splint
A:Virtual design;B:3D printing of the splint.

17.6 Common Surgical Procedures of Orthognathic Surgery

There are many types of dentomaxillofacial malformations and the clinical manifestations are varied with patients. It should be aware that not all dentomaxillofacial deformities need to be treated with surgery. Some mild deformities can be solved by orthodontic treatment. Some involve only the maxillary or mandibular deformity, it needs only a single-jaw osteotomy. More serious or complex deformities require a combination of multiple surgical procedures. The commonly used surgeries of modern orthognathic surgery are maxillary LeFort I osteotomy, bilateral sagittal split ramus osteotomy, and genioplasty. A reasonable combination of the three surgeries can be used to correct most dentomaxillofacial deformities.

17.6.1   Maxillary LeFort I osteotomy

17.6.1.1   Indication

(1) Maxillary deformity

Maxillary retraction, maxillary protrusion, maxillary asymmetry, etc.

(2) Bimaxillary deformities

Maxillary retrognathsim and mandibular prognathsim, maxillary prognathsim and mandibular retrognathsim. Long or short face syndrome, bimaxillary prognathsim, secondary dentomaxillofacial deformity, etc.

17.6.1.2   Surgical procedure of LeFort I osteotomy

(1) Anesthesia: general anesthesia with tracheal intubation combined with local anesthesia in the operation area.

(2) Incision: an intraoral labiobuccal incision from distal aspect of the maxillary molar to the the opposite side.

(3) Expose the anterior and lateral wall of the maxilla, the pyriform aperture, the maxillary tuberosity. Dissect the nasal floor, the lateral nasal wall and the septum.

(4) The osteotomy line should be at least 5 mm superior to the root apices of the maxillary teeth (Figure 17-7a). Perform the osteotomy with a reciprocating saw and special chisels. Separate the nasal septum and vomer are from the maxillary bone and separate the pterygoid plate from the maxillary tuberosity with chisels.

(5) Downfracture the maxilla with digital pressure by placing the thumbs on the bilateral canine fossa. The maxilla should be fully mobilized with Roweforceps and be passively placed to the designed position (Figure 17-7b).

(6) Place a prefabricated intermediate surgical splint between the maxillary and mandibular dentitions and perform intermaxillary fixation with steel wires. Reposition the maxillary segment according to the surgical plan(Figure 17-7c).

(7) Stabilize the maxilla with bent microplates and screws at the buttresses(Figure 17-7d).

(8) Suture the incision.

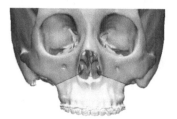
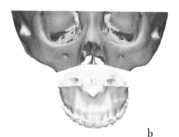

a   b

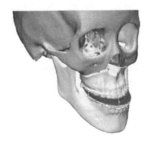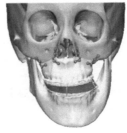

c   d

Figure 17−7　Illustration for the surgical procedure of LeFort Ⅰ osteotomy

a:The osteotomy line;b:Designed position;c:Reposition the maxillary segment;d:Stabilization.

17.6.2　Bilateral sagittal split ramus osteotomy(BSSRO)

17.6.2.1　indication

(1)Mandibular retrognathsim.

(2)Mandibular prognathsim.

(3)Mandibular deviation deformity.

(4)Long face or short face syndrome.

(5)Open bite.

17.6.1.2　Surgical procedure of BSSRO

(1)Anesthesia:general anesthesia was performed by nasal intubation,and the incision area was anesthetized with lidocaine containing epinephrine.

(2)Incision:incision from the vestibule corresponding to the buccal groove of the first molar,along the oblique line and the anterior edge of the ascending ramus,and upward to 1−2 cm above the mandibular occlusal plane.

(3)The anterior border of the mandible and the outer surface of the mandibular body are exposed. The medial surface of the ascending ramus is revealed by separating between the sigmoid notch and the mandibular lingula.

(4)Make the horizontal osteotomy line at 3−5 mm above the mandibular lingula,to the posterior of the mandibular foramen. The osteotomy is extended along the medial side of the ramus,and then along the oblique line to the buccal side of the first molar to complete the sagittal osteotomy line. The vertical osteotomy line is performed on the buccal side of the first molar and perpendicular to the lower edge of the mandible(Figure 17−8a,Figure 17−8b,Figure 17−8c).

(5)Complete the mandibular osteotomy with a series of special osteotomes. Gradually separate the proximal segment and the distal segment. The proximal tooth−bearing segment should be repositioned into final splint with no obvious resistance(Figure 17−8d).

(6)The mandibular and maxillary dentitions are placed into the final splint,and intermaxillary fixation is performed.

(7)Place the condyle at the physiological position and use mini titanium plates and screws to fix at the vertical osteotomy line(Figure 17−8e).

(8)suture the invision.

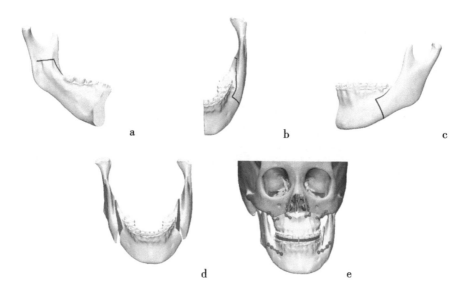

Figure 17-8   Illustration for the surgical procedure of BSSRO

a、b、c：The vertical osteotomy line；d：Osteotomy；e：Intermaxillary fixation.

17.6.3   Genioplasty

17.6.3.1   Indication

Genioplasty can be used to correct chin retraction, chin protrusion, long or short chin, and chin asymmetry.

17.6.3.2   Surgical procedure of genioplasty

(1) Anesthesia：general anesthesia with tracheal intubation combined with local infiltration anesthesia.

(2) Incision：the vestibular incision between the bilateral mandibular canines, retaining part of the mentalis muscle on the bone surface to facilitate postoperative suture.

(3) Perform a subperiosteal dissection and reveal the bony surface of the chin.

(4) Make the osteotomy line about 5 mm below the bilateral mental foramen and complete the osteotomy with a reciprocating saw(Figure 17-9a).

(5) According to the surgical design and intraoperative observation of the aesthetic effect, the chin bone segment is moved to the desired position(Figure 17-9b) and fixed with two microplates(Figure 17-9c).

(6) Suture the muscle and mucosa respectively.

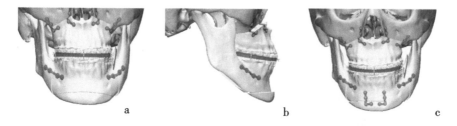

Figure 17-9   Illustration for the surgical procedure of genioplasty

a：Make the osteotomy line；b：Mored to desired position；c：Fixed with microplates.

He Wei, Tian Kaiyue

Chapter 18

The Relationship Between Oral Diseases and Systemic Diseases

❯ *Objectives*

To understand the clinical manifestation of systemic disease in the oral cavity.

To familiar with the effect of oral diseases on general health.

❯ *Introduction*

Many systemic diseases have manifestations on oral cavity, and some oral disease manifestations can also be used as clues for the diagnosis of systemic diseases.

18.1 Systemic Disease in the Oral Cavity

18.1.1 Blood and hemorrhagic disease

18.1.1.1 Leukemia

(1) The characteristics of the disease

Leukemia is a disease of unknown origin. It is characterized by a large number of special types of abnormal white blood cells in the body. The clinical classification is based on the development stage of the disease, the leukocyte system involved and the cell maturation. Oral manifestations can be found in all types of leukemia. Early diagnosis of a large number of cases is discovered by Department of Stomatology doctors. Correct understanding of oral manifestations and complications of leukemia and timely prevention and treatment are of positive significance for the treatment and prognosis of leukemia.

(2) Clinical manifestations

Oral manifestations of leukocyte disease:

1) Gingival hyperplasia and swelling: in addition to gingivitis and periodontitis, the color of the gums is pale.

2) Gingival and oral mucosa bleeding: gingival bleeding, mucosal ecchymosis, ecchymosis or blood blister.

3) Gingival necrosis: mucosal ulcer or erosion, no obvious inflammatory reaction near necrotic ulcers.

4) Gingival swelling, hypertrophy, sore throat, facial mass.

5) Toothache and tooth loosening: the infiltration of white blood cells into the pulp can cause severe toothache and leukocyte infiltration in the gingival tissue, which can make the teeth loose.

6) Lymph node enlargement: bilateral lymph node painless enlargement is more common.

(3) Diagnosis points

Its oral representation, some of the precursor symptoms of the disease, is of great value for early diagnosis. Department of Stomatology doctors should have a deep understanding of the disease, maintain a high awareness of the above performance, early detection, early diagnosis, and early treatment.

18.1.1.2 Anemia

(1) The characteristics of morbidity

Anemia refers to a common clinical symptom of human peripheral blood red blood cell volume less than normal limits. Because of the complexity of red blood cell volume, the concentration of hemoglobin (Hb) is often used in clinic. Chinese hematologists believe that in China's sea level, adult male Hb < 120 g/L, adult female (non pregnancy) Hb < 110 g/L, pregnant women Hb < 100 g/L anemia. Anemia with different etiologies has its unique oral presentation.

(2) Clinical manifestations

1) Iron deficiency anemia: pallid oral mucosa, glossy filamentous papilla and bacterial papilla atrophy, glossy surface, atrophic changes in the tip of the tongue, irritation of lip, cheek and tongue mucosa, which can form ulcers. The mucosa and tongue have burning pain, and there are inflammation or chap in the corners.

2) Giant naive cell anemia: early oral symptoms are painful glossitis and burning sensation of the tongue. There is ulcer on the tongue, atrophy of tongue papilla, bright red tongue, and fire like plaques, especially on the edge of tongue and tip of tongue. In severe cases, the tongue is smooth, waxy and tongue tension was lost. Many patients have difficulty in denture and can not be explained by poor denture.

3) Anaplastic anemia: the paleness of the oral mucosa, the continuous bleeding of the small gingiva, the bleeding of the mucous and the skin, with the slight trauma of the skin can cause ulcers and necrosis, which are common in the gingival margins, buccal mucosa, and hardships. Many patients are accompanied by tonsillitis and pharyngitis.

(3) Key points of diagnosis: according to history, clinical manifestation and local examination, the patients with high suspicion can be diagnosed by blood biochemical and immunological examination.

18.1.1.3 Hemorrhagic disease

(1) The characteristics of the disease

Hemorrhagic diseases including thrombocytopenic purpura and hemophilia.

(2) Clinical manifestations

The main oral manifestations are obvious bleeding tendency, which can be caused by brushing teeth, biting food, biting mucous membranes and bumping against trauma. It should be emphasized that any oral and maxillofacial surgery, such as tooth extraction and dental pulp surgery, can cause serious bleeding. The healing of oral trauma is delayed.

(3) Diagnostic points

According to the history, clinical manifestations and local examination, suspicious persons can be diagnosed by blood test in time.

18.1.2　Nutritional diseases

18.1.2.1　Vitamin A deficiency

Vitamin A deficiency reduces systemic and plasma cells, decreases local resistance, causes gingivitis, gingival hypertrophy, and periodontal disease in the mouth. Severe vitamin A deficiency can develop enamel and dentin hypoplasia. Due to the slow process of ossification, jaw bone can be poorly developed, and permanent teeth have delayed eruption and uneven dentition. The following jaw is more obvious. After vitamin A supplementation, the development of the disease can be terminated and the symptoms can be alleviated.

18.1.2.2　Vitamin B₁ deficiency

Vitamin B_1 deficiency in the mouth of the performance of the lips, tongue and gum mucous membrane abnormal smooth, edema, purple rose color, the tongue edge of the tooth scar, gums bleeding, lose spot color. There is a small blister at the junction of the skin and mucous membrane of the lip, containing serous fluid and small cleft. Peripheral neuritis in the trigeminal nerve area can result in oral mucosal hypersensitivity and tongue burning. After supplementation of vitamin B_1, symptoms can be rapidly improved.

18.1.2.3　Vitamin B₂ deficiency

The oral characterization of vitamin B_2 deficiency: ① oral angle inflammation, wet and white rotten in the mouth, the crack is about 1 cm by the angle of mouth, which can cover the yellowish eschar and both sides are symmetrical. ② Cheilitis, lip mucosa red, peeling off erosion, lip longitudinal split increased, deeper, especially upper lip, with dry desquamation, lips swelling, burning sensation. ③ Glossitis, red tongue mucous membrane, filamentous papilla atrophy, bacterial papilla hyperemia increased, conscious pain, tongue dorsal mucosa in a spot color or Myrica like, bald tongue, molting, a map like, severe tongue swelling, lingual dorsal longitudinal fissure, lingual edge teeth marks. The diet improved to maintain normal digestive function and symptoms quickly subsided.

18.1.2.4　Folic acid deficiency

Oral acid deficiency is characterized by severe glossitis, extensive stomatitis and gingivitis. Tongue margin congestion and edema, filamentous nipple atrophy or even disappear, with fire red, color tongue margin, and root can appear superficial ulcers, with obvious pain. Oral mucous membranes and gums are swollen, epithelial shedding, burning sensation, superficial erosion or small ulcers, increased saliva secretion and dysphagia. Vitamin B deficiency can aggravate the symptoms. Vitamin B supplementation, large amounts of folic acid and water can be cured.

18.1.2.5　Vitamin C deficiency

It is also known as scurvy, mild lack of oral symptoms are not obvious, severe cases are gingivitis, bleeding and bone development disorders. The gums are red swollen and hypertrophic, with the most obvious tooth tip papillae, purple red, soft texture, easy bleeding, spontaneous bleeding. Local stimulation, such as stones, plaque, incomplete dentition and trauma, often aggravates the bleeding and infection of the gums, the destruction of the connective tissue of the periodontal ligament, the absorption of the alveolar bone, and the loosening of the teeth and even the loss of the teeth. When adequate vitamin C is added, oral local treatment can achieve good results.

18.1.2.6　Vitamin D deficiency

It is also known as rickets, common in children, oral and maxillofacial characterization, square head, enamel dysplasia, prone to dental caries, tooth eruption delay and misalignment. X-ray examination showed that the trabecular structure of jaws enlarged, thin bone and alveolar bone became thinner. Vitamin D supplementation can control the progress of the disease after diagnosis, and measures should be taken to prevent caries.

18.1.3   Endocrine system disease

18.1.3.1   Diabetes

(1) Among the diseases of the endocrine system, diabetes is most closely related to the oral cavity. It is reported that the incidence of periodontitis in patients with non insulin dependent diabetes is 3 times about to have periodontal disease than normal people. The possibility of total mouth free diabetes in diabetics is 15 times higher than healthy people, and the periodontal infection of diabetics is more common and more serious.

(2) The oral characteristics of diabetes: ① gingivitis, periodontitis, gingival red and swollen, bleeding, gingival edge granulation tissue hyperplasia, easy to develop periodontal abscess; ② tongue color dark red, swelling, teeth marks, and can occur cleft, tongue tingling, mouth with sweet or rotten apple taste; ③ cavity mucous dry, congestion and transparency under dry, transparent, transparency The red lip is dry and cracked; ④ parotid glands are enlarged, showing bilateral painless and diffuse enlargement.

(3) Diagnostic points: according to history, clinical manifestations and local examination, with blood and biochemical examination can be diagnosed.

(4) Treatment plan: the diabetes patients should pay attention to the general condition of the body and the control of blood sugar in total treatment. The patients should be given anti infection before the operation, such as low resistance to bacterial infection, tooth extraction and deep curettage, and the operation should be performed in the morning. Strictly aseptic operation to minimize the trauma.

18.1.3.2   Hyperparathyroidism

The main manifestations of the oral and maxillofacial region: ① the polycystic lesions of the jaw, the patients complained of bone pain, and the X-ray showed that the trabecular bone is reduced, the image is blurred, the bone cortex is thinner, the bone marrow is replaced by the fibrous tissue, and the pathological fracture can occur in the severe cases; ② recurrent gingival tumor, gingivitis and periodontitis. The alveolar ridge is extensively absorbed and loosened, displaced or even dropped.

18.1.4   Specific infection

(1) The characteristics of the disease

Tuberculosis, candidiasis, syphilis and so on. Syphilis is more common and representative.

(2) Clinical manifestation

Its oral representation is listed below:

1) Syphilis gum swelling, good hair in the middle of the hard jaw, also in the lips, tongue, gums and tonsillar, in the beginning of the hemispherical swelling, hard as rubber, quickly caused by necrosis and bone destruction, perforated, also a perforated nasal cavity.

2) Syphilitic ulcers, which can cause oral ulcers in various stages. A hard chancre with shallow ulcers and a hard infiltration on the edge and bottom; mucous ulcers can occur simultaneously during the period of two stage syphilis; the 3rd stage of the gumma center breaks and forms deep ulcers.

3) Syphilis glossitis, only occurs in men, tongue nipple atrophy, smooth surface, hyperkeratosis, appearance of syphilis leukoplakia, surface hard knot, formation of fissure.

4) Abnormal tooth development, seen in the late tread syphilis, the anterior teeth were neck wide cutting edge process, the cutting edge was half – moon shaped, the incisor had a larger gap between the incisors, called Hutchinson teeth, the first permanent molar of the mandible was inclined to the central point, like mulberry, so it was also called mulberry teeth, the permanent teeth were not well developed, erupted late, teeth were inhomogeneous.

(3) Diagnostic points

According to history, clinical manifestation and local examination, blood syphilis antibodies can be diagnosed.

(4) Treatment scheme

Oral and maxillofacial syphilis, both fetal and acquired infection, are local manifestations of systemic diseases. Therefore, systemic treatment should be performed, deformity caused by late syphilis, repair and orthopedics of tissue defects, must be carried out after regular treatment.

18.1.5 Skin and mucous membrane diseases

18.1.5.1 Chronic discoid lupus erythematosus(CDLE)

(1) The characteristics of disease

CDLE is a kind of connective tissue disease, mainly with skin and mucous membrane damage, and about 5% of patients can turn into. The cause of the disease is not clear, most of which are considered autoimmune diseases. Patients may have congenital susceptibility factors, such as daylight exposure, cold stimulation, endocrine disorder, bacterial virus infection, mental nervous tension, drug irritation, the formation of the body's own antigen, the loss of recognition ability of immune active cells and the imbalance of self stabilizing function, producing a large number of anti self groups. Weave antibodies. Autoantigens are combined with autoantibodies to form antigen antibody complexes, which are deposited in tissues and cause lesions.

(2) Clinical manifestations

1) Skin lesions: it occurs in the prominent parts of the face, such as the forehead, nose and zygomatic region. The skin of the auricle, trunk and extremities can also occur. It is characterized by clear edges, pink spots, central depressions, covered with scales, surrounded by radial dilatation vessels, and typical lesions are butterfly spot.

2) Oral lesions: the following lip is most common, followed by tongue and mouth. Fresh lesions showed bright red spots, central atrophy, erosion from the atrophic area, surrounded by keratinous desquamation, telangiectasia radial. The lesions spread to the skin and the mucous skin boundaries are blurred. Old lesions show atrophy, scarring, keratinization, white radial stripes, mucosal decolorization or pigmentation.

(3) Diagnosis points: according to the medical history, clinical manifestations and local examination, the suspicious people's erythrocyte sedimentation, R globulin, a variety of tissue antibodies such as rheumatoid factor, anti nuclear antibody can be confirmed.

18.1.5.2 Drug allergic stomatitis

(1) The characteristics of the disease

It is the drug through oral, injection or local erasure, gargle and other different ways to enter the body. It is allergic reaction to allergies caused by the mucous membrane and skin of the inflammatory reaction. Allergy is the main cause of drug allergy. As a semi antigen, the drug enters the body and produces corresponding antibodies or sensitized lymphocytes. When once again the same person is exposed to the same drug, the body produces allergies.

(2) Clinical manifestations

1) The pathological reaction is complicated in clinical manifestation, and there are various parts, forms, and damage degree of the lesion.

2) The oral lesions are mostly seen in the front of the mouth, such as the lip and cheek, the upper jaw, and the anterior 1/3 parts of the tongue. The mucous membrane is hot and distended, congested, followed by red spots and blister, after the blisters, the erosion, pain, exudation, and the formation of gray or gray white fake film on the surface. Saliva increases in the mouth, often containing blood, and is accompanied by lymph node enlargement and tenderness.

(3) Diagnostic points

Diagnosis is based on history, clinical manifestations and general or local signs.

(4) Treatment

For allergic stomatitis, try to identify sensitized drugs and avoid re exposure. The use of suspected sensitizing substances should also be stopped. Antihistamine drugs, corticosteroids, vitamin C can be used all over the body. The severe patients are given support treatment, and local drugs can be used locally for anti-inflammatory, analgesic, astringent, anticorrosion, and myogenic drugs.

18.1.6   AIDS

18.1.6.1   The characteristics of the disease

AIDS is a highly dangerous infectious disease caused by HIV infection. HIV is a virus that attacks the body's immune system. It takes the most important T lymphocytes in the body's immune system as the main target of attack, destroys the cells in large numbers, and causes the body to lose its immune function. Therefore, the human body is easy to infect various diseases, and can cause malignant tumors with high mortality. The incubation period of HIV in the human body is 8−9 years on average. Before suffering from AIDS, it can live and work without symptoms for many years.

18.1.6.2   Clinical manifestations

Oral presentation mainly includes the following:

(1) Oral Candida albicans infection, the symptoms and signs of type four Candida albicans infection can appear, most appear before the onset of AIDS, often the symptoms of AIDS. The minority appeared in the middle of the disease. There are white lesions in the mucous membrane of the tongue and the tongue, and there are flaky erythema or leukoplakia in the mucous membrane of the oral cavity. There are white cheese like exudates on the surface, dysphagia, pain and burning sensation, and smear microscopic examination of Candida albicans.

(2) Oral hairy leukoplakia, in the bilateral tongue, the bottom of the mouth, cheeks, and other parts of the mouth can also be involved, showing a white patch with unclear boundaries, slightly uplifted, blurred boundaries, range from a number of millimeter to several centimeters, and the lesions sometimes fold or increase blanket.

(3) Oral Kaposy's sarcoma, which can be single or more frequent in any part of the oral mucosa. It is the most common with hard, soft, and gums. It shows a patch of purple and red size or a flat and high mass. It is soft, undefined, and bleeding easily. The clinical manifestations are similar to hemangioma, and sometimes pain can occur. Besides, oral malignant tumors such as lymphoma and squamous cell carcinoma can also occur.

(4) Gingivitis, periodontitis: gingivitis involves free gingival, gingival papilla and attached gingival. Gingival swelling, hypertrophy and hypertrophy can cover the tooth surface; free gingival margin crescent red

line and attached gingival spot red spot, a characteristic change; early gingival papilla necrosis, ulcer, pain; periodontal attachment and alveolar bone rapid destruction, and all the teeth are involved; the periodontitis was repeated.

(5) Oral herpes, in the oral mucosa appear with small blister formation of painful lesions, may be herpes simplex virus or coxsackievirus A virus.

(6) The cheek lymph node enlargement, common ear, ear behind, neck behind and submandibular lymph node enlargement.

(7) Salivary gland infection, parotid gland, submandibular gland swollen, often bilateral, diffuse mass, soft, some with dry mouth, dry eye, joint pain and so on, similar to the symptoms of Sjögren's syndrome. Some of them are parotid cysts, often accompanied by enlarged cervical lymph nodes.

18.1.6.3　Diagnostic points

According to history, clinical manifestation and local examination, suspicious blood immunoassay can be used to diagnose.

18.1.6.4　Treatment program

AIDS has a high degree of infectious, oral operation caused by bleeding can lead to patients and medical personnel and patients and patients with cross infection, so it needs serious isolation and disinfection work.

18.1.7　Syndrome

18.1.7.1　Krohn's disease

Formerly known as localized ileocolitis. In addition to a series of gastrointestinal symptoms associated with granulomatous inflammation of the intestinal tract, about 20% of the patients can be accompanied by granulomatous lesions of the oral mucosa, characterized by oral mucosa ulcers, small nodules and gingival hyperplasia. The predilection sites were buccal, lip, gingival and pharynx. The ulcer on the buccal sulcus is linear, and it does not heal for a long time. There is a small nodule hyperplasia, which is similar to the granuloma of denture. When it occurs in the lip, it can be diffuse swelling. The proliferating gums are red and sometimes grainy. Oral granulomatous lesions can be the initial symptom of this disease. With the aggravation of intestinal lesions, oral ulcers are also gradually aggravating.

18.1.8　Pigmentation–intestinal polyposis syndrome

This disease is obviously familial and is a dominant hereditary disease. It is characterized by mucous membrane, skin pigmented spots, multiple gastrointestinal polyps and familial inheritance. The clinical manifestations are as follows:

(1) Pigmentation often occurs in the skin around the mouth, eye, palm, plantar and toes. The red lip and oral mucosa can also be pigmented. The pigment is multiple, black but not brown. Looks like black spots, many patients have been born since childhood. The pigmented spots on the lips and skin can disappear gradually after puberty.

(2) Gastrointestinal polyps occur mostly in the small intestine, and can also be seen in the stomach and large intestine, causing gastrointestinal symptoms, such as abdominal pain, diarrhea and bleeding. Multiple polyps in the colon have a tendency to change malignancy.

18.1.9　Cutaneous leptomeningeal angioma

It is a special type of cerebral vascular malformation, characterized by facial hemangioma and epileptic seizures. The clinical manifestations are as follows:

(1) There are fresh erythematous nevus in one of the trigeminal nerve areas. It can expand gradually, increase color, or appear nodules on the surface. It often involves the hemi facial skin and the ipsilateral oral mucosa. Sometimes the same side head, neck and trunk can also be involved, occasionally the skin lesions occur on bilateral or midface.

(2) Infantile convulsions often occur, beginning on the opposite side of port wine stains, after the whole body convulsions. Contralateral spastic hemiplegia can occur in some cases after a considerable period of time.

(3) About half of the patients had eye damage, mostly on the same side, the eye is larger than the opposite side, external convex, increased intraocular pressure. The eye often glaucoma, conjunctiva, iris and choroidal hemangioma with retinal detachment. A few of it occur the optic atrophy.

(4) Mental retardation.

(5) X-ray examination showed a linear or spotted calcification in the ipsilateral gyrus, and a venous hemangioma in the pia mater.

18.1.10　Multiple basal cell nevus syndrome

Familial and autosomal dominant hereditary disease. It is characterized by multiple basal cell nevus or basal cell carcinoma, multiple jaw cyst, rib deformity and intracranial calcification. The clinical manifestations are as follows:

(1) Odontogenic keratosis of the jaws, with more mandible than the maxilla, single or multiple, often involving bilateral involvement.

(2) Nevus basal cell carcinoma occurs mainly in the face, neck, upper trunk, orbit, eyelids, nose and zygomatic processes. The upper lip is the most common part of the face and is usually unilateral. Most of the lesions are in a state of rest.

(3) Rib deformity includes bifurcated rib, fusion rib, incomplete or partial absence of rib.

(4) The most common intracranial calcification is cerebral falx calcification, followed by calcification of tentorium cerebelli.

18.1.11　Hereditary ectodermal dysplasia

An invisible genetic disease related to the X chromosome, characterized by less sweating, less hairy hair and hypoplastic teeth. Clinical manifestation:

(1) Most of the oral and maxillary incisors are missing, and the upper central incisors and canines are cone-shaped crowns. The number of teeth is missing or even full denture.

(2) The skin because of the sweat gland partial or all missing, even without sweat or lack of sweat, the patient can not tolerate high temperature, dry skin. And the lack of hair, hair sparse, eyebrows, axillary hair, and pubic hair.

(3) The forehead of the face is prominent, the bridge of the nose collapses, and the face is like a saddle nose. Pigmentation in the eyes.

The above diseases suggest that patients with special oral and facial features may be encountered in the diagnosis and treatment of oral diseases. These special representations may indicate that the patient is suffering from a certain disease. Only the Department of Stomatology doctors have a full understanding of these diseases can guide the suspicious cases in time and correctly. In order to make further diagnosis, the overall diagnosis and treatment level can be improved.

18.2 The Effect of Oral Diseases on General Health

18.2.1 Caries

18.2.1.1 The characteristics of the disease

Dental caries is the main cause of missing teeth. Loss of teeth will inevitably result in low masticatory function, affecting food digestion and absorption, leading to malnutrition. For children with more caries, the body shape is more skinny and it seriously affects development. Infectious arthritis is caused by the sensitivity of the synovium to the Streptococcus, and the endotoxin in the dental foci constantly triggers the chronic glomerulonephritis caused by the stimulation of the tissue.

18.2.1.2 Clinical manifestation

If dental caries are not treated in time, it can develop into chronic periapical abscess, gingival fistula and repeated purulent, and can become a localized lesion with pathogenic microorganism infection. This infection may spread to nearby tissues or organs, and may also cause diseases of distant organs and tissues, such as infection of teeth that can cause arthritis, endocarditis, and nephritis. Tooth extraction, tooth scaling and other oral procedures can cause temporary bacteremia, but generally do not leave behind. For patients with organic lesions of the heart valves, bacterial endocarditis can be caused, and the most important bacteria are Streptococcus group. The blood carrying these bacteria settle on damaged or abnormal heart valves, causing bacterial endocarditis to buy endocarditis. Therefore, preventive measures should be taken for oral operations that may cause infection, such as chlorinated mouthwash or oral antibiotics, and preventive injection of antibiotics to patients with high and moderate risk before and after operation. Other diseases such as neuritis, respiratory tract, gastrointestinal diseases and oral lesions have also been reported.

18.2.1.3 The main points of diagnosis

Timely detection of dental disease and early diagnosis is of great importance to health care and prevention.

18.2.1.4 Treatment plan

There are research reports, after removal of dental foci, many kinds of ophthalmopathy can be cured, such as siphon, iris ciliary body inflammation, retrobulbar optic neuritis, retinitis and so on. Sometimes the symptoms of oral diseases including erythema multiforme, herpes, measles, eczema and other skin diseases can be alleviated. Removal of dental foci prevents renal damage.

18.2.2 Periodontitis

18.2.2.1 The characteristics of the disease

There are various sources of infection in the oral cavity, such as various kinds of inflammation, abscess and infected cysts. Generally speaking, the infection of dead pulp and periapical periodontitis is not as great as periodontitis. This is because periodontitis involves multiple teeth and the area of infection is large. At the same time, because of loosening of teeth, when chewing, the teeth will be compressed to the root tip, and the microbes and toxins will be squeezed into the blood vessels and lymphatics. The incidence of transient bacteremia in patients with severe periodontitis after tooth extraction is 86%. The microbes in the bloodstream do not have any clinical symptoms, but bacteremia may be a cause of subacute endocarditis in patients with congenital heart failure or rheumatic heart disease. Recent studies have shown that periodontal disease is a risk factor for some systemic diseases and is related to general health.

18. 2. 2. 2   Clinical manifestations

(1) Cardio cerebral vascular disease

Experts in the patients with acute myocardial infarction in general examination, the majority of patients have different degrees of oral disease, of which the most common is periodontitis and periodontal abscess. There are a large number of pathogenic bacteria in the oral cavity. These bacteria can produce endotoxin and invade the blood, causing changes in the mechanism of coagulation and the denaturation of the platelets, and can also directly stimulate the blood vessels leading to the spasm of the small arteries. If the coronary artery is involved, the contraction spasm and the effect of micro thrombus will lead to the occurrence of acute myocardial infarction. Epidemiological studies revealed that dental infection and periodontitis were independent risk factors for atherosclerosis and acute myocardial infarction. Other findings indicate that about 8% of infectious endocarditis is associated with periodontal disease and dental disease. A study of the elderly showed a significant relationship between the plaque index and oral hygiene habits(the frequency of brushing, dental floss and professional clean teeth) with cerebrovascular accidents. Those who could not live independently could not have cleaned their teeth once a year. The possibility of cerebrovascular accident is 4. 76 times that of the control group.

(2) Pregnancy (relationship between mothers with chronic periodontal disease and low birth weight premature infants)

The concept of low birth weight(LBW) : birth weight is less than 2,500 g. Short pregnancy and LBW are the primary causes of infant mortality. Many studies have confirmed that premature birth and low birth weight are related to mothers' periodontitis. Some researchers found oral microbes in amniotic fluid and amniotic membrane. The most common bacteria are oral nuclear fusiform bacteria. Transient bacteremia from the mouth is transmitted through blood and placenta infecting amniotic fluid. Opportunistic pathogens and/ or inflammatory products in the oral cavity can play a role in premature delivery through blood. Biochemical examination of the periodontal status of mothers and oral microbiological status are related to LBW.

(3) Diabetes

Periodontitis and gingivitis patients are 7 times more likely to suffer from diabetes. There is a two-way relationship between periodontitis and diabetes. Diabetes control is also an important prerequisite for improving periodontitis. Non insulin dependent diabetics may have periodontal disease 3 times more likely to suffer from periodontitis, more severe periodontal infection, or disease, and a chronic periodontal disease that affects the control of diabetes. The reason is that periodontitis increases the susceptibility to infection, damages the host response, and produces too much collagen. Enzymes, all of which have adverse effects on the control of diabetes, and periodontal therapy can reduce the level of TNF-A in blood, increase the sensitivity of insulin, and help to reduce blood sugar and glycated hemoglobin levels.

(4) Gastrointestinal diseases

Helicobacter pylori (Hp) is an important pathogenic factor of chronic gastritis and peptic ulcer, and is closely related to the occurrence of gastric cancer. The oral cavity may be another gathering place of Hp. The detection rate of Hp in subgingival plaque is significantly higher than that in the subgingival plaque. Some scholars have found that Hp still exists in the oral cavity after the use of drug therapy to eradicate Hp in the stomach. It is suggested that oral Hp may be a risk factor for collecting and collating the reinfection of gastroduodenal Hp and the recurrence of digestive tract diseases. It is also found that the detection rate of plaque Hp in periodontitis patients is significantly higher than that in healthy controls, which is also significantly higher than that in gastritis group. The depth of periodontal detection in patients with periodontitis decreased significantly after basic treatment, and the detection rate of subgingival plaque Hp is also significantly lower than that before treatment, thus reducing the possibility of gastric disease.

(5) Respiratory disease

Plaque in the dental plaque, especially in periodontitis, may be a habitat for respiratory pathogens. Epidemiological investigation showed that the oral hygiene index of patients with chronic respiratory diseases was significantly higher than those without diseases. Many factors such as age, race, sex, smoking status and oral health index were analyzed by multiple factor regression. The results showed that the incidence of chronic respiratory diseases in patients with poor oral hygiene is 1.3 times that of those with good oral hygiene. Another 25 year longitudinal study of multiple factors regression analysis of factors such as smoking, alveolar bone height, age, education, drinking and other factors, found that increased alveolar bone absorption increased the risk of chronic obstructive pulmonary disease.

18.2.3　Main points of diagnosis

In view of the close relationship between oral diseases and general health, two aspects should be paid attention to when diagnosing.

(1) On the one hand, the oral disease is a simple oral disease, or the general disease related, or the general disease in the oral expression, because the treatment is very different, simple oral disease only do oral local treatment, if it is a manifestation of systemic systemic disease, often need to cooperate with the general treatment. The treatment, even the whole body treatment.

(2) On the other hand, taking into account what influence oral diseases will have on the whole body, such as whether or not the cancer of the oral and maxillofacial region has a distant metastasis, the severe oral and maxillofacial space infection is likely to occur in sepsis, sepsis, and cavernous sinus thrombophlebitis. If there is, it is not only a local treatment that is so simple, it is necessary. It should be combined with general treatment.

18.2.4　Treatment plan

In the treatment process, we should pay special attention to the relationship between the local and the whole body. Sometimes, in the case of local lesions, treatment may be very simple, such as a small oral tumor, it is easier to excision, but the patient may have serious cardiovascular and cerebrovascular diseases, which can not be hit by the operation, requiring relevant medical treatment, conditions for operation, and close observation of the heart and brain during or after the operation. Changes in vascular lesions. There are some lesions of the oral cavity. After timely and proper treatment, the lesions of the whole body can be eliminated or reduced.

Xue Peng

References

［1］吕慧欣,王卓然,高愉淇,等. 3724 例唾液腺肿瘤的临床病理分析［J］.中华口腔医学杂志, 2019,54(1):10-16.

［2］杜一飞,陈宁,李大庆.机器人辅助手术在头颈肿瘤外科中的应用进展［J］.中华口腔医学杂志,2019,54(1):58-61.

［3］尹圆圆,李飞,龙镜亦,等.颞下颌关节紊乱病疼痛患者脑功能磁共振成像的研究进展［J］.中华口腔医学杂志,2019,54(5):350-355.

［4］伍成奇,谢锋,谢振军,等.游离组织瓣修复半侧颜面萎缩 19 例［J］.中华显微外科杂志,2018,41(2):142-144.

［5］高宁,刘颖蒙,付坤,等.折叠腓骨瓣修复下颌骨缺损后种植修复的疗效观察［J］.中华口腔医学杂志,2018,53(1):26-29.

［6］王恒阳,代昕,刘洋,等. 202 例正畸患者的再矫治原因分析［J］.中华口腔医学杂志,2018,53(3):205-208.

［7］魏冬豪,赵一姣,邸萍,等.上颌中切牙即刻种植即刻修复后唇侧软组织形态三维变化的定量分析［J］.中华口腔医学杂志,2019,54(1):3-9.

［8］贾雪婷,黄晓峰. 84 枚支抗种植体周围颧牙槽嵴区解剖结构的锥形束 CT 分析［J］.中华口腔医学杂志,2018,53(1):8-12.

［9］LIX,SUN Q,GUO S. Functional assessments in patients undergoing radial forearm flap following hemiglossectomy［J］. J Craniofac Surg,2016,27(2):e172-e175.

［10］SILVA L C,SACONO N T,FREIRE M C M,et al. The impact of low-level laser therapy on oral mucositis and quality of life in patients undergoing hematopoietic stem cell transplantation using the oral health impact profile and the functional assessment of cancer therapy-bone marrow transplantation questionnaires［J］. Photomedicine and laser surgery,2015,33(7):357-363.

［11］FU K,LIU Y,GAO N,et al. Reconstruction of maxillary and orbital floor defect with free fibula flap and whole individualized titanium mesh assisted by computer techniques［J］. Journal of Oral and Maxillofacial Surgery,2017,75(8):1791. e1-1791. e9.

［12］XIA J J,SHEVCHENK O L,GATENO J,et al. Outcome study of computer-aided surgical simulation in the treatment of patients with craniomaxillofacial deformities［J］. J Oral Maxillofac Surg,2011,69(7):2014-2024.

［13］BROWN JS,SHAW RJ. Reconstruction of the maxilla and midface:introducing a new classification［J］. Lancet Oncol,2010,11(10):1001-1008.

［14］FERRI J,CAPRLOLL F,PEUVREL G,et al. Use of the fibula free flap in maxillary reconstruction:a report of 3 cases［J］. J Oral Maxillofac Surg,2002,60(5):567-574.

［15］PENG X,MAO C,YU GY,et al. Maxillary reconstruction with the free fibula flap［J］. Plast Reconstr Surg,2005,115(6):1562-1569.

［16］WANG S,XIAO J,LIU L,et al. Orbital floor reconstruction:a retrospective study of 21 cases［J］. Oral Surg Oral Med Oral Pathol Oral Radiol Endod,2008,106(3):324-330.

［17］YIM KK,WEI FC. Fibula osteoseptocutaneous free flap in maxillary reconstruction［J］. Microsurgery, 1994,15(5):353-357.

［18］LEVINE JP,PATEL A,SAADEH PB,et al. Computer-aided design and manufacturing in craniomaxillofacial surgery: the new state of the art[J]. J Craniofac Surg, 2012, 23(1): 288-293.

[19] ZHENG GS, WANG L, SU YX, et al. Maxillary reconstruction assisted by preoperative planning and accurate surgical templates[J]. Oral Surg Oral Med Oral Pathol Oral Radiol, 2016, 121(3): 233-238.

[20] REICH W, SEIDEL D, BREDEHORN M T, et al. Reconstruction of isolated orbital floor fractures with a prefabricated titanium mesh[J]. Klin Monbl Augenheilkd, 2014, 231(3): 246-255.

[21] RUSTEMEYER J, MELENBERG A, SARI R A. Costs incurred by applying computer aided design/computer-aided manufacturing techniques for the reconstruction of maxillofacial defects[J]. J Craniomaxillofac Surg, 2014, 42(8): 2049-2055.

[22] ZHANG WB, MAO C, LIU XJ, et al. Outcomes of orbital floor reconstruction after extensive maxillectomy using the computer assisted fabricated individual titanium mesh technique[J]. J Oral Maxillofac Surg, 2015, 73(10): e1-e15.

[23] MURPHY BA, RIDNER S, WELLS N, et al. Quality of life research in head and neck cancer: a review of the current state of the science[J]. Crit Rev Oncol Hematol, 2007, 62(3): 251-267.

[24] ROGERS SN, SCOTT J, CHAKRABATI A, et al. The patients' account of outcome following primary surgery for oral and oropharyngeal cancer using a quality of life questionnaire[J]. Eur J Cancer Care, 2008, 17(2): 182-188.

[25] ZHENG J, WONG MC, LAM CL. Key factors associated with oral healthrelated quality of life (OHRQOL) in Hong Kong Chinese adults with orofacial pain[J]. J Dent, 2011, 39(8): 564-571.

[26] COX DP, MULLER S, CARLSON GW, et al. Ameloblastic carcinoma exameloblastoma of the mandible with malignancy-associated hyper calcemia[J]. Oral Surg Oral Med Oral Pathol Oral Radiol Endod, 2000, 90(6): 716-722.

[27] LI WL, LIU FY, XU ZF, et al. Treatment of ameloblastoma in children and adolescents[J]. J Hard Tissue Biol, 2012, 21(2): 121-126.

[28] FARHADI J, VALDERRABANO V, KUNZ C, et al. Free fifibula donor-site morbidity: clinical and biomechanical analysis[J]. Ann Plast Surg, 2007, 58(4): 405-410.

[29] ZIMMERMANN CE, BORNER BI, HASSE A, et al. Donor site morbidity after microvascular fifibula transfer[J]. Clin Oral Investig, 2001, 5(4): 214-219.

[30] ROGERS SN, LAKSHMIAH SR, NARAYAN B, et al. A comparison of the longterm morbidity following deep circumflflex iliac and fifibula free flflaps for reconstruction following head and neck cancer[J]. Plast Reconstr Surg, 2003, 112(6): 1517-1525.

[31] URKEN ML, BUCHBINDER D, COSTANTINO PD, et al. Oromandibular reconstruction using microvascular composite flaps: report of 210 cases[J]. Arch Otolaryngol Head Neck Surg, 1998, 124(1): 46-55.

[32] 邱蔚六. 口腔颌面外科学[M]. 上海: 上海科学技术出版社, 2008.

[33] 徐启明. 临床麻醉学[M]. 北京: 人民卫生出版社, 2006.

[34] 宿玉成. 现代口腔种植学[M]. 北京: 人民卫生出版社, 2004.

[35] 姚江武. 口腔修复学[M]. 北京: 人民卫生出版社, 2009.

[36] 邱蔚六. 口腔颌面外科理论与实践[M]. 北京: 人民卫生出版社, 1998.